HOSPITAL

Hospital

AN ORAL HISTORY OF
Cook County Hospital

Sydney Lewis

FOREWORD BY
Barbara Ehrenreich

THE NEW PRESS · NEW YORK

PUBLISHED IN THE UNITED STATES
BY THE NEW PRESS, NEW YORK
DISTRIBUTED BY W. W. NORTON & COMPANY, INC.,
500 FIFTH AVENUE, NEW YORK, NY 10110

LIBRARY OF CONGRESS
CATALOGING-IN-PUBLICATION DATA

Lewis, Sydney, 1952–
    Hospital : an oral history of Cook County Hospital / Sydney Lewis.
      P.   CM.
    ISBN 1–56584–138–7
      1. Cook County Hospital (Chicago, Ill.)—History. 2. County
hospitals—Illinois—Chicago—History. 3. Cook County Hospital
(Chicago, Ill.)—Employees—Interviews. I. Title.
      [DNLM: 1. Cook County Hospital (Chicago, Ill.) 2. Hospitals,
County—history—Chicago. WX 28 AI3 C5L6 1995]
RA982.C452C665 1994
362.1'1'0977311—DC20
DNLM/DLC
for Library of Congress   94–21775
                                      CIP

AUTHOR PHOTO BY JANET RODERICK

BOOK DESIGN BY CHARLES NIX

ESTABLISHED IN 1990 AS A MAJOR ALTERNATIVE TO
THE LARGE, COMMERCIAL PUBLISHING HOUSES, THE
NEW PRESS IS THE FIRST FULL-SCALE NONPROFIT
AMERICAN BOOK PUBLISHER OUTSIDE OF THE UNIVER-
SITY PRESSES. THE PRESS IS OPERATED EDITORIALLY IN
THE PUBLIC INTEREST, RATHER THAN FOR PRIVATE
GAIN; IT IS COMMITTED TO PUBLISHING IN INNOVA-
TIVE WAYS WORKS OF EDUCATIONAL, CULTURAL, AND
COMMUNITY VALUE THAT, DESPITE THEIR INTELLEC-
TUAL MERITS, MIGHT NOT NORMALLY BE "COMMER-
CIALLY" VIABLE. THE NEW PRESS'S EDITORIAL OFFICES
ARE LOCATED AT THE CITY UNIVERSITY OF NEW YORK.

Printed in the United States of America

94 95 96 97   9 8 7 6 5 4 3 2 1

FOR MY PARENTS,
JOYCE AND FRED

Contents

Foreword

BARBARA EHRENREICH

HEALTH CARE REFORM, AS WE KNOW IT FROM THE CURRENT debate, is a cold and bloodless affair. Health care itself may be something real and meaningful in our own lives, but health-care *reform* seems to have vanished into a fog of financial and bureaucratic complexity. Too often, we forget what is really at stake—human suffering and disease.

There is one setting, though, where no one can lose sight of the human drama of medicine. Big-city hospitals—such as Chicago's Cook County, the setting for this book—were established more than a century ago as holding pens for the contagious, the indigent, and the mentally disordered. As medical technology advanced in the twentieth century, the public hospitals expanded their mission to include curing, as well as merely containing, the misery of the urban poor. Cook County Hospital, New York City's municipal hospitals, and their institutional peers around the nation became huge, overcrowded, receptacles for pathologies—social and individual—in all their heartbreaking, bizarre, and fascinating forms. Night and day, urban emergency rooms treat gunshot wounds, grossly neglected chronic conditions, cases of malnourishment and lead poisoning, as well as sore throats and aches of people who cannot afford a private doctor or find one in their resource-poor neighborhoods. The public hospitals have come to bear the brunt of all our epidemics—AIDS and tuberculosis, domestic violence, industrial accidents, homelessness, hunger, and overexposure.

The very drama, the unrelenting tragedy, of the public hospitals has given them a special role in medical training and research. In a private hospital serving more affluent patients, a young doctor encounters a much narrower range of injury and disease, and finds his or her authority severely circumscribed by the older, attending physicians. But in a place like Cook County, where the majority of patients do not have private doctors of their own, young interns and residents assume broad responsibility for patient care. At the same time, the conditions they are likely to encounter include not only diabetes, cancer, and heart disease, but the diabetic with cancer *and* heart disease—all perhaps severely neglected and nearly out of control.

Traditionally, young doctors have taken an almost macho pride in the life-and-death challenges of big-city hospitals. A few years of "battlefield medicine" in a place like Cook County or New York City's Bellevue Hospital is a prized rite of passage on the way to a comfortable private prac-

tice. In a perverse way, it has helped that the public hospitals are so miser-
ably underfunded. A good private hospital provides its house staff with the
latest technology and abundant resources. The public hospitals, on the
other hand, provide opportunities for desperate and heroic improvisation.

So places like Cook Country, chronically understaffed and erratically
equipped, have been a crucial linchpin of American medicine. The conditions of ghetto life—including poor housing, stress, and violence—help
generate a rich proliferation of medical pathologies. Poverty, abetted
by the racist politics of many private hospitals, guarantees that these
pathologies will flow almost exclusively to hospitals such as Cook County,
where they play a central role in the education of each new generation of
doctors. Thus the urban poor, meaning usually the urban black poor,
effectively subsidize the medical system for the rest of us, and they do so
with their own bodies.

The injustice of this situation inspired a wave of genuine "health
reform" in the 1970s. A new generation of young doctors, many of
whom had been radicalized by the social movements of the 1960s, found
little glory working in the nightmarish conditions of the public hospitals.
Hospital workers, energized by the civil rights movement, wanted
respect and an opportunity to provide decent and respectful care.
Patients were becoming less willing to be treated as "teaching material."
In Cook County and in municipal hospitals throughout the county,
coalitions of doctors, hospital workers, and community groups organized to upgrade their hospitals into high-quality, accountable, community resources.

This was health reform with heart and blood and soul. Angry community residents staged confrontations with hospital administrators and
public officials. Doctors, nurses, and other health workers went on
strike—not only for bread-and-butter gains but for better patient care.
Places such as Cook County and Lincoln Hospital in the Bronx became
centers of radical activism, concerned not only with patient care but with
environmental sources of disease such as dangerous workplaces and
vermin-infested housing. For a few minutes of historical time, the old
hierarchical divisions—between professional and nonprofessional,
patient and provider, Black and White—were swept aside by the new
energy of reform. There was, however briefly, an overriding determina-
tion to get the job done.

At the heart of *Hospital* is the story of that reform effort as it has
unfolded in one place, Chicago's Cook County Hospital. It is a story
involving dramatic tactics and real risks. At one time, for example, exas-
perated medical staff dramatized the inequities of the health system by
transporting their emergency room patients en masse to a private hospital
that would normally have barred or "dumped" them. It is a heartening
story, with real victories to celebrate; at Cook County, for example, it is

now possible for patients to have their own doctors, who are responsible for their total care, instead of seeing a different doctor on each visit.

But it is also a story that illustrates the limits of reform within any one institution, and in the absence of a national commitment to health care for all. No matter how valiantly the reformers inside Cook County struggle to improve patient care, they are hampered by inadequate funding, a crumbling physical structure, and understaffing so severe that patients must often wait many hours to see a doctor or have a prescription filled. This is health care for the poor and uninsured, and it painfully underscores the larger American inequalities of class and race. Very simply, in a society that fails to provide universal health coverage, some people's lives are valued far less than others.

No one can read *Hospital* and still think of health reform as a remote and tedious abstraction. Here are real, living people, diverse, sometimes tired and nearly burned out, always deeply engaged: the doctor who breaks into tears as he discusses his patients, the housekeeper whose life of hard work is more than redeemed by the opportunity to serve others, the community residents who treasure Cook County as "their" hospital no matter what its faults. Somewhere in this mix of hope and frustration, exhaustion and altruism, so vividly reported by Sydney Lewis, lies the key to genuine health reform.

Perhaps the real lesson of this compelling book is that genuine reform is not likely to be a product of elite task forces operating at a safe remove from the problems. Real reform takes sweat and tears, organizing, agitating—years, perhaps, of effort. The heroes of *Hospital*, from housekeepers to department heads, are not too different from you or me. Their message is that the struggle for health reform and for greater social equality in general has to start with determined grass-roots political effort—meaning, with us. And to judge from the conditions described in the pages that follow, it might as well start right now.

Acknowledgments

A SPECIAL THANKS TO HOSPITAL DIRECTOR RUTH ROTHSTEIN, whose permission was essential to this book's existence. Thanks also to those in the Public Relations Department; their non-interference, and patience with my pesky phone calls was appreciated. My gratitude extends to all the County people who contributed in important and numerous ways to the shaping of this book. Among them: Dr. Adolfo Carvajal, Mary Driscoll, Joan Duda, Dr. David Goldberg, Rose Houston, Dr. Taki Matsuda, Dr. Rosita Pildes, Dr. Rob Smith; and a few reluctant-to-appear-in-print doctors, who shall remain nameless.

My earliest leads came from folks outside the world of County, and I offer my thanks to: Bob Horn, Frank Melcouri, Marilyn Rice, Pam Sourelis, and Eileen Valentin. Thanks to Crystal Glass and José Narvaéz for their cooperation in securing elusive release forms, and to Jack Clark for his knowledge of Chicago.

My gratitude to Denise DeClue and Tim Kazurinsky is boundless: they hauled me out of the dark ages and into the world of computers with their generous gifts and loans of equipment. Their enthusiasm as well as that of my writing teacher, Carol Anshaw, helped convince me I could do this book. M'Lou Kogan aided with the gift of a good typing chair for a bad back. In town, my dear friends Lucy and Lenni Bukowski, Lois Baum and David Krupp, and all the Redheds, made sure I kept my sanity and sense of humor; from a distance, the same task was ably handled by Elissa Guest and Ben Sandmel.

It is my good fortune to have had André Schiffrin as my editor and publisher. He and his associates at the New Press, Jodie Patterson, Akiko Takano, and Matthew Weiland were gentle, genial and of enormous assistance in guiding this work into print. My appreciation to Ted Byfield for editing copy with great skill, sensitivity, and respect.

Finally, for a multitude of things—their grace as humans most especially—my thanks to Ida Terkel and her husband Studs, the maestro.

Introduction

FOR THOSE OF US WITH HEALTH INSURANCE, KNOWLEDGE OF our public hospitals is often vague or non-existent. In Chicago we have one public hospital—Cook County Hospital. For many years my awareness of County was limited to what I read in the newspapers or heard on the evening news: County, the hospital for poor people; County, the hospital of crisis; County, a big old building over there somewhere on the Near West Side.

But nearly ten years ago a close friend of mine was in a terrible chemical accident and suffered serious facial burns. Because of the severity of his injuries County's renowned Burn Unit was the best place for him to be. (Oh, and also, he had no insurance.) I visited him often during his thirty-eight days in the hospital.

That was my only experience of Cook County Hospital until spring 1993, when André Schiffrin asked me—based on my years of working with Studs Terkel—whether I'd be interested in talking to people who work in hospitals. Given the burgeoning talk of health-care reform, he thought it would be a good time for an oral history portrait of life at a city hospital. I agreed, and wanted to do the work. Both my mother and her mother were nurses and I've always felt at ease in hospitals. Though I'd never been a patient in any Chicago hospital, I had visited people in several of them. I remembered my favorable impressions of County's Burn Unit and thought that of all the hospitals in Chicago, Cook County Hospital, whose existence and future seem alternately taken for granted or up for grabs, would be the one most intriguing for a reader to frequent.

Public hospitals are a gauge of the cities in which they sit; the walls separating a public hospital from the street are permeable, and the public hospitals have become, in effect, a national health-care system. A visit to Cook County Hospital is a living, breathing illustration of the trouble our society is in. The human toll taken by poverty, racism, violence, and despair is clearly seen at County. The effects of poor access to education, jobs, health care, and decent housing are etched on the thousands of bodies pouring through the hospital doors each and every day. In the medical world County is known for many things, but it's best known in Chicago as the place that won't turn you away.

County's Burn Unit is on the fifth floor of the Children's Building, one of 13 buildings that make up the hospital complex. What I remembered

xv

most about those earlier visits to the Burn Unit was the extraordinary sensitivity of many of the nurses and clerks. I asked a nurse on the unit how she managed to go on, day after day, in her job. She said, "This beats oncology. Here every day you come in you're seeing progress. Every day someone's getting a little better." Except for those who don't make it. I sat in the visitor's lounge one evening, talking with a woman whose brother had been helicoptered in from Indiana. He'd been assaulted with a can of gasoline and a match. He was in such bad shape she said she almost hoped he wouldn't live.

My own badly burned friend shared a room with four people. A gas heater explosion, an apartment fire, and then there was the John Doe— a Hispanic man found in an abandoned and then burned building. No one was certain if he spoke or understood English; once conscious he wouldn't speak at all.

Since then much work has been done in the Burn Unit and elsewhere in the hospital, but at that time the shabbiness of the large rooms, the old-fashioned crank-up beds, the stark simplicity of the wooden wheelchairs, all evoked images of World War I, of black and white photos, of times long gone.

I came to this book with only these preconceptions. I didn't actually set foot in what is known as the Main Building—a truly Goliath structure— until I began interviewing people. Because of the building's age—eighty years as I write this—it has been referred to as a medical museum, and it does indeed resemble one. I knew nothing of the hospital's history, had no idea that it was at one time the premiere training ground for doctors in this country and that it has been, in a sense, Chicago's version of Ellis Island—a shoal for the waves of immigrants who once came seeking work in the hub of the Midwest.

Ruth Rothstein, Hospital Director since 1990, kindly—some might say courageously—gave her permission for me to interview anyone willing to talk to me. I then spun the dial of my own acquaintances until I hit on the names of a County-employed nurse and a doctor. They each generously—and again, perhaps courageously—gave their time and knowledge, and pointed me toward yet others. "Oh, you gotta talk to..." is the phrase at the heart of this book. Chance played a great role in my interview roster, and that is reflected in the wide range of voices, attitudes, and concerns offered in these pages. The hospital has almost 6,000 employees; and there is no such thing as a typical County worker.

For the most part people were eager to talk about their County lives, but getting them to steal time for a conversation often took weeks. Once or twice I had to throw myself on the mercy of supervisors willing to ferret out interview subjects among their staff, and there were employees who wanted no part of this book. This was more true of the non-medical staff, but several doctors either turned me down, or after speaking, decided they didn't want their interview used because they, in the words of one, "don't want to get in trouble." About half of those interviewed wanted to see their transcripts. Some were shocked by how strongly their mood at the interview dictated the tenor of their words. Others were appalled by how relaxed they had been, how much they had said. Everyone fretted over bad grammar.

Most of the interviews took place at the hospital. Stand still anywhere on the complex and within moments you're likely to hear phrases in Spanish, Polish, Tagalog, Urdu, English, and occasionally, since recent changes in immigration, Chinese. County may very well be the most integrated turf in Chicago.

The staff is integrated as well, although in a stratified manner; the majority of attending physicians are White, while a large number of the residents—doctors in training—are from other countries; the nursing staff is increasingly Asian although there are still many Black nurses, as well as some White; and most of the support staff—patient care attendants, transporters, housekeepers, dietary workers, etc.—are Black. This is, in more ways than one, *their* hospital.

I'd often pause in front of the Main Building and look across the street—past the statue of Louis Pasteur that stands in the park of his name, past the low, flat oblong of Malcolm X College—to where truckloads of money were busily metamorphosing into a brand new stadium to be used for conventions and athletic events. There has been talk of building a new County Hospital off and on for decades, but priorities are variable and the clients of County are not known for their clout.

These interviews took place between spring and late fall of 1993 and the streets around the hospital were always teeming with life. Workers taking a break, having a smoke; people waiting to be picked up, waiting for the bus, a cab, or just waiting. There's an odd small-town, campus feel to the place. (County shares the immediate neighborhood with the private and well-appointed Rush Presbyterian St. Luke's hospital, as well as the University of Illinois.) But it is as urban a campus feel as you are likely to find. The County community is jazzed, vibrant, energizing, awesome and disturbing.

Most hospitals have security guards, but not County—they've got police. A nurse laughingly told me, "Don't be calling them security. You got to call them police officers or they might not help you." One afternoon, with an hour or so to kill between interviews, I sat in the rear triage area of the emergency room. County police officers stationed in the ER gathered around the TV at the police desk—the White Sox were in the play-offs. During that hour I saw a young boy hobble in, arm slung over a friend's back—gunshot to the thigh. (A nurse later told me he must have messed up on a drug deal.) I saw a frail man, end-stage AIDS, wheeled in from the cab that brought him. A woman who'd nearly sliced her finger off in a door chanting a mantra of pain, "It hurts, oh, it hurts." A young man, catatonic and pale, with his befuddled parents. A prisoner from the county jail, bloody face, bloody chest, hands and ankles cuffed. A middle-aged woman, moaning, screaming, incoherent. I was told it was a slow day, and that anyhow, the front triage area is where the real action is.

But walk over toward Fantus, the building which houses the ambulatory patient clinics, and you see mothers and their restless children, elderly men and women patiently waiting for a check-up, young men uncomfortable and anxious to get moving. And sometimes lately, people who look vaguely middle-class and ill at ease. People who have lost their insurance.

While conducting these interviews talk of President Clinton's health-care reform plans accelerated from pure speculation to evaluation. Everyone at County desperately wanted to see health-care reform—and single-payer was the unequivocal choice of all who mentioned it—though most felt that the impact of any reform would be slow to reach County's patients. That there is a health-care crisis is not in dispute at 1835 West Harrison Street.

Also not in dispute is that patients are immensely loyal to and have great faith in the hospital. For some workers County is a place from which they can't stay away. "It gets under your skin," I was told. And over and over, "I'm a County person." There is a sense of family at the hospital—a feeling that there exists such a thing as a County clan. They may and do squabble with each other, but don't you even think about coming after "The County" or you'll have them, arms linked, to answer to.

"There's just something about this place," I was told. And there is. Come sit next to me. Listen.

Lives

Dr. Steve Meeks

A THIRD-YEAR RESIDENT *in Emergency Medicine. Under his fashionably old-fashioned wire-rim glasses are thick-lashed Egyptian eyes. He is animated, his stories embellished with mimicry and a keen sense of drama and timing. "I have friends at private hospitals, and they're working really hard. But these are people who would not survive at a place like Cook County. They would get frustrated, quit, go crazy, whatever. But I love it."*

I GREW UP IN SOUTHERN ILLINOIS, ABOUT FIVE HOURS DUE south of Chicago. A small town. Five hundred people, rural, blue-collar—a mining town. It was a predominantly Black town.

My mother's brother is a radiologist, and he trained here at the County. He's the Chief of Radiology at a small hospital in Carbondale. My uncle was actually a pretty big inspiration. I always thought that I wanted to go into medicine: it's a challenging career, it's a steady career, it's something where I can interact with a lot of different kinds of people.

I went to Harvard as an undergrad, and came back and went to Washington University in St. Louis for medical school. Washington is a private, wealthy institution, and most of the people who I went to school with thought I was a complete nut for coming to a place like the County. But hearing the stories I heard from my uncle, I knew it couldn't be anything but a good learning experience. He had good and bad stories, but even the bad stories made me think, Wow, if I can make it through a place like that and deal with that, then I can do anything.

I remember him telling me one story: He was a medicine intern here, and he said he was up on one of the floors working, and there was a psychiatric patient who had a boyfriend who was in the hospital; apparently he jilted her or had been out with another woman or something. He said this woman got in to visit her boyfriend—and, mind you, my uncle is three or four months into his internship. This woman gets into the hospital, goes into her boyfriend's room, and slices his throat. *Hello?!* Okay? [laughs in disbelief] Now, you're three months out of medical school and you're not expecting...And this is somebody coming to visit a patient who's there for something else. And she...did him in, basically. I was thinking, Now, just that kind of thing—if I can deal with that kind of stress and get through it and manage it, then there is nothing on this earth that will scare me.

3

I've seen the effects of that already. I went back down to visit him a couple of months ago, and I poked my head into the emergency room at Carbondale Memorial. There was a woman that had come in, and she was a diabetic with a blood sugar of 600. The person that was running the ER was like, "Oh my God!" He starts yelling at the nurses, "Get this, do this." I was like, what the hell is he getting all freaked out about? People come into the County two and three at a time with blood sugars of 800, 900. So…it just prepares you for anything. And in our ER you see tons and tons of primary care, because a lot of the people in the inner-city, they don't have access to a pediatrician for the kids, and to an obstetrician for mom, and to clinic doctors. I mean, they have to go through gang neighborhoods to get to their clinics, and they just won't do it. So they come to the ER.

The County is world famous: everybody just about everywhere knows something about Cook County Hospital. It's such a big, crazy place. At the end of my internship I was talking to my uncle about the fact that I still wanted to go into the Peace Corps and he was like, "What the hell are you thinking? You're doing Third World work basically now." And I thought, You're kind of right. I'm doing a lot of things for a lot of people who really need it right here.

My point about the residents is that the type of residents who choose to come here are the type of people who really want to do something good for people who need it the most. I look at my class, and these are people who have gone off to other countries and done things and have had some really interesting and neat life experiences, so their perspective is much different than your standard—which is what I am, personally—college to med school to residency…It tends to be a little looser-type person. It depends on the department, I guess. When you get into the more competitive specialties—Emergency Medicine is competitive, Optho, Radiology—you tend to find people who came here because this is where they got in. But if you look at the Internal Medicine group, the family practitioners, the pediatricians, these are people who really want to do some good. They tend to be your more left-wing sort of crowd.

I don't want to generalize, but I'm going to because…I'm just going to. A lot of the surgery residents tend not to want to be here, because it's hard work. They gripe and they complain, but it's also part of being a surgeon. I don't know if that's so different here than anywhere else. It's a personality type; and if you get worked like a dog you're going to be tired and cranky. But some of the comments that I hear from them—like, *these* people, and *they* don't take care of themselves, and *why* don't they make their clinic appointments, and *why* don't they these, those, that.

These are mostly White residents talking about County patients in general. They say the same thing about the Black patients, the White patients, the Polish patients. I'm sure that race has something to do with it, but intertwined with that—and maybe even a bigger factor, probably—is class-consciousness. I think if you look at the makeup here, whether you're Black, White, Hispanic, or whatever, you tend to be working-class or unemployed poor, or even working but no insurance. So you've got a group who the people who tend to be in medicine have not had a lot of contact with. I looked at my medical school class, and 85 percent of these people had a relative—either a mother, a father, an uncle, or an aunt—in medicine, and it's funny, including myself. [laughs] But I grew up poor so I don't think of myself as being part of that class.

Most of these people were and are, and they tend to look down on people who don't have what they have. There was one surgeon who was down in the ER who was trying to stick a needle in this lady's knee with the door open. She's screaming her head off. I went to him and I said, "Would you do that at Rush?" And he looked at me, and his cheeks turned red. I said, "Right, you wouldn't, would you? Close the damn door when you examine a patient." But that's the kind of thing you see among those people who didn't choose to be here. They tend not to care as much. I don't want to say that that's true of all of them.

Lots of the clerks and other support staff have been here many, many years and seen residents come and go and they let you know that: [laughs] "I was here before you, and I'll be here after you, so..." Well, it changes. It's changed over the period that I've been here.

When I came as an intern, yeah, you come as an intern to any new place and first of all you don't know anything. You graduated from medical school, and I don't care if you were the top of your class, you don't know a thing until you have done a year of patient management. You can answer any question anybody asks you, but when you have a patient that's crashing in front of you, you don't know anything, so you're intimidated by that. You come to a hospital that has, I don't know what, 900, 1,000 beds, you're intimidated by that. You come to a hospital where you see young brothers walking down the hall with Gangster Disciple tattoos, and they're flashing you the signs.

I had a guy flash me a sign one day and I was like...[turns head to left and right, wild-eyed, and laughs] I had on jeans and a Malcolm X T-shirt and a baseball hat, and I had on a beeper. I was checking up on a patient and I turned my head, and I was like, Naaa—I just kept right on walking. I didn't look like a physician; but that doesn't matter, because I had somebody come up to me and try to sell me drugs here one time when I *did* have on my white coat. This was somebody who was here to visit a patient. He was like, "Man, I got some—" And I was like, "Let me tell you something: you better take that outside, because you could get in a helluva lot of trouble for that." Isn't that something?

So I mean, you come to this place, it's big, it's crazy, you don't know anything: you not only have to deal with the Black patients here, but Indians and Hispanics—it's a fishbowl. And I'm not only talking about patients, I'm talking about staff too. So you have to come in and immediately start interacting with a wide variation of races, socioeconomic statuses, religions, attitudes. I mean, you have to come in here and be ready to deal with just about anything.

You mentioned the clerks. Well, when you first get here you really are sort of overwhelmed and intimidated. The way I dealt with it, and the way I see a lot of other interns dealing with it, initially you're Mr. Nice Guy. You come in and you're the new kid on the block, and these are people have been here for years. They see you coming, and some of them I think are purposefully mean to you, just to see how you're going to react, okay? Once they find out that you're not one of these people who's fresh out of medical school and has the attitude and all that, they back off—in fact, they even start being nice to you and start helping you. But first they kind of try you. As you learn what this place is like, you're more able to deal with it. You have to know when to be Mr. Nice Guy, you have to know when to get angry, and you have to know when you're dealing with something that you are not going to change, so you leave it alone.

I think that some of the Black staff actually, for whatever reason—maybe because they identify with us—they're more likely to be nicer to me sooner...But if you don't show your colors then they'll treat you right. It's probably easier for me to warm up the Black clerks and whatever than it would be for a White person. It's a fact. I don't have to jump as high a hurdle as someone who's White might have to. I mean, it also depends on your attitude, because if you're a Black American and you come in here with a funky attitude, they will treat you as badly as anyone else. It's more whether you're a nice person, so I don't want to say it's really a race thing, because it's not; it's more how they perceive you. I see them treating a lot of the White residents that way too. If they're nice people, they treat them right.

I think most of the staff who work here are reasonable people. Now, you have some complete idiots, but you have some physicians who are complete idiots too. [laughs]

In terms of my social life? There is that doctors-and-nurses soap opera myth, and there's truth in all myths. There is a certain amount of fraternization. Not a whole lot, actually—not as much as people would like to think. As a resident, I'm so busy trying to get my work done and trying to get people to do what I would like them to do that I don't even have time to think about trying to date and hook up. I mean, my personality is such that I'll laugh and talk and have fun. But as far as really dating somebody with whom I work, I don't do it. Because it's too...it can get too complicated, and what if it doesn't work and you get mad at each other.

In fact, I've dated two people that work here. You don't have a lot of time to meet a lot of people outside of Cook County so...you know. Although I vowed after this time I'm not going to do it again. But I vowed the last time so...People would like to think: Oh, Dr. So-and-so and Nurse So-and-so. But the nurses, oftentimes, they will not have a thing to do with you. There's a lot of funny dynamics here with nurses and physicians. With physicians and *everybody* here.

You always hear about the nurse-physician relationship. Especially as an intern, you have a lot of that head-bumping, because you have the headstrong intern and the nurse who's been here, or even the young nurse who's not going to put up with your shit. Because now nursing is a respected profession, and they're not taking any shit anymore—and they, in fact, oftentimes will try you too. They're with the patients twelve hours at a time, so there are a lot of things that they're going to know about the patient that you're not. If you don't act right they can really hang you out to dry. They can sit back and...they will know if somebody is going bad and they will tell you, or they'll call you at the last minute.

By the same token, my second month here I was in the Intensive Care Unit and there were things that came up I just had no idea how to handle, and the nurse would kind of sit back and be watching. She'd say, "You don't know what to do, do you?" They'd say, "Well, such and such is going on, what do you want to do?" I'd say, "What do you think?" or "What do you guys usually do?" [laughs] They'd say, "Well, we usually do thus-and-such." I'd say, "Okay," and I'd write the order down. Um-hmm. Dr. Meeks says...[laughs] and go on back to bed.

Another thing a lot of my fellow interns would get is they would get beeped in the middle of the night: Mr. So-and-so is having pain, he wants some Tylenol. "Give him the damn Tylenol," you know? "Why are you calling me for that?" I personally didn't have so many of those problems, because I was nice and I tried to deal with people. But other people get frustrated easier and so they yell and scream and go on—and so you pay for it.

Nurses aren't supposed to take phone orders, and that became an issue in the middle of my internship year. At the beginning there was no problem giving phone orders, but I think they had a patient go bad. Something bad happened when somebody gave an order over the phone—and I think that the doctor denied that he said that, so it became a big stink. The new policy is, "We're not going to be taking phone orders." It makes you want to tear your hair out. As an intern, when you're on call—*if* you get a chance to get into your bed—okay, *you* come over to Karl Meyer Hall [a residence for interns and residents]. For you to have to get up and wait for the elevator and go down fourteen floors and walk all the way over and get up to the sixth floor in the main building, all the way on the east side, *just* to give somebody two Tylenol...I mean, it pisses you off. And you find that some of the nurses actually will take phone orders, but they make sure they say, "When you come over here tomorrow at seven you make sure you write this order or you sign it." But they're not supposed to do that, and they could get into a lot of trouble. But if they like you they'll take care of you, I've found.

These men and women who have been in nursing for years, they can manage patients better than any intern and better than a lot of residents. The only problem is they don't have M.D. by their name, so legally they are not able to do all these things. I learned in medical school that you better listen to the nurses. I'm serious. They can really make your life much, much easier, or make it complete hell.

I was in the ER the other day, and I was working in the GYN [gynecological] section and it was incredibly, incredibly busy. When you get back there you're trying to move patients, you're trying to get things going and keep the flow, see as many and treat them effectively...At the triage desk they'll oftentimes bring people back who are looking bad. One of the nurses brought the patient back and she said, "You better see this one now." I looked at the girl, she didn't look too bad. I looked at her vital signs, everything was normal. I said "Look, we're busy crazy back here, take her back and I'll see her later." One of the nurses in the ER, a really sweet lady who's been there for years, she came back—and she's somebody that I really respect a lot. She said, "You know, Doc, I know you just sent this lady back, but she's really starting to look kind of bad. Would you please see her?" And even though I thought to myself, There's no reason to see this lady right now, I said, "Fine, bring her on back." She said, "Let me put the IV in her." I said, "Go ahead, go ahead."

So the girl really started complaining about pain. I said, "Just go in and take a peek at her." I went in and did the speculum exam and her os [hole in cervix] was completely open—in other words, she was miscarrying *right there*. I got the IV in, got the fluids open, and there was no indication; her signs were still fine, but she was just having more pain and bleeding and I thought, *Whoa*. I got her upstairs immediately. So that's experience for you: when these people tell you something it's not because they want to be the doctor, it's because they tend to be patient-care advocates, and they know when something is going bad. She saved my butt. If this lady had started to bleed really vigorously and we weren't able to resuscitate her...There you go. I would have been standing in front of the department on Thursday morning going, "Ah, well, uh, I thought that...uh, uh, uh."

Part of my love for Emergency Medicine is also a love for County. I mean, I really like this place. Although some days I get *so* mad and *so* frustrated. Today was one of those days. It was just like, things aren't going right.

I was in Fast-Track, which is where you see the bumps and the bruises and the broken bones and sprained ankles and cut fingers. So these are people that you're supposed to get in and out quickly. Mondays and Tuesdays and Wednesdays are notoriously busy in the ER, especially in Fast-Track. You know, when you're on the West Side, folks go out on the weekend and they come in Monday morning with the weekend shoulder that's been hurting and the arm that they fell on this weekend when they were playing basketball. So it's just crazy.

From midnight to eight it's relatively nonbusy. People aren't going to come in in the middle of the night for something that's minor. So people start coming in around seven, eight o'clock. We started seeing patients at eight, and they just kept piling in and piling in. Whenever something more acute comes in—like I had a lady come in with her thumb, it was all cut in half pretty much, one part was falling off—so that kind of thing, you have to see her right away, sew it up and get films or whatever.

By the time four o'clock rolled around we were seeing patients that registered at ten o'clock. If I had to wait in the ER for a cyst on my behind for eight hours, I would be *pissed* by the time...And so people get really mad. It's hot, it's crowded out there, you're hungry. If you're not a County patient you don't know to bring your lunch or to bring a book, because you're going to be waiting. So people get real, real pissed. And as the day goes on, you've got an attending who's coming up and saying, "Well, what's going on here?" *You* start to get really pissed. [laughs] Just because you're frustrated, you're seeing as many patients as you can.

I forced myself to stop for ten minutes to grab a bite to eat. I had to, because I was too hungry and too tired and too frustrated. So, it was just a really, really, busy, crazy day. Ten minutes. That's all I stopped for today. Just enough to eat, and I stopped once to pee. [laughs] That sounds crude, but...Like Friday for instance, I went from eight o'clock to six o'clock without...I didn't even stop to pee Friday! [laughs] I didn't stop to eat. It was just go, go.

Friday I was in the center, where you see the more acute patients. As a third-year resident you're responsible for all the resuscitations, which are people who come in with really abnormal vitals, or people who need to be seen right away—people with acute heart attacks, cardiac arrest, hypertensives whose pressures are off the wall, people who are stroking out. Whenever there's a resuscitation you have to run back there and get things going. These things come in every fifteen minutes.

I had three people who were end-stage AIDS, all of whom came in with cystolic blood pressures of 80, and they were IV drug users—so there was no venous access—so I had to try to get central lines. I almost stuck myself with a needle, and that's when I said, okay, relax. Nothing is that serious for you to stick yourself with a needle. I don't care if you know if they're HIV-positive or not. You don't know. This man I knew was end-stage, so it was that much more scarier. But when I left Friday, when I left today, I still felt good. Isn't that weird?

It takes, I think, a certain amount of toughness to survive at a place like this. Not only do you have a really tough patient population, in the sense that a lot of these people who come here are really sick, but you're in a hospital where there are only a limited number of unit beds. As an intern I manage patients who at any other hospital would have been at an Intensive Care Unit with one-on-one nursing and monitors, and we just don't have the resources here to do that. You keep them on the floors and you manage them as best you can.

What frustrates me the most? You know, I think I probably get much more frustrated with staff, as opposed to the patients. The patients...me, personally, I can only get so angry with them. If you're in a situation where you have to make all kinds of arrangements, you have to have somebody watch your kids, then you have to get the money to take the bus to the train...I mean, it's not easy to get here, to make your appointment.

I had a guy come in here today, and I was reading in the chart and it said, "missed ortho appointment." I went back and said, "So you missed your ortho appointment." I didn't yell at him or anything. It turned out his grandmother had died. Usually it's more like, I didn't have anybody to watch my kids and I didn't have the money. I mean these are real issues in these people's lives that a lot of us don't even think about. So I don't get too mad about that. But when you find staff who are not happy with their jobs, and who don't care about the patients, that's what frustrates me the most. I'm going to use Radiology as an example. You go to the Radiology Department and you say, "This guy is having real bad pain, he's throwing up fecally smelling stuff. I think he's obstructed. Where's his obstruction?" [imitating snotty attitude] "I don't know." "Has the X-ray been done?" "I do not know. And, girl, I said, blah-blah-blah." *And they're on the phone.* Ohhhh, I just wanted to grab the phone, ohhh, that makes me madder than anything else—because they're here work-ing, making money on a job that a lot of people would be glad to have, and they won't even get up off their asses to do it. That's what makes me most angry about this place, when you have people who work here who don't care about their job or the patients.

I think it's important for our patients, who are predominantly Black, to see Black physicians here. I cannot count the number of times where people have asked me, "Are you a doctor?" They say I look too young to be a doctor. I had a twenty-three-year-old guy today look at me and he said, "You really a doctor?!" Meanwhile I'm sewing up his finger. I said, "Yeah, man, I'm a doctor." He said, "You are the first young, Black doc-tor that I have seen." They're proud, they're impressed, and they also get the sense that, wow, it can be done.

I remember when I was at Harvard—85 percent of the Black people in my class were either African or West Indian. These weren't American Blacks. And these people come from countries and societies where they grow up with Black teachers, they grow up with Black mayors, Black doctors. So they have the sense that this is something that they can achieve, that it's normal. A lot of people who grow up in the inner-1city don't even have the concept that this is something that somebody can do. I think it's of utmost importance. Not only because you're probably much more in touch with them and you can identify easier—because they will probably relate to you easier—but also because you want to give them the sense that this is something that can be done.

I had a little gangbanger one time, about seventeen. He came in with a dislocated shoulder, and I gave him about 100 of Demerol: and he's sitting there…he really started just running off at the mouth. He was like, "Man, a doctor, huh, wow! I wanna be a doctor." Meanwhile this poor boy hadn't been to school since he was fourteen, fifteen. He was just yakking, yakking. "Wow, man, so you can do that, huh? Maybe I'll get back into school. Maybe I'll, maybe I'll…" And that was impressive to me, to think that this guy who's like, I'm one of the real tough guys on the street, but maybe I want to do something like this some day. And if you plant that kind of a seed in this little boy's mind, who knows what could happen? Just giving him the sense that this is something he could do, that it is achievable. It's good for him and it's good for me. It's good for Black society.

I think there's a real schism that's forming here in Black America with the 10 percent that have and the 90 percent that don't have. I think it is important for some of us to hang around and spend some time—do your time, as it were. It's good for the patients who are here, it's good for the other Black residents.

You know, being Black and getting through medical school…it's stressful for everybody. But as a minority you oftentimes perceive this as, Well, they're racist and they don't want me. So I look at Michelle Grant, for instance, who is now chairman of the Department of the Emergency Medicine Program at Howard University—she was an attending here. I'm like, Wow, she's thirty-six and she's chairman of a department at a major university-affiliated teaching facility. I'm like, well hey, I'm twenty-seven, maybe in nine years…Just the same way that gangbanger is impressed with me, I'm impressed with her, and it's a continuum. And I think it's important for us to be visible in the community and say, "Yeah, I made it, you can make it. Sure it's tough, but it's not easy for anybody."

I feel a little resentment toward those Blacks who take the training and run. I tend to resent them, not because they leave—it's more of an attitude…not even what you have, it's more the way you think: people who tend to separate themselves from their community tend to think that they're better than everybody else, and they tend to be the most narrow-minded, egocentric, and on and on and on, star and asterisk, curse word, curse word. [laughs] So, I don't have much respect for those kind of people in general, whether they're Black or they're White. But I think it hurts me a little bit more when I see Blacks who are like that, because they should have a little bit of a sense of responsibility to their community. But again, if you think about it, a lot of those people, they never dealt with that. They grew up with money, and so, I guess, you can't really blame them. Maybe some people feel they've already paid their dues and now they want to collect. But that's a little selfish, I think, because you can collect and still do some good, you know? I plan to.

Diana Dosie

EXPRESSIONS DON'T SO *much appear as flash across her face. A scowl in a second becomes a great gleamy smile. "When I was small, you know how your parents ask what do you want to do when you grow up? Well, I wanted to be a doctor. I had my first baby at sixteen, and got married—we're still together—so that kind of deterred me from being a doctor. But I still had my sights set for the medical profession, and nursing was the next best thing, I thought." She was born at County.*

WHEN I WAS AT MALCOLM X COLLEGE, IN THE NURSING PROgram, we got our practicum [clinical experience] at County, and I thought I could go to County and wouldn't have to move out of County to get any kind of experience I wanted: I want to be multifaceted. I might even go back to school for nursing—like a masters or something—and teaching. But right now I like the Peds ["peeds": pediatrics] ICU, I like the fast pace. It's not boring. Never boring.

I wanted to come back to County after I got out of school. I had roamed those halls on the basement level—it's a fallout shelter too, and it's huge. You can go to any other building in County underground, so I know the whole tunnel system: I can do it blindfolded.

I've been at County seven and a half years—in Peds the whole time. We range from newborns to sixteen. Sometimes we get older kids, like cardiology patients, we do cardiology peds, we do critical care peds, we do trauma peds: we get the whole gamut. I think I like working with the kids better, they seem to bounce back better as far as illness is concerned.

Of course, I can't stand to see it when they die, but that's the same with all of us. Sometimes you have to have a meeting on it to sort everything out: Was I doing the right thing? Could we have done something different to change the situation? And then sometimes you understand and it's better for the patient to go. Better for the patient. *You* might not want them to go as much as they want to go. They might not want to die, but they're tired: "If this is all I have, then I'm tired." I've worked with adults—their spouses die, and they say, "I don't want to live anymore," and they die two weeks after their spouse is gone. You say, "How did they do that?" From being a well person and dying in two weeks, how did they accomplish that? Broken heart? But that's all I can think, because they do go.

People say, "How can you work with these kids, seeing them so sick?"

You know, they get sick just like adults, and somebody has to take care of them—and it should be people that like kids, want to be there, and right now that's me. I think I have a good rapport with kids, even the rough ones that come in. And rough ones do come in there. There's the traumas like motor vehicle accidents; the rough ones are the gangbangers that come in with gunshot wounds. Most of them can relate to me. We've had 'em, like two young teenage boys, fifteen and sixteen, they don't know each other. One was beat up real bad, and he was laying in the bed, semi-comatose. And then there's this other one, gunshot wound to the stomach—first day, post-op, but he was awake and alert and everything. He turned over and looked at the other guy and said, "What gang is he in?" OK? I said, "It doesn't matter, you're in our gang now—Cook County's gang, and I run it. All right?" Oh, he couldn't get out of the bed. I said, "You cannot get out of the bed, and you're wondering what gang he's in?! Give me a break, OK? Fix yourself up."

They're terrible. You know, they have the tattoos on them, gang sign—and they say, "Oh, that's just something I did." I say, "Come on, I know what that is—I know what gang you're in. I just asked to see if you'd tell me the truth. So let's start on the same level." And once they realize that we're not as naive as they want us to be, they usually break down and tell us what happened: who did this, and what happened. They might not talk to police like that, but they tell *us*.

Sometimes they even break down and act like scared kids. We had one kid, he broke into somebody's house—and it happened to be a policeman's—and the policeman shot him in the back. Paralyzed from the waist down, OK? Fourteen. The boy had a gun too, and he turned and fired before the policeman shot him. Somebody had to be at his bedside all the time: "Fix my pillow, I'm not comfortable. Turn me around. What's this, what's that?" And we were just saying, "Hey, you're a big guy. I'm sure you wouldn't want the people you're dealing with to see you acting like this. Why you do it?" He was scared. He cried a lot. His parents weren't very supportive either—they were mad at him. They'd come to the bedside, and they were fussing, not to him but to each other. It got to the point where we would say, "You guys cannot be arguing at the bedside. If you're gonna argue, you're gonna have to take it outside. You want to come in here and visit, you have to be cordial." So they visited less because of that. It was so depressing.

I try not to judge young people, but it seems they could do better. I was sixteen, I had a baby, I graduated from high school. If I can do it, *anybody* can do it. Maybe I'm a little critical—in the sense of saying, "You can do it"—but I want them to, you know? I don't want to see them on the corners, I really don't. I *know* they could do better. And me being harsh to them sometimes...I'm trying to bring them down to reality, that's all. I do whatever I can to make them happy. To make them comfortable and everything. I understand that the parents are in a horrible situation too. Their kid is paralyzed, they feel guilty. The only thing I can do is just deal with the patient. I guess they thought we were saying, "Stay away from the bedside." We were not saying that. We were saying, "Don't argue around him, he's already feeling bad."

Sometimes we're taken the wrong way, and I don't know what to do about it, I really don't. We had a critical case, we were working feverishly on him—there were two or three nurses, three or four doctors. He was crashing—his heart rate was going down, he was turning blue—we had to do some real quick things to save him. And we had two parents at the door, they wanted to see another patient. Our unit is small, so all these people, and other people too...When we have an emergency, we *always* put the visitors out of the room. But they were standing at the door, they walked in, and I told them, "You can't come in, we have an emergency." And they said, "Well, it's not with my kid, so I'm seeing my baby." So I said, "No, you're not! You got to get out. I told you we got an emergency." So they said, "I don't see no reason why. You can do whatever you want over there, I'm going over *there*." And so I told them, "If you don't leave the room—I don't have time to argue with you—I'm calling security." They told me, "Fuck you, bitch! Who do you think you are?" And then I said, "I don't have no time for this," and I told the clerk, "Call security on them."

It was a big mess, OK? We talked in the hallway—they accused me of saying other things that I didn't say—you know? [laughs]—making it worse than what it was. I just told security maybe I could have handled it another way, but I was in an emergency and I was trying to get them out of there. They were standing in the middle of the door, screaming and hollering at me, and I needed some assistance to get them out of the door. Security told them, "If the nurse in charge tell you you have to leave, you have to leave. If we have to come up here again the only time you'll be able to see your baby is with security." I never called security again. They rolled their eyes at me, called me all kinds of names under their breath. I'm like, "Forget it, okay? [laughs] Leave me alone."

All our kids are on monitors, and they need our help. They are very critical, the peds laying up in our beds, and I feel like I'm needed. It's very fulfilling to see those kids from coming in comatose, responding only to pain, to when they start talking to you. It's a big thing. We had one little girl, a car crash—I'll never forget. She was comatose for about a week: she was intubated, all kinds of lines, and it was just a matter of her healing. As she improved, the lines started disappearing, and it got to the point where we could extubate her. She was a pretty little girl, about six or seven. It seemed like a long time for her to start talking. I was working with her one day, giving her a bath—I talked to her every day—and I said, "I'll be glad when you just say 'hello.'" I had my back turned to her, and she said, [small voice] "Hello." [laughs] I ran and got the other nurses, I mean, it was a big thing: just for her to say that. Everybody came in, everybody wanted to talk to her. It was so nice—and she recovered.

Once they leave peds ICU, most of them don't come back. We ask them, "When you go to the clinic, come back and see us; we'd love to see you." But just a few of them come back, and we are *always* glad to see them—always. We take pictures of them if they want us to, and we have a board that we put the kids up on.

Some of them are so young and their accidents, their trauma was so severe, that they don't even remember. Their parents say, "You don't remember them? They've been with you for weeks." They say, [kid voice] "I don't remember her." I say, "That's okay, because I remember *you*. I'm glad to see you."

It's not only the traumas. We have kids that come in with tumors and chronic illness. The parents that are really, really concerned—they ask so many questions that when the patient is ready to go home, they know almost as much as we know. They seem to do better—the patient and the parents—if they're informed.

We get kids in because of abuse, too, beat up, sexually abused. I think the worst case was a little baby that was sexually abused by her natural father. She was three years old—I think that's a baby. He was like six-two. He brought her in, was in a hurry to get to work—but she was sick, and he felt like she had to be in a hospital. Which she did: she was sexually abused by this guy, scared to death of him. She had stomach pains, throwing up, high fever. Her diagnosis was syphilis—*syphilis!* She had been sodomized and her hymen was broken, all kinds of bruises down there.

He dropped her off, and he would not wait. Somebody snuck around the corner to get to a phone. We called a child abuse expert, and she was on her way. We had him in the back, trying to get assessment from him— he said, "I don't know none of this stuff, you have to ask the mother. I don't know how much she weighed when she was born." Like he was dropping her off at a baby-sitter! We couldn't hold him, and he left. The baby, she started getting lethargic and her stomach started getting distended. It was just horrible.

The next day I came in, she didn't look like the same baby we admitted. She was just *swollen*. I don't know how long she'd suffered with that infection. We quickly got rid of it, but it was too late; she had suffered too much at home. She recovered—it was a long time—but the mental scars on that baby. You could tell: she was very depressed, she didn't talk much. They arrested the mother and the father. The other relatives that came in were angry—they didn't know this had been going on. [sadly] I just felt like she was being victimized because of what had happened. She lost a mother and a father. The father was no good, no way...but it seemed like she was all alone, no support.

Those kids, something has to be done. Anybody that's abused…I don't care who it is, it should not happen. I've seen a two-year-old—this baby didn't even get to our floor, he was on the regular unit. His mother and grandmother were prostitutes living in a crack house *selling him to men in the crack house, OK?!* He had no help. He was on Ward 46 and 66 for months. We had to give him a bag…You know, I'm so upset I can't even remember what it's called: we had to bring his intestines to his stomach so his rectum could heal. He was self-abusive. He would bite on his hands, bit his toes to the nubs. He wouldn't let anybody see him do it. He'd get in a corner somewhere in the dark. Once you got ahold of him he'd be bloody from head to toe from biting and scratching on hisself. We put mittens on his hands and everything. But he was like *Houdini*—he got out of all of *that,* OK? So he could do what he wanted to do to hisself. His eyes were so haunting—it's like he was looking right through you, saying, "What are you gonna do to me?" I said I wouldn't want to see him at twenty. And it's not his fault. [on the verge of tears] It's not his fault.

Do I ever get discouraged with the human race? I think they can be helped. I'm talking like I'm not in 'em. We have to think that way, or else we're going to blow up in smoke. It's got to be across-the-board education: don't give it to some and not give it to others, *everybody* deserves this. We *all* will benefit. If you educate all of us, then they won't be so likely to hit you in the head in the morning when you're going to work, because they'll be busy doing something productive. And that's what we have to start doing, is helping each other.

Some of this stuff should not have a price tag on it: health care, education, food, and clothing. And the people that's in power, that can change these things, they got to start looking at it. I think they're still going on that racial edge. Education, health—it's got to be across the board so there's certain things people just *don't* have to fight to get, or feel isolated or different because they don't have these things.

I don't know what age to start at, because the young ones are getting into it younger and younger: little kids shooting other little kids and not knowing what's going on. We had a three-year-old—her brother was seven or eight, and he had *shot* her. He came to see her, and he smiled at her, but was gone—she was brain dead. He didn't know what was going on—you could look in his face—*he did not know.* But I think at ten or twelve he's going to know that he killed his sister. It was the father's gun, it was under the bed, they were at home alone. The mother and father had went somewhere, and the kids got the gun and he shot his sister in the head…

It's the nurses who work with the patient at the bedside the most. The doctors write orders and do labs and stuff like that, but we're the ones who're there. Before, when we'd be there on rounds, we had input and they used it; now they insist that we be on rounds, and they say that they want our input, but if we *do* say something—and it's happened several times, not only to one nurse, but several nurses—they say, "No, that's not right—we won't be doing that."

It's gotten to the point where we are *experienced* nurses up there on that ICU; most of those nurses have been there for years. I don't like pointing my finger and saying, "See—you see what you did? And didn't we say something about that?"—but it's gotten to that point. That's the only satisfaction that we can get, is pointing the finger. I don't like that. And vice versa, too, they're pointing the finger at us for something we do that we shouldn't have did. And it's stressful, it's a lot of tension. Whereas, before, it was a team effort: if the patient came through and it was smooth, no problems, we all felt good. Now it's like, "See what I did. Look! The patient's great." It's awful.

And we have had meetings, you know. Certain things like a cancer patient, and we say, "This kid is not being managed painwise—I think we need to give him more *pain* medicine." And then, on rounds, the patient isn't as critical, or he's not in a crisis of pain at that moment, and they say, "Oh, it don't look like he needs that. Let's do this: we'll get him a TV, get him a radio." Or if he's itching, "Put some of this lotion on him," instead of giving him some Benadryl or something, you know, to *knock that itch out*. OK? The lotion *will* do it in the long run, but how long do we have? I'm talking terminal. I don't think there's anything shouldn't be done immediately for those kind of people. And the kid was a noncomplainer. He was nine and he knew he was dying. He talked to his parents—they were very close. It made me want to cry sometimes. When he died, we all, the nurses all felt real bad—we got so upset, we said, "We need a meeting, we want a meeting *today*." And what we addressed was this kid dying without being managed as far as pain was concerned.

We have a lot of foreign doctors, Black doctors, Indian doctors. It's pretty much mixed for regular services; the specialty services, they usually are majority White—Ear, Nose, and Throat, Orthopedic, Surgery. Some of them are nice, some of them empathize with the patient pretty good—and then you get your idiots. Everywhere, right? That's just a way of life. It's not a color thing; you can find them in all races.

I had an Arab doctor that even poked me in my chest because I hung up on him. He was being very belligerent to me, and I didn't feel like I had to listen to all of that and I hung up. He burst through the doors: "Who is the nurse I was talking to on the phone?" I said, "Here I am." He said, "Who do you think you are?" [imitates him jabbing at her with his finger] I just backed off of him; I was calm, because I knew he was out of control, didn't know what he was doing. [laughs] Maybe he was in surgery twenty-four hours, you know? So I said, "Listen, *don't* put your hands on me. I'm a married woman—I have an evil husband. Do *not* do that!" "I'm going to write you up! You disregarded my orders completely." And as he was talking I was calling security, because I didn't know. [laughs] He might have wanted to hit me. And he was calling me stupid and all kinds of things, so I felt like, Let me get somebody up here to get in the middle, because I can hold my peace for a *little* while. Not long, though, with somebody calling me stupid.

So I got the supervisor up there, I got security up there, I told him they'd take him to jail if he didn't apologize—and I said, "And that means *in writing*." We got the situation straightened out. He admitted he poked me and that he was out of control. He said, where he came from, the nurses followed the doctors orders all the way down the line and didn't give them any flak. And I said, "You're a first-year resident. Where else have you been practicing medicine?"

And the way they teach you in nursing school, in my experience, they encourage you to be meek and keep your mouth closed. They give you what you need to function, but they don't prepare you for the real medical field—you have to get that on the job. They don't prepare you for the decisions that you have to make, to be able to say, "I know that's not right and I'm not going to do it." We need to start changing the way we teach people and not make everybody—all these doctors or lawyers or priests—like gods. And that's the way we have been trained to feel towards these people: they can do no wrong. But idiots are *everywhere*.

People say that if there's health care reform there won't be a need for County? That's bullshit—they'll need it even more. The people that run County Hospital, they're going to have to be the ones that implement some of this stuff: *they're* going to have to be the ones that make a plan and carry it out. How is it going to close us down? [angry] Close me down, okay? *Close me down.* You know, that's great. If they don't need as many nurses as they need now, for the stuff that we see. I'm tired of taking care of three- and four-year-olds, gunshot wounds to the head, stab wounds for teenage girls. I'm tired of that. There's enough diseases out here that will keep us busy for the rest of our life.

Dr. John Barrett

DIRECTOR OF THE TRAUMA *Unit and the President of the Medical Staff. "In my neighborhood in Ireland there was one family from India who were so unusual that people would stop and point at them as they walked down the street. America was all strange. You get off the airplane in New York and, man, it smells different, people talk in strange accents, they're abusive and they yell at you, no one holds open the door. The whole society is so different. So I never really appreciated the issue of most of the patients being Black. Yeah, they were culturally different from me, but so was everybody else."*

I WAS BORN IN 1945 IN CORK, IN IRELAND. UNTIL THE FINAL year in medical school my vision of what I wanted to do was very clear: I wanted to be a family practitioner in West Cork and stay in Ireland, live and practice in Ireland. Even that was fairly ambitious, because Ireland at the time, as it does now, has a national health scheme. Just because you're a doctor doesn't mean you get a job. There are a certain number of general practitioners, and they were all given districts. You were paid a per capitation—like, you had two and a half thousand people and you were their primary health care provider, and the government paid you. If they had a person in that slot then they didn't need any more. If you wanted to go out into private practice, fine, but no one was going to come to you because they all had national health.

In my final year of medical school I was attached to the old professor of surgery in a hospital called the South Charitable Infirmary. Surgeons in Ireland are called "Mister," so this was "Mr. Kiley is coming to make rounds." And then we'd all troop along, and he'd stop and he'd turn to me and say [pinched, nasal voice]: "OK, Barrett. Name the seven spaces of the hand." He liked me a lot and at the end of the rotation he called me aside and he says, "Barrett, what are you going to do with the rest of your life?" I said, "Well, Professor, I'm going to be a general practitioner out in West Cork." And he says [squawking "nyeh" sounds], "There's the makings of a fine surgeon lost in you."

Medicine in Ireland is different. The Irish attitude toward life in general is different. It's, well, you do whatever you can and if you can't, you can't, and if people die, they die. For instance, later, when I was an intern in the North Charitable Infirmary, we had a guy who was riding a motorcycle and he struck a horse. He had a very badly mangled leg. The surgeon was looking at the leg and he was going [thick brogue] "'Tis very badly broken. 'Tis all dirty and 'tis infected and all. We should cut it off, we should really take the leg off." The senior registrar—who would be like a senior resident—said, "Ah no, we can clean this up." Then he turns to me and says, "What do you think, Barrett? Shouldn't we just take it off? He'll be better off without it." Then he turns to the anesthesia and goes, "Don't you think we should take it off?" And he finally talked everyone into it, and we amputated the guy's leg. I remember he went down to talk to the family and explain that he had to amputate the leg. He said, "Sure, he's better off without it. He'd always walk with a terrible limp." [laughs] And people accept that in Ireland. They go, "Yes, of course he would."

The North Charitable Infirmary serves an area called Graunnabrathar, and the people were tough. They were lower socioeconomic groupings, and they were pretty violent as far as Irish people go. So I would happily sit there on Saturday night as the bars closed—they'd wheel in all the drunks who would get involved in bar fights, and they'd have facial lacerations and cuts from beer bottles, and I'd just stitch 'em up. At the end of that year I was convinced that I was going to be a plastic surgeon—because that's what plastic surgeons do, right? They stitch up people's faces.

There was a very good plastic surgical program in Norfolk, Virginia, and I went there in July of 1970. But it rapidly became very clear to me that plastic surgery had nothing to do with trauma. What it had to do with was cosmetics, and I just couldn't stand that stuff, so in '71 I returned to Ireland. I'd decided that what I wanted to be was a general surgeon with a special interest in trauma. That was pretty much unheard of in Ireland at the time: every surgeon did trauma, it was not specialized stuff. I decided to spend some more time in America in a surgical training program. I recall I came here, and I was shown the Trauma Unit, and I couldn't believe it. The Trauma Unit at County was internationally famous and it's a tiny, small, dingy little place.

So July 1st in 1975 I start my rotations at County. My first rotations were on the Burn Unit and then on the Peds Unit. It was interesting, because I was pretty much trained, but it really didn't help a tack. The attendings were these creatures that came in once or twice a week, kind of generally looked things over. But the senior surgical residents really ran the services, and you were a workhorse and you did the work; they didn't want to hear your opinions until you'd been here for a couple of years.

I didn't go into medicine to make money out of it, so the fact that we weren't getting paid a lot and it was hard work was incidental. It was the volume of work that was done here—there was just so much of it. It worked well insofar as the technical ability of the surgeon to develop your own technical ability: we learned a lot.

People say, "You're a surgeon. My God, you must have a steady hand." Steady hands have nothing to do with surgery: you could teach educated gorillas to operate. It's the *decision* to perform the operation. And I think that it was a very aggressive bunch of people in this hospital; I think that they really pushed indications to the limit. I'd come from a much more conservative approach—"Let's wait and see—let's wait until they get peritonitis, and then we'll operate." Whereas the approach here was, "No, let's pick these things up early. And if we do some negative operations then we do negative operations, but we don't want to miss anything."

The difference between Irish medicine and American medicine is this: In America the patient has an anticipation of being cured—they automatically think they're going to be cured rapidly, without any pain. They want to come in and be given one pill, you take the one pill and you're cured. Whereas in Ireland they anticipate that maybe the doctor can help you but, God help us, he's only doing the best he can—and if you go into hospital of course you're going to die because it's your time.

But the people who came to County were different types of people—and, increasingly, those people became more and more difficult to recruit. Part of the reason I got here was because there wasn't a lot of competition. I was a foreign medical graduate, and in my class at County there were two other foreign medical graduates of the eight of us.

In 1980,the director of the Trauma Unit asked me to stay on as an attending. And at that stage I decided that was it: I was clearly going to stay in America. That was when I decided to get married, to move toward permanent immigrant status and, ultimately, citizenship. Ultimately, my ambition was to run my own Trauma Unit—that I would go from here to somewhere else. The director was diagnosed as having cancer, and he died in February of '82. He was sort of my mentor. I had not thought that I was going to run the unit, because I was not the most senior surgeon—and I was certainly not the best surgeon. I didn't know anything about administration, and what I knew of it I didn't like. I wanted to spend my time doing the fun stuff—looking after the patients and operating and teaching. They finally convinced me to do it. I think they took an enormous chance. To my total amazement, I loved it.

Most surgeons hate going to meetings and want to just concentrate on the patient care. The patient care is the most important thing, and the second most important thing is teaching, and the third most important thing is research. But you can't do any of them unless you've got a structure to do it in. Most people just bitch and moan about: "Well, we can't do this because it's all screwed up." Well, why is it all screwed up? I mean, there's a corresponding administrative structure that doctors in general and surgeons in particular don't want to touch. Surgeons are self-centered, aggressive, dogmatic, authoritarian. They stick out their hand and say, *"Gimme a knife."* And they expect a knife to be put into their hand—they don't want someone to say, "Well, knives are very expensive this week. How about we give you a meat cleaver instead?" But you can't divorce yourself from what's going on around you. You work in a health care system.

It was a surgeon from Cook County Hospital who established the concept of trauma systems: getting the seriously injured in. Cook County's Trauma Unit was the very first one that was ever established, in 1966. But we never truly implemented the system in the city of Chicago. We had designated Trauma Centers in the city of Chicago, but there was no one who said who should go where. So in the early eighties, even though we were a designated Trauma Center, the Chicago Fire Department took the injured patient to the closest hospital, which was the wrong way to go.

Trauma systems consist of the appropriate patient at the appropriate hospital in an appropriate time frame. The average patient is triaged, but what you're supposed to do in trauma systems is to *over*triage, get more than you actually need, so that you don't miss anyone. The problem with that is it means that patients are going past the doors of *your* hospital to come to *my* Trauma Center. Well, people weren't too happy about that: "Why should he pass my door?" *Especially* if they were paying patients. Ha ha ha ha. So we had to tighten the criteria—very, very tight. Everybody and their mother wanted to be a Trauma Center: nineteen places applied to be Trauma Centers. We really only need about six. They were sure there was money in it, and they were sure there was prestige in it. Their administrations saw it as a marketing business, they *had* to have this designation. So the original system went into effect in '86 with ten Trauma Centers.

After two years several things became obvious. One, there was no money in it—in fact, you were *losing* money, because trauma systems in the inner city deal primarily with penetrating trauma, lower socioeconomic groupings. And before, those losses had been spread out throughout the entire community of hospitals, which were now concentrated in the trauma system. By '88, four of the hospitals withdrew. That's still a major problem for us because of the geographical distribution. There's no trauma center on the entire South Side—people have to go either to County or to Christ Hospital, which is very far south, and then County takes care of the West Side as well. But the good news is, there are six trauma centers still in existence, and at five of the six units the Trauma Center directors have worked here at County—and we all know each other, we help each other. If the patient can withstand the extra few minutes, we'll send him this way and we'll protect him that way. Patients that are being referred to you from other hospitals, send them to us: teamwork, mutual help.

My original interest in trauma was from a surgical point of view, because it fulfills all of the criteria that surgeons really love. Surgery was really developed from following armies around. The first surgeons operated on military casualties, and that's what we're doing. We're essentially operating on people who are shot and stabbed and mangled and beaten and thrown out of motor vehicles and who fall from high places. They tend to be young, they tend to be male, they tend not to have preexisting disease. You have to make a rapid decision—I mean, really rapid. Sometimes within a minute or two you have to decide what to do. Mostly, you have to operate. Of the patients who arrive on our unit who are alive, 98 percent leave alive. And they're young: in terms of preventable years of life lost, there are more preventable years lost due to trauma than to cardiovascular disease, hearts, strokes, and cancer combined.

So that's the initial challenge for a surgeon: it's immediate, it's dramatic, it's kind of sexy. You operate, they do well, you've saved another life. Trauma surgeons are adrenaline junkies. They just love this stuff. In fact, they're very similar in personality to Emergency Medicine physicians. They have the same sort of need to have the excitement. They have close companionships with paramedics and firefighters, police officers, the same sort of personality.

But as time passed, it became clear to me that there's more to this than just cutting. What we really need to get across—and here we have failed—is that trauma is a *disease*. It's a disease like any other disease. The words we use don't help us. We say, "She was involved in a motor vehicle accident." *Accident* implies, well, there was nothing much you could do about it—it was the will of God, blah, blah, blah. Well, that's not true. An accident happens, of course, because something went wrong: you were driving too fast, you were drunk, your car was not in proper repair, the road was badly designed, inadequate lighting. Something *happened* that caused an injury. Injuries are not accidents. So we need to get that across that this is a disease, and we should deal with it as we deal with other diseases.

The most important way of dealing with a disease is prevention. So the concept has expanded from "Let's just operate on them" to "Let's prevent it from happening." And that's where I think most of our effort needs to go in the future. When you talk about injury-prevention strategies, most of them are orientated toward blunt trauma: automotive wrecks, drunk driving, seatbelts, airbags, safer vehicles, and so on. I'm much more interested in the tougher one, and that's penetrating trauma or what is called intentional injury: gunshot wounds, stabbings, personal assaults.

Now, we can do some things relatively quickly. Gun control is one of my favorite things. You know, we don't have rights to have semiautomatic weapons. In 1982 when I became director, of the twenty-five hundred patients we saw, about five hundred of them had been shot. Of the five hundred that were shot, only 5 percent were struck by more than one bullet—they tended to be low-caliber Saturday night specials, .22 caliber bullets. They're great fun from a surgeon's point of view: you operate, you stitch up all the holes, they do fine, they go home.

Last year we had forty-five hundred admissions—over *a thousand* of them were gunshot wounds! [with amazement and horror] Over a thousand gunshot wounds! And, of that number, 25 percent are hit with more than one bullet. And they're not .22 caliber slugs anymore, they're 9mm automatic weapons—those kind of bullets do *far more* damage. It used to be you'd open them up and stitch up the holes; now you have problems as to *which* cavity to open. He's shot in the chest, he's shot in the belly—where do you go *first*? And then, when you go in, it's such devastating injuries you can't just stitch them back together—and they're more likely to develop complications, require repeat operations. Much longer periods of time in Intensive Care, more susceptible to infection, and a much longer recovery time. In fact, our major problem right now is not that we don't have enough surgeons or we don't have enough operating rooms—although the operating rooms do get tight occasionally. We don't have enough Intensive Care beds. We constantly play this game of "Who's the least sick?" And if there's someone more sick in our Resuscitation Area, then bump the guy in the bubble and send him over to the wards.

The surgical techniques that we use on these patients are techniques that were developed in Vietnam. We're fighting a war out there, *now*. It's more than the guns, though, and this is my current soapbox. If you and I had an argument, I probably wouldn't shoot you for two reasons. First off, I don't have a gun; and second, if I had an argument with you, I would somehow cope with it. I would say, "You're really annoying me, and the reason you're really annoying me is this, and I wish you wouldn't do that, and do you think in future you could..." We would come up with some sort of solution, some sort of coping mechanism. The short-term problem is that people have access to guns; the *real* problem is that they don't have coping mechanisms. You get angry, you resort to violence. And that's what I think we need to change. I think we need to be out, right now, in the schools teaching children about drugs and safe sex, but I think we also need to teach them that violence is not an acceptable social behavior. Smoking is not acceptable, violence is not acceptable. You *do not* hit people. And we will have to teach them coping skills, behavior modification skills. We should try, I think we should. But I'll be honest with you, I think that when you're eighteen, nineteen, twenty, twenty-five, it's too late. I think we've lost an entire generation here. This violence is going to continue on for another twenty years. But if we can start educating a new generation of people that just say, "They were crazy. They used to go around shooting people, and they would beat each other with baseball bats because they had disagreements."

What I'm trying to do is to create a box—that's how I refer to it—with all these people in it. I have on my staff a person who has their master's degree in public health, who's very interested in injury prevention. We have emergency medicine people who work with us. We have rehabilitative people who work with us. We have surgeons with a particular interest in intensive care. And all of those people need to be coordinated, all together, in order to get anywhere with it—the nurses, the social workers, the occupational therapists, physiotherapists, everybody. We've all got to sit down and talk to each other. No more of this, "I'm the doctor, you're the nurse, you do it because I'm the doctor." We all have professional capabilities, and we all mutually expect and respect each other for what we can do. And therefore the whole team gels together as a *team*. And that's really, I think, the ultimate challenge. When things go wrong, we all sit down and we analyze it: we say, "Well, yeah, he died, but you know, we actually did the right things, we made the right calls"—or, "We really blew that one. Next time we'll have learned something." That's challenging.

I don't know what's going to happen in terms of health care reform, but I think there will always be a need for County-type institutions. I don't think we're ever going to get to the stage of saying that everybody is covered for everything. I don't think you're going to get a plastic card that entitles you to walk into any hospital and ask for a liver transplant. You'll have some things that they'll do for you; but there will be some patients that other hospitals don't really want.

Trauma is a good example. Trauma patients in the inner city tend to be poor, they tend to be Black, they tend to be penetration cases. Of all of our patients, 4.7 percent are infected by the HIV virus, 7 percent of them have hepatitis. Of patients who present with penetrating trauma requiring operation, 10 percent are HIV positive. And blood is all over the place with these patients—so they're high-cost, high-risk, high-volume, high-intensity. Other hospitals don't want these patients, just as they don't want the AIDS patients, don't want the TB patients, don't want the diseases of addiction. And I think even if they were paid money they don't want them, because it's disruptive to them. They want to do their liver transplants or their in vitro–fertilization or their cardiocatheterization. And at the University of Chicago there are hundreds of doctors who are discovering the cure for cancer.

I feel an incredible sense of loyalty and commitment to *this* institution. I've been offered jobs at other places—they'll come and they say, "Can't you do this?" It's interesting: they don't truly understand it when you say, "Well, I'm at County, why would I go?" I stay here because I think I'm needed here. I think there's an enormous need here that I'm fulfilling. Also, I'm so egotistical that I think if I was pulled out, no one else would do it quite as well. That's not true: other people would probably do it just as well. But I don't feel the same sense…I mean, when someone comes to me and offers me other jobs for more money and more academic prestige…

I consider myself an academic surgeon. But academic surgeons are totally horrified that I don't get paid by the university, and I work purely in a county hospital. It's as if, "Well, there must be something wrong with you." It's like the old conception of military surgeons: [snootily] "Well, if he's a doctor in the army, he can't be a really good doctor. He couldn't get a proper job. He couldn't go out there and compete in private practice. Ha ha ha ha—wouldn't want to go to him." That's very bothersome to me, especially for the young surgeons who come here; because we are *the* academic trauma—we are *it*.

The role of the surgeon is changing enormously—ignoring trauma— because surgery does things that medicine fails at. In other words, if you have a cancer, what we should do is cure it—and if we can't cure it, then we cut it out. Well, cutting things out is kind of medieval, you know? You draw a circle and then you cut it out. Operations on the stomach, for instance, for ulcers, are rapidly disappearing, because we're curing ulcers. Ultimately, someone will figure out a way of dissolving gallstones, so then we won't be operating on gallstones anymore. But there will *always* be a need for trauma. In my lifetime no one is going to come up with a pill to give you when you're shot in the abdomen, to take care of the bullet wound. Increasingly, where surgery came from—the followers of the armies—is where it is going in the future.

I think there will always be a role for county hospitals. I think the poor will always be with us, and they will always have unique needs. I think those unique needs will be met by institutions that are essentially public institutions.

Let me say this: There's a real problem in the way that we train physicians in this country. And a lot of it is the fault of people like me. When a medical student rotates on my service, this is high-glamour stuff: snatching them back from the brink of death, blood and guts and television cameras. But we are highly specialized. The country doesn't need specialists. The country needs primary health care physicians. We should be graduating 80 percent of our people and putting them out there in community health. We're only actually putting about 20 percent into community health; 80 percent of the graduates in this country, even today, want to go into subspecialization. And we've got to change that.

A lot of it is financial. In fact, if you talk to a plastic surgeon, for instance—there's a training program in plastic surgery, they rotate here at this hospital, and I've talked to some—how many do you think have as their life ambition to stay in the inner city and look after the plastic surgical problems of the sick poor? None! Zero! *None*. They're all going out to white suburban communities. Well, that's wrong. And I think it's especially wrong that they're trained at a county institution and take advantage of their learning and take it elsewhere. I think that is wrong.

I came from a system in which, granted, I had to pay to go through medical school, but it wasn't that much, and it was actually covered by a scholarship...But when I came out of medical school, I didn't have enormous debt. I was fine. I think we need to have a quid pro quo there: I don't think people should become doctors because they anticipate making a lot of money. I've heard people say, "He must be a fine surgeon, he makes $250,000 a year." There's no correlation between the two. I'm not sure how you change that, but I think we really have to.

People need to go into medicine for reasons other than financial reasons, and they need to be primary care orientated. And that means going all the way back to medical school training and changing the entire attitude among medical students. The way that medical students are trained, rotating them through speciality units, maybe that shouldn't be how it's done—maybe they should be spending all their time out in community clinics, talking about prevention. To me, there's something fundamentally wrong with an attitude of mind that says, "You're sick, pay me." The ancient Chinese had it much better—they said, "When you're well, you pay the doctor; when you're sick, the doctor pays you." That's a much better system—*now* you're talking prevention.

Jewell Jenkins

SHE'S LIVED ON *Chicago's South Side all her life. She is tall and thin and strong of will. Pioneer-tough. She sits in my yard in her housekeeper's uniform, speaking her mind. "Some of the nurses say you got to do this, do that. I say, 'I don't got to do nothin' but stay Black and die!'"*

COUNTY, WHEN I FIRST WENT THERE, THE NURSES THAT I WORKED with seemed to really care. I started working there in 1989 as a housekeeper: I was given a ward in the main building. It was all right, but at first I was told that I would have to work P.M.s [evenings] or nights, and I had just come off a night job which I did not like—it curtailed all my activities at night. [laughs]

So the AIDS Ward opened up, and I could get a day shift because, at the time, nobody wanted to work up there. I volunteered, and then I later found out that my nephew had AIDS—and it gave me a chance to be close to him. He was grown, and he had told my sister, "Oh Mama, don't tell Aunt Jewell. Don't tell her." You know, [laughs] he was my special kid. When he got sick and confined, she called me and told me. I said, "Yeah, I noticed his name was on the board for transferring." At that time he didn't even know exactly where I was; he just knew I was working in the hospital. I guess he thought, Maybe there's a possibility she won't find me up here. And he comes up and I was the first one that greeted him at the door—I said, "Hey, Mike, how you doing?" [laughs]

I wasn't scared—you know, I didn't even think about it. The little bit I had heard was that you could contract it through IV drug abuse or sex, OK? I had just divorced my husband, but we were still messing around, so I figured I was fairly safe—and I'm not a drug user. We had a lot of gay guys up there, and everybody was teasing me. I said, "First of all these guys have done what they wanted to do in their life, OK? Nobody stood up and said, 'Here I am, come get me, AIDS! Here I am, come get me, I want to be sick!' It's something that happens." I had gotten to know quite a few of the fellows and they seemed very nice, despite them being homosexual. The girls was teasing me, "Girrrl, everybody up there is gay." I said, "Well, you know what? I could care less what people think about me. If this bothers somebody and they don't want to associate with me—bye." To me, these guys are gay, and they are here looking for the same thing I'm looking for—a good man! I said, "I'm not going to jump

28

into bed with none of them, so I ain't worried about catching it." They said, "Well, you can get *stuck.*" I said, "So I get stuck. Me, within myself, I have the feeling that I've lived fifty years, if God has given me a half century, then I have been blessed. Now the rest of it I'm going to take one day at a time, because none of it has been promised."

My job involves me in cleaning. I've been written up several times for being too friendly with the patients—written up and suspended. One boy, he had been there a total of six months. His parents had kind of said, "Oh, gee whiz, no, not him—my only son, and then he's gay." So they stood back. Nobody came up to see him, nobody wanted to be bothered with him. He annoyed the nurses all the time, because he stayed on the buzzer—he wanted attention. I paid him some attention. I used to talk to him. I would bring him things from home: food, books, whatever he asked for. [slyly] Cigarettes. I asked the head doctor, which was Dr. Shearer at the time, "If we put him in the wheelchair, could I take him out on my breaks and my lunch? Because he's getting tired of these four walls that he's looking at." All I was concerned with was, is it safe enough to take him out?

All I did was put him in the wheelchair, took him downstairs, and rolled him around the complex. I don't know exactly who told, but I know several of the supervisors saw me, and it was reported. I got reprimanded for it, and I think I got three days off. They said I was in housekeeping and "I was not supposed to bother the patients." When I was called into the office about it they told me, "This isn't what you do, this isn't what you're here for." I said, "You're telling me that I'm working in a place where I'm supposed to be a human being, *and I can't be humanly?!*"

What I had started to do is when the new patients came and were up and about, in a wheelchair or something, I would try to show them around—tell them about the lounge room that we have with the TV, and books, and the quiet room, the washroom, the way I try to keep it...the soiled utility room where, if they get up overnight and want a urinal emptied and the nurse don't get to it, where to take it—and not to take it back in the bathroom and empty it. We have a dining area where, if they don't want to sit in their room and eat, they can bring their tray out and set it on this dinette table. I was told I wasn't supposed to do this. I would welcome them when they came in: "Hey, this is Ward 65, this is the special ward!" I had the time to do this, because the ward was new, and it didn't take that much to keep it up. I would do my cleaning, say, seven until about eleven-thirty, and from then I would have time to stop: "Hey, how you doin'? Did your mother come see you yesterday? How's your son? Did your friend bring you something?" Something to keep their mind off their illness.

I tell them certain things on how to make the food taste a little bit better. The Ensures [a high-protein drink] that they try to make all the patients up there drink, I started taking them home and drinking them. I started gaining weight. I come back and I tell them, "Oh, I hate it, but—you know what?—if you drink them in between your breakfast and your lunch it'll put the weight on you." I would stand up and say, "Look at me. Look at my hips. I'm getting *big.*" [laughs]

I've had the dietician come up and ask me, "Did So-and-so eat?" I say, "Yeah, but he don't like that." "Oh, he doesn't like that?" I say, "No, give him a larger portion of something else and just a little bit of this, and you can get him to eat." Last week, a guy had told the dietician he was eating. I told her, "No, he ain't eating." I step back in the room and I said, "Why do you want to lie to her? The only way they can help you is if they know what you're doing."

It's the same way with the medicine. I found one of the little cups of oral medicine. The boy was stashing it, he wasn't taking it. I went in and I told the patient, "If you're not going to take the medicine then refuse it, because they're writing on the chart that they gave it to you! The doctor is reading the chart, assuming you took it, and assuming is making an ass out of him." I said, "By this being something new, they have to know exactly what is going on. They're still learning." I went to the nurse and I said, "Do you know he's not taking his medicine?" She said, "Oh, yes, I gave it to him." I said, "Oh, no, he's not taking it." "How do you know?" [takes hand from behind her back] I said, "Here, look. Does this look like he took it?"

We've had a few nurses there before who did not like it. I got called down about that, how I'm up there trying to do *they* job. I said, "Well, I'm the one that's slopping up all of this—y'all giving out pills and writing down on the chart these patients is taking this stuff, but I got a bucket full of medicine melting in my water." I was told, "You're taking over our duties, this is not for you—you are in housekeeping." I said, "Yes, I am in housekeeping and I will do housekeeping work, OK?" So then when they start asking me I say, "I dunno. I dunno." The way it was said it was like, "You don't have the education to do anything but scrub floors." It really pissed me off. I let them know: "I am a college graduate. I have a B.A. [real loud] I am doing this because it pays money and since I have gotten into it *I like it!*" I told them, "I'll shovel shit for money, long as it pays."

There are a lot of things, according to the union and the hospital, that we are not supposed to do. I have broken every rule, OK? I done broke them *all!* [glaring defiantly at the tape recorder] I have broke every rule, but in breaking the rules I hope that I have made someone's life just a little more happier—specifically, the patient's.

Now, I have a made a few nurses miserable, and I know this. I'll do this again as long as I've got that job. [laughs] But I *like* being the type of person that, when I'm off, when you walk in the room: [excitedly] "Where were you yesterday? We missed you!" It's like nobody came in with a pleasant smile.

I don't know why I, all of a sudden, really am dedicated to this thing. I made up in my mind in the last week, I'm going to nursing school. I give myself three years, four if I'm unlucky. I know it's a lot that I've got to learn, but this is what I want to do because I want to help more. But I want to work from the registry and come into the hospital. I don't want to be a County employee, because County is full of shit. I mean they've got so many bosses telling so many people what to do—and the people that's telling you what to do don't know what is supposed to be done.

I have gotten into it with the nurses. I have found IV tubings, I have found *needles* laying around. I mean, these things are *dangerous*. If you don't think about the patient, he's already sick, he's going to die, what the fuck? OK, who cares? But *I've* got to come back through there, *you've* got to come back through there, your co-worker, another nurse, a visitor…Then the hospital is sued. We go through all of this just because, [simpering] "I was gonna get it." You're *grown*—you're supposed to have a mind. You want to play the big cheese here, you done passed the state board, so that makes you more intelligent than me—OK, I can buy this. You can be more intelligent than me, I wouldn't care. But *if* you are, and I *tell* you about it, *don't* tell me I am doing your job or telling you your job. If you know your job, you would do it. So this is why we have had so many clashes with me and the nurses.

Some people, it's like, "I don't have to rush" and "I don't have to do that, somebody will remind me," or "I'll get it done later." When to me, OK, you can just about walk out of a room and turn around—and one of those patients could have a seizure and die. While you're *thinking* about doing something for 'em, they can *die*. I told them, "If I fall out, put me out here on the street, OK? Don't service me at all in this hospital, because I will get quicker service out there in the street. Somebody probably will bend down and say, 'What's wrong?'"

I mean, we've had patients to fall out the bed! And I go tell the nurse and they take their time about getting back down there. One in particular fell out the bed, and I'm calling the nurse—I done picked him up and put him back in the bed before she got to me. "Well, we got to document this," she says. "How *you* going to document this? You ain't seen *nothin'*." The nurse asks me, "How did he fall? Where did he fall?" [disgusted] I said, "He fell on the floor. You think he fell out the window?"

They'll move me around because 65 is only a half a ward now, so you don't have to spend the whole day up there. I've worked 35, 45, 55, 65, 75, I've worked 15. The ward that I worked on today was 25, which is dialysis. And I've gotten friendly with two of the fellows down there. One of them, he had grits and egg and a biscuit. He had jelly, he had butter, he had coffee. He didn't want the grits. He said, "Gee, if I had me some cold cereal, I'd be into something." I said, "That's what you want?" He said, "Yeah, I sure want me some cold cereal." I said, "Hold on one minute." I went back to my cart. Occasionally, they give them those little packages of cold cereal—I had some on my cart. I went and got two packages, and I went back and I gave it to him. He said, "Oh man, that sure was swinging."

It made me feel good to a certain extent. But you know what? I don't glory in *them* making *me* feel good. I glory in the fact that I've done something to please somebody. It's not an ego trip for me to do for them. It's like, you wanted it and I was able to give it to you. I was thinking about saving it and taking it upstairs and eating it on my break, but I'm not starving—and it was something *he* wanted. It was important that he ate, for his health. Mine is pretty good. I'm not in the bed—it was him in the bed.

I never went to County as a patient, but my sister was born there. When my kids were small, I used to take my kids to County. I used to call County Hospital, and they would send doctors out to my home. This was back in '57, '58. They made house calls—they had my kids' records. I would call, and the doctor would call me back and question me, and then he would know what medicine to bring. County was all right then. As my kids got older I used to tell people, "You get past the first floor— that's Emergency—you got it made." The few times that I went out there, I knew to get up early in the morning and pack me a lunch, you know, like I'm going on a picnic. Bring you a couple of books and some knitting, something to sew, because you're going to be a while.

But since I'm on the inside looking out, I wouldn't go back up in there now—and it's horrible because it's the only county hospital in the city. I keep trying to tell the nurses this makes no sense: it's Black-orientated, it's Black-worked, the majority of officials, the administrators are Black, darn near all of the patients are Black. How come it couldn't be A–Number One? You should *want* it to be A–Number One. But what happens? All the other hospitals…it's like a dumping zone. County is like a trash catcher—they dump all they trash on us. And it's either because they're short-handed, or they don't want the patient or…To me, I'm the last one to look at a money situation when a person is sick.

The residents are not orientated to be a doctor to the patient. They're orientated to learn something and get up out of there. You go all over the city and you see all these doctors who practiced at County, but what did they do for County? They didn't make County better, they left it the way it was. And it's very unfair.

The first thing I would let them know is, "You're going to learn *every*-thing that goes on in this hospital." We've got doctors that don't know how to fill out slips to get medicine, to get blood drawn. They can't draw blood. They can't do certain tests. They don't even know how to fill out the paper. Now, when you come in and you can't fill out a paper to get something done and you don't know how to do it, what do you do? You leave it. So, a lot of things that really should be done for the patients are not done. The residents don't know. These doctors, they go through, every four weeks they're at a different location. And every four weeks these same patients is going through the same tests because the doctors prior to, in front of them, didn't ask for certain tests that should have been taken.

We've got girls that draw blood that don't know how to draw blood. They're *sticking* them—and then when they call somebody else up, from the IV team, to do it again, the patient says, "Nuh-uh." And they write it down that the patient don't want to take the test. Then *everybody's* got an attitude toward the patient. The blood drawer is mad because she had to come upstairs. [testily] "If I'd a known he didn't want no blood drawn, I wouldn't even have come up. Why didn't this doctor find out whether he was going to let me draw blood?" The doctor didn't know, because he didn't find out whoever he was supposed to have had do it before, did not get it. He ain't got the papers. And the nurse is upset because all she did was come in to tell the patient it was a different person to take the blood and she's got something else to do—so *she* cops an attitude…This makes no sense whatsoever.

These doctors don't know shit from shinola about where those patients come from, what their lifestyle is, what they're used to, what they might do, what they won't do. One of the patients told me their doctor was asking leading questions: "Do you feel all right?" That's not asking how do you feel. They have to learn how to talk to people and to patients. If somebody said, "Do you feel all right?" it's like you're supposed to feel all right. The residents treat me fine. You know what? They could treat me like shit, I wouldn't care, as long as they treat their patients right. Don't misuse somebody that's helping you. And those patients are helping them get an education so they can make twice as much money…

When they finish their residency they're gone. A lot of them don't even want to see me. Me, as a Black woman, they don't want to see me, they outta here. They going back to their country or another city where they can set up a practice and make some money. Nine chances out of ten they're not going to remember half the people they treat here. The ones they learned off of—they ought to be grateful! Grab any one of them that's been up there six weeks ago and ask, "Name one of the patients that was up there on the floor," and I bet you they couldn't give you a name.

If they cut down on the intake of the patients to where they would be able to know the person when they see them, be able to stand up and hold a conversation with them. It's like the dietician: she knows them, but she don't know who eats, who don't eat, who likes what. She's not allowed this much time to spend with one patient. She's got too much ground to cover. It's on paper that the hospital is working this year;

everybody is getting their salary. You know, big deal. Money is not gonna take us to God.

I don't have all the answers, I know. I just keep getting up in the morning and…Like I used to get in and I'd go to the ward and say, "Let's see what God is doing out here today. Let's raise the shade." I do this even when it's raining, and I'll stand there and say, "Hmm, boy, it's wet outside," to call their attention to what's outside. My thought is like this: I am glad to wake up. I didn't have to wake up. I tell them, "There's so many things that's happening, there's so many people that's dying." I mean, kids are being shot and they haven't spent *any* time on this earth, so be thankful for what you got. They're like, "How can you be so happy all the time?" I say, "Well hey, that's me. I don't find nothing to be sad about."

Dr. Lorena Jauregui

SHE IS TWENTY-NINE AND *has just finished her first year as a resident. "I'm from Mexico. I grew up in a city, Mexicali. I was between being a veterinarian or an M.D. I liked both, and I liked astronomy. I said, astronomy, I don't know. What would be something I could apply more, especially in Mexico? So I decided to go into medicine. We don't pay for university in Mexico. That's why we have what you call a social service, and once you finish medical school, you do a year of social service. You go to a rural area where there are a lot of poor people and do free service for one year, twenty-four hours a day. What I did was a rural community, basically. Pickers that come every year to pick tomatoes, strawberries. I was the main clinic in the community. You're there by yourself."*

WHEN I GOT HERE TO THE HOSPITAL, THE MAIN ENTRANCE, that was my first time in Chicago. I was like, am I in the United States? You know, like, *whoops!* This huge, big old hospital? It was weird, because I was used to seeing new hospitals. That's the first impression that I had of Cook County Hospital. But there are a lot of things that I like at the hospital, especially because I'm used to working with poor people.

At first it was strange, but not hard. I don't have anything against Black people or Chinese people or whatever, but that was kind of weird. I've gotten used to it now. The culture is different. But I call—maybe it's not the right word—the poor people, they're not complicated people. Sometimes, if you go to a private hospital where everybody has their own doctor, it's: "Oh, you're a first-year resident, I don't want you, I want my doctor." So I wanted to be more free to work with the people.

I want to do family practice. Maybe in the future I would like to live by the Mexican border and go back and forth, give free service there, whatever. Here it's more difficult, because of legal stuff. And here you can make a lot of money if you're a specialist, but I'm not sure that's right or fair for the other people. But there are a lot of things in the medical system that I think are not right in the United States. What makes the medicine so expensive is technology and all these things—plus the malpractice insurance. I don't know how to say it, but...I don't feel comfortable. Everybody likes to live okay. I've got my daughter and my husband, and we want to build a future for her.

But sometimes the doctors become very insensitive. I have seen it here.

For example, I just finished Labor Line; the way it works is a patient gets into the admitting room, usually in labor pain, and there's a nurse, a clerk, and at least a couple of doctors. The patient is here on the bed in pain, and they come stick the patient, and everyone tries to put in the IV, and it's [aggressively] "What's your name, what's your name?" The poor patient. They cry very often there. What I did is just let everybody finish, and I'll do it later, or I try to do it first, to talk to the patient, in between contractions. You have to get the medical history and whatever. They're having contractions, and you're asking them, and they're screaming. But that's the way it is because everyone wants [snaps fingers rapidly] to finish fast.

You get this way because you have a lot of work. You get one admission, you have to finish as soon as possible—because if you don't finish, then you will be stuck, and it will be the whole night trying to finish the patients. But I think at least spending five or ten extra minutes with the patient, it would make a big difference. You're talking to a person, not to a patient. I always ask them, "How do you want me to call you?" If they are Mexican I know, because I am Mexican—I know my culture, and I call them by their name. I call them Jose, or whatever is the name, or Don—we use that a lot. And then they feel like there is no barrier, there is a communication.

Sometimes it's hard, because there are a lot of patients. I had one case three months ago, in family practice ward. He was an HIV-positive patient. He had a lot of problems, and he didn't want to talk to anybody. So you ask, "Why you came to the hospital?" "I don't want to talk about it." It was like this every, every, every day. He signed out AMA [against medical advice]. Then he came back a week later, he was more sick. He was still the same, not talking to me. One day he talked, he was very mad, screaming at me. He thought he was going to be discharged. The social worker was talking to him, and she told him that we were planning to discharge him—but he didn't have a place to go, so we kept him for an extra week trying to find a place for him. With him I almost lose my patience. It was like, That's it, no more. I kind of looked at him and said, "You don't know me. You have been seeing me for a month, and you don't know me yet. I want to help you." And I was looking at him straight—I said, "Believe me, I want to help you." And since then, the next day he was smiling to me. That day I was very happy.

Most of the doctors around here are residents, and they don't care, because they are just temporary here. I think a lot of people are in medical careers because they want to make a lot of money. That's my thinking. Especially when I see these people—selfish.

The thing about foreign doctors is, it's very hard. You are discriminated against all over. A foreign doctor, especially going to the West, you will have a lot of trouble getting a residency. Places where you can get into a residency like New York, Chicago, those places, where they need foreign

doctors because they have people from all over the world; they need bilin-
guals, they need all of that. I sent probably sixty applications for interview,
and I just got three back. That's what you have to do. Once they read
where you graduated from, oh, from Mexico, they...[throwing-away ges-
ture]. I have a friend, he was in the review committee of a hospital in Seattle and he told me, "Once we see an application is from a foreign doctor,
we just put it in the garbage—we don't even open the envelope."

I interviewed at another hospital here, and I didn't like the hospital, it
was more private, nice. I didn't like it. It's kind of a feeling, you know?
But here, I liked it.

One of the things I was a little nervous about was—because English is
my second language—I never wrote even a single note in English, a medical note, nothing. And my first day was very hard, because it took me forever just to write a note like this [indicates a small space with her hands].
So I thought, Well, I'm not going to be the only ugly duckling. If I go to a
private hospital with all White doctors, I would be the ugly duckling.

Sometimes it's very, very frustrating. When you're on call and you order
a CT [cat scan], and then it's STAT—like you need an emergency X-ray or
an emergency CT—and then it's two, three days after and nobody knows
about the CT. Or whatever you ordered, blood work, and they didn't
come, they didn't do it, and so you have to draw the blood and send it. And
then it never gets to the lab, it gets lost. And you get very...[sighs] "I sent it,
I sent it." And then you have to do it again. "I'm sorry, but I have to do it
again." And you have to stick the patient again. Everything.

There are a lot of things, but everything has something positive. You
learn to do a lot of things. Sometimes I would call it a dysfunctional hospital, because you have to work as a doctor, as a clerk, transporter, everything. You work a lot. On call sometimes you don't sleep for thirty-six
hours. And we are human beings, so sometimes it's like, No more. But
then you rest, you get energy. But that's the positive thing: you're able to
do a lot of things. And my goal is to get a very good training.

There's a lot of people, they have had a lot of problems. They are on
call, and they fight with this and with this. A lot of stories. Like they
ordered these things and it wasn't done, and then they're still working, so
it's like we're slaves here and nobody cares. And that sounds like a slave,
right? Working more than thirty-six hours. But when you are working
like that, you're not thinking you are doing public medicine, that this is a
public hospital. You think that everybody is using you and nobody cares.
I feel that way too, but as I said, I try to think positive.

There are good clerks, there are bad clerks. You know, there are clerks
that you go and ask them something and it's "I don't know."
They...[drops head abruptly] cut communication. Like, "Don't ask me
more." That's it. Ohh, okay...There's a lot of people around here. Like
people in the elevator. There are nice people in the elevator, and

then…[shrugs] Because we're in contact with everybody, not just with patients. So there's people very, very nasty, and people very, very nice. And there's very good nurses and then there's people like *woof,* you can't even talk to them, they get very…[makes barking noises] There is a lot of lazy people. They just come and spend the shift and, *whoosh,* disappear.

There are good people also. But we don't see those things, right? That's the way we are. The bad stuff, negative. It's like, if you are a doctor and you work thirty, forty years of excellent medicine, but then you make a mistake and you go to court, nobody would say, "Oh, but he was a very good doctor." The good thing is nurses here are used to working with a lot of foreign doctors, a lot of accents, colors, everything. Some people are just always in bad moods. But it's hard sometimes.

Some of the personnel…Like if you ask the transporter, say, "We need this patient picked up at a certain time, they need a test or X-ray"—and the way they answer to you. Not because you are the doctor, but you have to be respectful…Like, I'm not going to treat you bad because you are a transporter, right? In the sense of human beings. They answer very, not the right way—"No, I'm going to do it when I want." And boom, they hang up. When they talk to you, it's not with good manners sometimes.

The patient, sometimes they don't treat them right. I think it's the system. I mean, like on Ward 45—that's the admitting ward—in one day you can admit up to sixty, seventy patients in one call, twenty-four hours. It's just one room. They bring the patient, put the IVs, stabilize the patient, assess the patient, and then they send the patient different places. So nurses are just working and working, and the clerks, another one, another one; nobody wants to talk to anybody, everybody wants to finish. Sometimes you get three, four at the same time. The clerk has to admit four patients at the same time.

This week I was on call on Monday. I got here at seven in the morning. We had a class with the attending; we discussed an article from eight to nine. Then we started clinic—that's from nine to five P.M. That's the whole day. We had a lot of patients, because the previous Monday was a holiday. So we were there up to six, seven o'clock seeing patients. There were people at ten in the morning and we saw them at three! There were sixty-three people in the morning and three in the afternoon, so maybe I saw like sixteen or eighteen patients. It takes time, because in GYN you have to take a pap smear and a pelvic exam and everything.

And then after the clinic we went back to the ward, and we had already five admissions, five patients waiting, and they're mad because they're waiting. You can't explain—they don't understand. I just take it, you know? "I'm sorry you waited." All of them were D&C, because they were bleeding—we dilate the cervix and kind of clean it. And we finish the last one about twelve-thirty [in the morning]. And then they paged me. We have our own patients, our clinics, and our own pregnant females. At about one they called and said I had a patient in labor, so I went up and admitted her, and came back to GYN. The patient did delivery about an hour later, so I went back and did the delivery and everything, with the paperwork. There's a lot of paperwork. We went to bed about three-thirty. We woke up at six-thirty, and we did the notes on the five patients we admitted the previous day. Then we met the attending at eight and went over the cases; and again we had clinic on Tuesday, the whole day. We finished at seven. I was like a zombie that day. I felt very weird. And then I got home and I wanted to spend a little time with my daughter, so I went to bed around nine-thirty.

And then, unluckily, they called me again for delivery for another of my patients. That was about three in the morning. So I came back to the hospital. You are not obligated to do it, because there is people in labor line—they can do it. But I feel like once you see a patient for seven, eight months every once in a while, you get very familiar to the patient—they like you, and you like the patient. She was sixteen years old, Spanish, she didn't speak any English, so she wanted me. Because nobody speaks Spanish there and sometimes, unfortunately the Spanish patients, they don't put a lot of attention to them. So it's, "Oh I want to pee"—but it's in Spanish, and they don't understand, so nobody pays attention on labor line. I was very often bringing the urinal to the patient. So I went there, and she delivered at about five, and I came to my room at Karl Meyer Hall and slept a couple of hours, and then again, a normal day. On Wednesday I had my family practice clinic from nine to one and that was it. Then I went home and slept.

And that's not really bad. On the Family Practice ward it's terrible. At least in GYN you are just there in one floor, but in Family Practice you start your call in the morning and then you have to come to Admitting Ward, to 45, and then you have patients all over the hospital. You have to go to fifth floor, second floor; you're on your feet the whole time. Sometimes you come to your room and you're getting your shoes off and *beep-beep-beep:* "Doctor, you forgot to sign." And then you have to walk all over again. You get very, very tired.

In GYN I was feeling not really tired, but because I didn't sleep enough my head was a little light. In Family Practice when you have to go on different floors, you get very tired—physically and mentally exhausted. The hospital would be ideally great if it were, like, fourteen, fifteen floor, and you just take the elevator, go up and down. With elevators that work.

But I'm really glad to be here. I'm learning. I have very, very good training. I like to do a lot of procedures, so when there's a chance to do a procedure or a delivery I want to be there. Like when I was in GYN I did—that was a record—I did forty-two deliveries in one month. And usually they do twelve, seventeen a month. And I got the Intern of the Year award.

Kathy Barrett

THIN LIKE A TEENAGER, *pretty and blond, she still looks like the small-town girl she once was. "I feel that I was successful in integrating myself and being open and learning about different peoples. You have to know how to fit in at County or you won't survive. And how do you do that? It's respect. You respect me, I will respect you. I will learn about you, you will learn about me. There's exchange. And we are equal." She is married to Dr. John Barrett.*

THE ONLY THING I EVER WANTED TO BE WAS A NURSE. PROBABLY because of my mother. When someone would get hurt, she did not know what to do and she would get very upset. We had all these family catastrophes—the time my three-year-old brother caught his penis in his zipper and had to be brought to the emergency room. My mother was running around in the back yard screaming with her hands over her ears, so *I* would call the doctor. And being the oldest of eleven, I knew how to change diapers and what formula to give to the baby and how to stop bleeding, what to do with scrapes and bruises.

When I was in high school, I had a job at the local, teeny-tiny hospital where I worked the switchboard and admitted people. I had experiences there that made me feel utterly helpless. I can remember two that were so sad. [she gets teary] I was sixteen when I had the job. I would admit you when you came into the hospital, and do all the paperwork, insurance papers and things like that.

One night we had a young boy come in by himself—*by himself!*—he probably wasn't much older than I was. He had an axe wound to his head; he came in with bloody towels wrapped around his head. The nurse that was on duty—God rest her soul in peace—was one of the coldest, most evil people I think I've ever met. When an admission would come in, she would determine what was to be done with the patient. She was a registered nurse, an older woman. That night she had determined that this patient was fit to sit in the office, and I had to sit there and ask him [voice still shaky] "What is your religion? What is your name? What is your next of kin?" And he was bleeding all over the place—it was really traumatic. Oh, I just hated that woman. I remember that boy's face. I kept saying, "Can we call the doctor now? Please?" I remember feeling so helpless, that this was inappropriate—and why would she do that? And thinking that if *I* was a nurse, I would make a different choice.

Another incident stands out in my mind. There was a very bad accident with lots of cars involved, and they brought in lots of people. They were lined up in the hallway on stretchers and they kept bringing them in. I was walking up and down the hallway, because it was my job to admit them: "What is your insurance number? Your name? Your age?" The big main emphasis I want to put on it is, "What is your insurance number?" I remember feeling so helpless and thinking that someday I would know what to do. I knew that asking them their insurance number was of no help to them.

I wanted to go to a place where I would learn how to be the best clinical nurse. I decided that I would go to Cook County Hospital, Bellevue in New York, or Charity in New Orleans. My parents were horrified. The wife of a physician in the town was an old Cook County School of Nursing graduate and my mother told me that she wanted to talk to me. This woman was active in the Alumni Association, and she told me that she had all the recent information on the Nursing School, and that it was going to become a Black nursing school—and that I *certainly* would not want to go there. I thanked her for her information, and I went to County.

I always, always wanted to be a pediatric nurse. Am I a pediatric nurse? No, I am not. [laughs] The nursing school was a three-year diploma, but we went all year long, right through the summer. I did my pediatric training at the very end of nursing school, and the whole thing was a nightmare—I could not do it. It was too painful. I remember in the Pediatric Emergency Room they had a room called the "shot room," and that's what you did—you'd give the children injections. When I would be assigned to the shot room I would lock myself in the bathroom, and I could hear my instructor calling my name: "Where is Miss Curzon? Our babies need injections—where is Miss Curzon?" And I would be in the bathroom with my hands over my ears, just as my mother had once done. I could not stick a baby.

The moment when I really decided that I couldn't do pediatrics was a day when a police officer came into the Pediatric Emergency Room. It was cold out; he had a baby in his arms who had nothing but a wet paper diaper on. The baby was a bag of bones. The baby had fallen out of a window, and the police officer was in shock: he was clutching the baby and he wouldn't let go. The officer was babbling, and they had to pry his fingers off the baby. And the baby was very, very dead. The instructor sent all of us home.

At that time, in the seventies, I was working as a nurse's aide on the Medical Admitting Unit, which was like a holding unit for patients that were coming from the Emergency Room. We had such a large volume of patients in the ER that you couldn't keep them in the ER to treat them. The patients would be triaged in the ER—very basic triage, assessment, and evaluation, very minimal treatment. If it was a medical problem, you would go to Medical Admitting. There they'd stay mostly no longer than twenty-four hours; it was an area where all the doctors could examine and work up the patient. On a Saturday night, if there was a concert, we might have eight patients, all overdoses, lined up in a row. And you would start at one end, do vital signs, arouse the patient, "Can you hear me? Wake up." And you'd get all the way down to the end and then start back all over again.

It was like a medical emergency room, but you could keep the patients long enough to see if they would respond to the intervention, and that was really gratifying. It was very fast paced, and we usually had more patients than we had beds: we had the patients in wheelchairs and on stretchers lined up in the middle row. A true County person is someone who can quickly make priorities and someone who can improvise. And if you couldn't do that, you wouldn't make it.

Any other place that I have ever worked at, I always felt at the end of the day as if it really didn't matter that I was there, that they would have done just as fine without me. But there's never been a day I worked at County that, when I went home, I didn't feel that I was really, really needed and that I made a difference. It sounds so corny, but that's how it is: the patients need us. A lot of nurses have co-dependency problems; we feed on people needing us. Well, this is a great place to act out a co-dependent personality, because you're *really* needed.

I got interested in taking care of cardiac patients, so I requested a transfer to the Coronary Care Unit, which was at that time Ward 15. It was an incredible nursing staff, everybody helped one another. That's one thing about County that I never found at any of the other hospitals where I worked: no one person is anymore important than any other. The nurses aren't anymore important than the person who brings the patient their food; the doctor isn't anymore important than the nurse who stays all night. It's a team. You can tell the senior resident, "I'm not giving this medication. I don't think that it's indicated," and we talk about it. You can't do *that* at a private hospital.

At that particular time they were opening up the Prison Unit, and they were unable to recruit nursing staff because nurses weren't flocking to work on the Prison Unit. It was the size of a regular ward, and it was quite an education: it was incredible—incredible bad, incredible bad, incredible bad. There wasn't any type of unit like this, it was totally new; no one knew exactly how to set it up. Previous to the opening of the Prison Unit, what we would do for the patients—I prefer to call them "patients" rather than "prisoners"—when they were injured or ill, they would come from the jail over to the Emergency Room. They would be triaged just like the other patients, and they would stay with a guard in the area they had been triaged to. The locked Prison Unit allowed a greater number of patients to be cared for with a much smaller number of guards. It was a mix. We had White patients, Hispanics, and Blacks. Most of the patients were young.

It was very frustrating to be locked in and locked out, to be in the nurse's station preparing medications, and turn around and look out the window and see a patient having a seizure—and you're pounding on the window, "Open the door, Let me in!" I learned what constituted contraband. You have to learn to be so careful: anything you might leave on the unit could be used as a weapon—a needle, a rubber tourniquet.

When you're a nurse, you're taught you're supposed to help the patients get well. Well, what do you do with a patient who does not wish to get well? It was much nicer to stay on the Prison Unit at County than it was to go back to Cook County Jail at 26th and California in lock-up. You would have patients who would have an operative procedure and be transferred back to the Prison Unit, who would spit in their wounds: they'd love to have an infection in their wounds, because that meant they could stay on the Prison Unit longer. It was virtually impossible to ever transfer a diabetic patient back to the jail. They would trade anything they had for a packet of sugar from another patient's food tray. [groans] That was frustrating.

Then I had a chance to apply for a job on Ward 15 in the Shock Room—it was officially called the "Procedure Room." We put in temporary pacemakers and special catheters. The equipment was huge. We did electrophysiology, testing on the heart. It was a great place to be with the patients: you could really help them, because they would be so petrified. This was all new technology. That's part of the nurse's job, that patients understand what is going on. They're supposed to ask questions: they're not supposed to be victims, they're supposed to be participants. We were taught in nursing school that the worst fear is fear of the unknown and that your patient should not suffer from that.

I think it's the public's perception that physicians are benevolent, all-knowing, and that you don't question the physician. I find that more with older patients. They don't question authority. If the physician came to them and said, "We recommend that your head be removed," they would say, "Yes, Doctor" and "Thank you, Doctor."

I think everything is cyclic. In the late sixties, early seventies, we had the hippy-type people coming into medicine to help people, for altruism. Then in the eighties where we had the invention of the preppy, and preppies don't want to come and train at Cook County Hospital. Now we're into the nineties, and I see us getting out of that "me me, I I, car phone, Brie cheese," and more into the doing for others. I think we'll see people coming back into medicine to help people, not for the big buck.

I left County in '79 because I needed to go back to school full-time and I needed my pension money to fund my schooling. I got married in 1981. I met my husband at County while he was doing his surgical residency at

County. John doesn't have the stereotypic surgeon personality, which is the ranting, raving, throwing the instruments, cold, dogmatic. I used to tease him and tell him that he had a "medicine" personality. A year after my son was born, I wanted to go back to County, but there was a hiring freeze. Instead, I went and worked somewhere else waiting for the freeze to be over.

In '86, after the hiring freeze was over, I went back to County and Ward 15. It had changed tremendously. It was no longer Coronary Intensive Care, it was now Medical Intensive Care, and we're talking totally different patients: the majority of patients were medicine patients, and there were very few cardiac patients. Now we had AIDS patients and it was horrible—it was a scary time at that time for the nurses to take care of the AIDS patients. I didn't have any trepidation about working with AIDS patients, because if you look at it from a scientific point of view, if you are protected...I had no fear that I would catch AIDS. But they're difficult patients to take care of. It is the most horrible death. It's hideous.

I had always thought the worst death to die would be an alcoholic death. At that time, a lot of the patients had the Karposi's sarcoma, and they had huge weeping, open lesions on their skin. They would have them in their esophagus and their stomach. They would be bleeding—pain. At least with alcoholics, towards the end, they have encephalopathy—there's a chemical depression of the brain due to an accumulation of toxins, and they become unconscious, or go into a coma. But AIDS patients didn't have that luxury: we would have to heavily sedate them, they would be on the ventilators. It's so hard to take care of those patients—and at that time, you knew they were going to die. There were some nights when I would feel as if I was doing nothing more than torturing them. I wished that what I was doing to them would make them better—I was wishing that I didn't have to suction them and cause them pain, even though I had to, to take out the secretions so they could breathe.

It was tremendously depressing for me to work there, and it happened that I was not enjoying going to work, so I requested a transfer. Then I felt that I had abandoned the patients on Ward 15; I had moral dilemmas. I didn't think that it was a great idea to be doing a full-court press on a patient whose chances of ever sitting up again were very poor—I had a problem with that. I transferred back to medical admitting. The patients could talk back to me, and I felt that I could help them.

Medical Admitting in the eighties had changed in that it was so huge, and there were so many patients that they made arrangements to accommodate Medical Admitting on two separate floors. It's an incredible place: you're having patients come in, you're transferring patients out to other floors. You have patients that become critical, they have cardiac arrests, you're resuscitating them, sending them off to the Intensive Care Unit. Sometimes we'd be sending patients off to surgery. It is in constant change—you do not sit down, you do not stop, and you are *never* done.

The position that I have now, the type of climate in the Department of Quality Assurance is incredible. I feel like I can help many more patients than the few patients assigned to me in direct patient care. And if I didn't feel that, I couldn't do this job. I have a support system reinforcing the fact that I can go around saying, "Wait a minute, this will not be—this is not appropriate." The one thing that you can never let happen is to stop being outraged. When something is wrong, you have to still be able to say, "This is not acceptable, this can't happen." And when you stop doing that...just hang it up, you're there just for the paycheck.

Working as a staff nurse on a floor, sometimes you don't have access to make long-term changes. You can make changes for your patient; maybe if you're awake, alert, and oriented, you could save a patient's life— that's a great thing to do. But you can't make any long-term, significant changes. And it's such a huge bureaucratic web, it's so difficult to get things done. As a peon staff nurse, you don't even have access to all the resources to make change. And if you did—please tell me, who is going to give your patient their medications, empty their bedpan, change their dressings, and take care of them while you're off making significant changes in policy?

I don't know what type of effect Clinton's health reform will have on County. Some people think that when that goes into effect, there will be no more County. I think that there are hospitals that don't want to take care of some of the patients we take care of—and I think that we take care of them well. We try to give nonjudgmental care. I don't know that other hospitals would want our patients, or be able to deal with the health problems that are associated with the urban poor population, such as substance abuse, violence, the infectious disease problems. And patients who are poor—I've taken care of patients who work and have insurance and come to County: "This is my hospital." I have had patients who were employed at other hospitals and had insurance coverage and come to County "because I've always come here, and they know how to deal with my problem. This is my hospital."

I'll be utterly devastated if they ever knock the hospital down. And our patients, they deserve a new hospital. They deserve everything to be sparkling new. To have their own clean, spotless, brand-new hospital. But I have a tremendous emotional attachment to the building. I wish the patients wouldn't have to wait as long as they do for things. I wish that the patients had some of the things that they had to offer at private hospitals: there's no TV, there aren't any telephones, private rooms. No one gives you a menu where you get to make choices. You get what is brought to you. But yeah, there is loyalty. And the patients will come back.

Dr. Ellen Mason

THERE IS A BREATHLESS *quality to her, a sense that she must speak swiftly, because there is so very much to be done. She was born and raised in Chicago. "When I talk to the people who live in my parents' neighborhood, in West Rogers Park, what everybody always says, when you say you're from County, is, 'Are you in training still?' You say "no" and then they say, 'Why are you there?'—as if no normal person would ever be there unless they were like Mother Teresa, Mahatma Gandhi, a raving lunatic, or incompetent."*

MY DAD WAS AT COUNTY DURING ONE OF THE MOST EXCITING periods of County's existence, which was during World War II. He was an Internal Medicine resident and fellow there. There was a lot of anti-semitism: it was a definite hurdle, something that nobody was even ashamed to talk about. It was hard to get into residencies, too, according to him: at that time, there were two good Internal Medicine residencies— Michael Reese and County—and everybody was competing for them.

So he was there during the war, and apparently it was just an unbelievable place. It's always had a history of being a crowded hospital, but during the war it was probably more crowded than it's ever been. In the stories he tells, there wasn't a single square inch of floor space anywhere. The hospital was different then: there was a separate hospital building for contagious diseases, there were TB wards, there was all this specialization.

Interestingly enough, the *training* was not as specialized. Everybody was a master diagnostician, but actually you couldn't do much for a lot of problems. Even intravenous fluids were not very common then. And antibiotics...they had sulfa and penicillin. During the war, penicillin was like gold: it wasn't manufactured widely, you couldn't get it—patients had to buy their own and bring it to the hospital to be administered by the doctor. The doctors administered drugs to themselves to see what kinds of effects...He was part of a team that was the first group of doctors to give these cancer drugs derived from nitrogen mustard—they gave the first drugs, they had no idea what would happen, no idea what the dose was or anything. There was no such thing as informed consent then, and they just sort of gave you these drugs. I don't think it was considered unethical, because they were willing to give them to themselves, and they were pretty open about it: "We have no idea, but there's nothing left to offer you—do you want to try this?" But there was no real process, the way there is now for strict control and evaluation.

Aside from drugs, there were shortages in everything, and the food situation was really bizarre—especially for the house officers. He said they would go for months where they would eat sheep's heads—they would have all these sheep's heads boiled and lined up. Or they'd have stewed red plums on the menu, every day for months. The dining room sounded really interesting—with china and forks, and then you sat down and women came and served you. The women servers were mostly young Irish girls, and they tended to favor White Anglos much more—and if you were Jewish or Black, you didn't get as much food or you had trouble getting served.

In those days they didn't have paramedics, so you went out in ambulances with the cops—and you could go into almost any part of the city and almost anything could happen. The impression I got was that it was a hodgepodge of every possible problem, and there were so many new immigrant groups then. I was looking at the labor and delivery log books from that period, and from the thirties, and I noticed an amazingly vast array of names, of Swedish names, and German, Polish—every ethnic group, southern people who had recently arrived.

It was this amazing time where there was an incredibly high level of learning about medicine and diseases. They all took it incredibly seriously: they worked day and night, they studied day and night, and went to the lectures of these great professors and listened to them as though they were gods. A lot of what we take for granted as knowledge that's been known for centuries was actually learned in this very short period of time—and a lot of it was learned at County. Also, things like developing surgical techniques and such—they were very proud of the advances they made there. Repairing hernias, even: I don't think most people know that for years and years, you just kind of walked around with these awful hernias and disfiguring bulges. A lot of stuff that was just taken for granted as the miserable lot of humans was addressed and worked on in this incredible period of learning.

You get the feeling it was like being in a "happy" war or something, an experience that very few physicians in training will ever have. It's not duplicated later in any way, shape, or form—maybe a *little* bit like MASH units in the Korean War or the Vietnamese War, where there's a very steep climb on the learning curve about surgery and surgical techniques as a result of a certain level of sophistication in anesthesia and training. And then you have this huge morass of people flowing in that you could try stuff out on, and nobody was too particular about how you did it because you were in the trenches—like they were in the trenches at County. So you developed, you made, you learned.

And my dad grew up in this tradition where all these great professors saw patients regardless of their ability to pay. Part of a doctor's job was

to donate time. I think that's something that's absolutely gone from medicine, the idea that without being a saint, without anything, you do that.
This was the culture in which he became a doctor.

When I first started at County, I said to my dad, "Do you want to come
down and see my office, tour around?" He said, "I couldn't bear to see it
disheveled, I couldn't bear to see it down at the heel, I couldn't bear to see
what happened—I just could not bear it." It really is funny: he talked
about it all the time, but he never could go back.

It wasn't just that the county didn't have the funds: there was no political will to maintain the building. County Hospital is such a football. For
most of the city, it's like having a retarded child hidden away in the bed-
room: you sort of know it's there, you wish no one would see it, you don't
want to deal with it, and—to the extent that you can—you're not going to.

It's always painted in such a bad way. At one point, I became really
depressed at the way you would always see these TV minicams in front of
the place; and it was hardly ever for anything good. If the local press is
going to do a story about something local, about AIDS or some other
medical thing, there's almost no chance they'll do it at County. *U.S.
News and World Report*, or one of the financial magazines, had this very
irritating issue devoted to the best hospitals in the United States. They
had it broken down by speciality and region. For AIDS in Chicago it
didn't mention County, even though County is, without a doubt, one of
the best places—not even a *mention*.

I'm an internist now. I finished my residency in '85, and I had been
imbued by this whole County myth, even though I had never set foot in the
place. It was part of the County system that I didn't get hired right when I
applied—so I went down and the chair of OB/GYN said, "Fine, you're
exactly what we're looking for." I started going through the County hiring
process, and it's unbelievable—it's *still* like that: things go to different
offices, and they just stay there. You have to be fingerprinted, you have to
go down to the County building. It's sort of like this Soviet bureaucracy
where there's absolutely no ability or interest to push things through. It
takes about three to six months to get hired: they lose your stuff and...

Meanwhile, I was moonlighting trying to decide whether to take
another job, and I was beginning to think, No, this is too crazy. How can
I work at a place where they're not sure where my papers are? They don't
know when I'm going to get hired, they can't schedule the physical. So I
said no, I didn't take the job—and on some level I really regretted it. In
'87 they called me back and said they'd never gotten anybody else, and
would I still be interested?

I came on board in January of '88. I'd been in almost every major
teaching hospital in the city and this was like nothing I'd ever encoun-
tered. Getting things done that you could presume to be straightforward
was not straightforward: I learned very quickly that something simple,

like getting somebody to get an X-ray or getting a result from a lab test, meant making a personal relationship so someone would give you that thing—getting it as a favor, not just ordering it…that nothing could be expected to happen for sure, pretty much ever.

I think that people would come and then stop doing any kind of clinical or research work, because it wasn't possible in this incredibly confusing place: there was no support, and there was no ability to get anything done, or keep records of anything—where you're lucky if you can have the chart and the patient in the same room at the same time…And if you want to get hold of that chart later, good luck to you. You don't necessarily get it, or if you do get it, you might have to make incredible friends with—and possibly bribe or bring food to—the medical records people.

One thing that's really cool about County is it's kind of a real people's hospital, meaning—literally—there are twenty million ways to get in, lots of open doors…After the baby was stolen, they tried to make it a little more secure.* But it's *impossible* to secure, and in some way it seems to me unjustifiable that it should be secured. Meaning if it really is—and it is—a place of last resort, then people have to be able get in: people who are confused, people who don't speak English, people who are coming on foot or from buses in every direction, they need to be able to get into the building.

I know it makes the place seem even more weird and fast and loose. You don't expect any security at County, basically. There are horrible incidents, but I don't know why people should be so shocked—considering that the level of crime in the city is high, and the West Side is not like Glencoe—by the fact that every now and then somebody is stabbed or jumped at County.

I had an experience in the elevator of the Nurses' Residence which was truly amazing, two or three years ago. I went there one weekend—it was wintertime—and I got into an elevator, and this unbelievable scene confronted me. This is a funny anecdote, in a very grim way. There were these two men—Black men, sort of disheveled looking—in the elevator, which was covered from floor to ceiling to walls with blood, like an abattoir. There was blood on the floor, blood dripping down from the ceiling like in a Stephen King movie.

Now, you would say, "Ellen, what did you do?" I got into the elevator. I still can't believe I did that. I thought, Well, what is this? These two men were standing there, both extremely drunk. One of them had a deep cut on his hand—he must have cut an artery, blood was spurting out like a pumper. I think he'd only lost about a unit of blood—but it was very dra-

---

* During the summer of '93, a mother handed her newborn to an older woman she assumed was visiting another patient on the pediatrics ward. While the mother went to use the bathroom, the older woman fled with the baby. A few days later, the baby was found, unharmed, and returned to its mother.

matically displayed. I said, "You're bleeding to death here! You have to come to the Emergency Room right now." He was like, "Uh?" I grabbed the man and started dragging him. We left a trail of blood all the way. It took them at least a week to clean the elevator.

I work for the Department of OB/GYN, and I take care of medically ill pregnant women, of which there's a fairly large number there. Most big hospitals in the city have similar setups, where there's some kind of special arrangements made for women who are medically ill and pregnant to get special care. The whole scene in Western countries has changed: older women get pregnant a lot more, medically ill women get pregnant. People with severe diabetes didn't used to think about getting pregnant—they were often just sterilized: "You'll die if you get pregnant, let's just take out your uterus." A lot of people get pregnant now who would never have gotten pregnant in previous eras, never, never, never—or would have done it only against great odds and maybe taking the risk of dying, or having little chance of bearing a healthy baby.

All the way into the sixties, the deliveries were among the highest number for one hospital in the country. When I started there in '88, they were starting to climb, and by '89 we were close to eight thousand a year. Then they fell to six and a half [thousand] and now they're four and a half, so they've dropped by huge increments in the last couple of years. That's because, in part, people like me and others have worked very hard to expand Medicaid eligibility to 180 percent of poverty level, so now women can deliver elsewhere.

Another thing that a lot of us have worked hard against is patient dumping. In the early years I was there, I remember we had cases, not infrequently, where somebody horribly sick and indigent would walk into another hospital's ER pregnant and they'd say, "Walk across the street." Even if it was life-threatening for her, she had toxemia of pregnancy, incredibly high blood pressure, bleeding, in labor. The COBRA laws—Consolidated Omnibus Budget Reconciliation Act of '85—cover things like inappropriate patient transfer, or "dumping." If you make the reimbursement money enough, hospitals will probably keep most of the patients. You'll never get rid of racism, and other hospitals won't always want all the patients. But what they did for delivery, in 1989 I think, was this: the Medicaid reimbursement for a normal vaginal delivery was four hundred dollars, which was hardly worth anybody's time, and they made it nine hundred. That was the year our deliveries fell by two thousand.

One thing I noticed was that we continued to take care of even more women in our high-risk prenatal clinic (for women who are medically ill and pregnant). The people in the community, these storefront docs or local docs, would sort of tell them, "All right, fine, you can deliver at Jackson Park or St. Bernard's or wherever you want, but go to County, get the care, be managed, and then come to me and I'll deliver you." So we see a lot of people getting prenatal care with us, and sometimes it's quite costly and intricate. I don't object to that, as long as County gets its share. If we were reimbursed for what we did and had additional resources—which we don't—if we take care of someone and keep her in a good status, she should be able to deliver in her community. But County doesn't get reimbursed for that kind of care, really, because actually the Medicaid reimbursement for pregnancy is a package. It's prenatal care and delivery. County is trying now to construct a system of patient encounter forms and tracking so they can submit to the state how many people we saw and get reimbursed.

The other thing that happened since I came is abortion. For the past year there's first-trimester abortion at County that's elective, but second-trimester is still only done for medical need. It's still a hot issue, because there are somewhere between ten and thirty thousand calls to the clinic line per month. County does about thirty a week. This is the *national* scene; we're not talking just the hospital. Women in this country have no access to low-cost abortion. Women aren't calling that hotline because they really want to come to County, they're calling it because they can't get abortions. My patients have to borrow, beg, and steal, prostitute themselves, to get the three hundred dollars that they would have to pay at a private clinic.

We don't know what happens to all the people that call the abortion line. On some level I feel firmly—and I'm the most prochoice person you've ever met—that it's not my problem, as a County doc, to make sure that every single person who wants an abortion gets one. I'm viciously against the Hyde Amendment—I'm incredibly disappointed with the Senate for voting down, again and again, federal funds to pay for abortions for women on public aid. It's just inequitable. It is *not* OK to say that this one thing is legal for them, but it's not legal for you. I cannot see how this can be in our country, how they can do that.

And if the antichoice people wanted to save money...I'm not trying to make this horrible, conservative right-wing case—but you *do* have to pay for those deliveries, those children, those WIC coupons, those everything. You have to find jobs for those teen youths. I don't want to be seen as a reverse racist, a genocidist or something, but I feel like all the problems of the quote-unquote underclass that everybody is talking about tie in to some extent with things like being able to plan your life, plan your childbearing. Family planning methods too—it's not just abortion.

Title X grants—those federal block grants voted by the Congress to set aside money to pay for family planning services in a variety of settings in this country—were cut to a tenth of their former size during the Reagan-Bush years. So people who were indigent were between a rock and a hard place: people hate them for being on welfare and they hate them for having more kids, but they really can't get contraception and they can't get abortion, and then conservatives talk about abstinence. It's not a question of abstinence, or that the women are surging masses of libido. I don't know if that's even a relevant fact to a woman who's living in a situation where her human relations are, partly, that you have sex with someone and they help you and give you money. I'm not talking about a prostitute as such, or anything—but it's just a different thing than what a White senator who went to law school knows about.

We're in a unique situation: unlike New York, we don't have fifteen public hospitals, we have *a* public hospital. We're being put on the spot to make up for the deficiencies of health care in the broader scope. Meaning, if there isn't affordable abortion that's accessible for women, and it becomes available at County, it's going to be totally snowed with requests. I mean, local providers send people with a note saying, "She needs an abortion, she has this or that terrible thing."

You can get into this awful situation with patients where somebody will show up in the middle of an incredibly busy clinic and say, "My doctor told me to come here, and he said you would take care of this right away." They'll be second-trimester and you'll say, "Well, actually we're gonna have to do these things, and you have to register," and blah, blah, blah—and then they'll get all upset. "He said I would just come here and you would just take care of it." Sometimes you feel unbelievably put up upon because you hate those other providers, you hate the patient, you hate them all. It's like, What do you think I am? What do you think I can do? I have a hundred people here today, and most of them have an appointment!

To be honest, I don't see it the same way some others do. All the medicines are totally free—and while I don't think people should have to wait a long time, and I think it *should* be made easier—you're not paying for anything so far, though the County Board is trying to change this, so you pay with your time. I sometimes feel like everybody is unfairly expecting us to be able to fill in every gap that there is in health care, meet everybody's needs all the time for everything that isn't taken care of someplace else, and do it fast, efficiently…And it's just not an efficient place. And then, if the scene changes, all of a sudden the resources are put elsewhere, then we're slow: all of a sudden you'll have the county commissioners, especially the ones that are unfriendly to the hospital, saying things like, "Well, look at how they're inefficient, they're not as busy as they were—and they have a nerve to ask for more resources!" So it kind of feeds on itself. And then, somehow, there seems to be this sine wave where things get bad on the outside and everybody comes back, requires that County be there. Like the University of Illinois runs out of its Medicaid days and, all of a sudden, patients are back at County.

Since I've been at County, there's been a major crisis every six months—to the point where you feel you can never make any plans or work on anything. There's been a residents' strike threatened, a nurses' strike, a disaccreditation, then the revisit for that...all these things keep happening, or they're going to close the hospital or...And during those crises, the bureaucracy—some of which is well-meaning, but most of which doesn't work so well—response to you when you needed to do something was frequently, "We're busy, leave us alone—we can't talk about this issue."

You have high expectations of trying to do things, of yourself, and you start to learn that if anything happens it will almost be by chance, or when you least expect it. It's like that weird conditioning that drives rats crazy, where they don't know whether a shock will come or a food pellet, so they don't function as good rats anymore. [laughs] I don't know what the Skinnerian term is.

Another thing I'm involved in is this program whose catchy little name is "New Start"—its federal name is Comprehensive Care for Pregnant Substance Abusers. Until very recently, there were almost no drug treatment services for pregnant women—in fact, programs were allowed to discriminate against pregnant women. We wanted to set up a program at County and we got research grants. County had a deliberate policy to stay away from treating substance abuse for many, many years, because they felt that it would open the floodgates, that they'd get *everybody.* It was hard getting our program started five years ago; it's hard to develop new models of care anywhere—but at a place like County, which moves at a glacial pace...

In six years I've learned so much about politics, micropolitics, the structure of politics, class, race. I think it's more than at other public hospitals. I think it's accentuated because the hospital is embedded in the political tensions of a Republican state government and a Democratic county government. Half the commissioners are White and come from White Republican districts where people can't even accept the idea that they might want to see things from the point of the view of the people they're serving; they sort of take the attitude that the people coming to County are lucky to get anything at all.

I think people shouldn't have to wait, especially if they're sick. The whole structure is faulty: it's not the hospital that's responsible for setting up that system, it's society that's responsible for setting up a system that makes an amputated, diabetic woman, waiting for her medicine, sit in a wheelchair all day after she sees her doctor. This is a patient of mine I'm talking about: she was sitting and drinking a soft drink in the lobby after clinic and I said, "What are you doing?! You're not supposed to have any pop!" She said, "I haven't eaten all day, and I'm not going to be able to eat until I get my medicine—but I can't take my insulin until I eat, and I can't go without eating, so I'm having a pop."

This attitude, this dichotomous thinking about society—"We have our society, and then there's them..." Somehow, they don't see that it's *one* society, and *it's* us all. This is a very polarized, racially divided city.

But I think when you work at County—even as a White person from a middle-class background—you *can't* see the society as two societies, you *can't* get this feeling that it's them and us when you're there. You're totally aware that, no, these people are not going to hide, and they're not going to die quietly at home—and actually their children are getting more militant and more up-front about their disappointments, their expectations, and their needs.

There are doctors who say that when the bureaucracy overwhelms them, seeing a patient restores them...But medicine isn't that easy either, it's just a different kind of headache. People are not cars, where you can just look at the diagram: there's a shamanistic quality to taking care of somebody. In some ways, yes, seeing a patient does restore you when you've totally had it with County in every respect. But seeing a patient doesn't necessarily always make it better—sometimes it just fills me with extra despair, because there are so many nonmedical things that the patients need that I can't get for them.

I'm on the Residents Admissions Committee, and one thing we try to do in OB/GYN is make a huge effort to attract African American and Latino people and women. Sometimes we have fights about it among ourselves; we have *some* doctor attendings who didn't see it that way...Luckily, most of the sexist White males have gone in these six years I've been there, the ones who used to say amazing things—not necessarily about Black people or minorities, but about women, especially older women—they'd say, "Well, she'll be on menopause before she finishes residency." We'd get an amazingly brilliant female candidate and they'd be like, "No, she's not even in consideration, because she's an older woman"—or because she's divorced, or because she has a child.

Now, our residencies are usually a third to a half minority and women. Most of them do their training, leave, make huge amounts of money in private practice, don't work in underserved areas—although we're always hoping to attract people who will. Of the doctors who stay at County, African American ones are far less class-divided than any other group you'll ever see. I think it's something to admire, and think about how everybody in this society could change. There's an African American woman who's an attending in my department, and you'll see her sitting and chatting and joking with the secretaries. I think that's one really good thing you can see at County.

Another thing I want to talk about is that there's a high instance of substance abuse across class and across race. Everybody's image of a cocaine baby's mother is a woman of color: almost exclusively, if you think "crack baby," you picture a little Black baby crying inconsolably. I think partly that's just the natural outgrowth of racist attitudes and our society, and partly it's fed by a White, male-dominated research structure.

There might be more problems in the drug-exposed children born to indigent women of color, but I think it's a much more multifactorial issue. It's not just that you use drugs: drugs hurt if you don't eat enough, don't get prenatal care, and don't have your infections attended to. Part of what our program is about is proving scientifically, to the extent we can, that the care makes a difference, the circumstances of one's *life* make a difference. For a dually diagnosed woman...a lot of them are depressed, or have post-traumatic stress syndrome, or have borderline personalities. A lot of women self-medicate to dull the pain of...So many of our women—not 100 percent, but well over 50 or 70 percent—were sexually abused as children; and for them, self-medicating makes sense, in a way. I think a lot of times when you talk about living in a violent, awful neighborhood that's scary, it would seem really weird if you *didn't* take drugs. It makes me sound like the kind of person Rush Limbaugh would be the first to machine-gun, but it *can* make sense to drink or take drugs. I mean, it's not a healthy coping mechanism or anything...

And then 100 percent of our women have been sexually and physically abused as adults—there isn't *anybody*, almost, who hasn't been raped at least once, if not many times. A lot of them have this weird disassociative thing, which our psychologist pointed out to me. You ask them if they've ever been hurt or attacked, and they say "no." Then, what I've noticed—because I do physical exams on all of them—is you say, "What's that scar from?" "Oh, my brother hit me with a bat," or "I got beat up once," or "Oh, I got cut with a knife." I say, "I asked if you were injured." And it's, "Oh, I forgot about that." It didn't happen in the last five minutes, or if they're asked a generic question about injury they just can't make that connection. I mean, if I was knifed I would remember it for the rest of my life, I would tell everybody I knew about it, it would be a central fact of my existence.

People aren't made of unusual stuff: people are made of people stuff, and people don't triumph above everything, they just kind of survive. I think there's a general societal moral condemnation associated with people who are unfortunate or indigent or whatever. So, intrinsically, if you're poor you must not be deserving—you must be lazy, bad, unlucky.

One thing that's awful about maternal addiction is the focus, always on the "innocent baby." I'm totally prochild, but it's not like it's the "innocent" baby and the "guilty" mom. To split it like that—people do it in AIDS all the time: there are "guilty" AIDS people like the IVDAs [IV drug abusers] and homosexuals, and then there are the blood transfusions or perinatally exposed kids, the "innocent" victims of AIDS. And it's that way for poverty and for people who don't embody what the country still chooses to call "American values." There's this persistent myth that the Bible-belt or White Protestants, whatever, is the *real* America, and everybody else just kind of got here, or is squatting here. If you look at demographics, given birth rates and immigration patterns, you'll see that in ten years it will be halfway away from that, and in twenty years more than half of America will not be White.

Regina Daley

A WARD CLERK. *She is pretty and vivacious. One minute she's talking about her passion: "Roller skates. I love it. Freedom." The next, the big picture: "So many times we're told that you can't get there, or you're not worth it. It really all depends on how you feel about yourself, and lot of people don't have the intellect, nor do they have the opportunity to be exposed to better things, or to even want them. They don't even dream..."*

I GREW UP IN CHICAGO ON THE WEST SIDE, AND I'VE WORKED here for seven years. I've been on Ward 23 for about four years. Most of the time when I come in in the morning, I try to get an idea of what the day is going to be like. Sometimes we can prepare ourselves—like a lot of times we know beforehand who's going home, who needs their medicine, or clothes or charity clothes.

This Friday was exceptionally bad because they had a water main break, and the hospital can't run without water. They had water brought in for patient care, and the water was supposed to be turned off in this section of the building; but miraculously they got it fixed. And we had a flood in the supply room. My legs were so tired from walking back and forth to Admissions and trying to get the patients' clothes. We had thirty-one patients, and—this is totally unusual—we had twenty-something discharges on Friday. And the labs still had to be done, patients weren't getting their trays—ah, it was ugly. We had one man working in the Clothes Room for the *whole* hospital. But they got the water fixed, so that was good...until it happens next time. [laughs] And there's inevitably going to be a next time.

I always say that if they made me a boss—put me in a position where I was able to hire and fire—I wouldn't be able to *drive a car* around here...There would be so many people I know who come here, early in the morning, seven o'clock even, and say, "I'm not going to do anything." You can't take that kind of attitude in a hospital. It's sad to hear them say that. It's seven o'clock in the morning: "I ain't doin nothin' today." This collective attitude of "I'm just here for a paycheck," I don't like that. Because it could work if we work it, it really could.

There might be someone else that's even more caring than I am; all I can deal with is me. I know I'm putting out there what I feel from my heart. And until I burn out, where I don't care anymore—which I hope never happens—that's all I can deal with. If more people just basically cared...because there are people that care here—just not that many.

I'll never forget one time...This lady was on the ward cleaning up, and she had the bed actually broken down to the springs and raised up. I said, "I should get a camera. I've never seen anybody do this." She said, "You know what? I might not be here tomorrow, and somebody I love could be laying in one of those beds." And that held with me: it *is* important. Even though her job is considered a menial job, it's a very important job. I think a lot of people, if they adopted that attitude, they might change.

Sometimes I have a problem holding my tongue. I don't think before I say things, and there's a way to say and talk to everybody. Some people, you just have to go get all the way ugly, you know? I'll take a lot until I see people doing things that're really uncalled for—like stealing brand-new linen off...Why would you want some linen that belongs to a hospital in the first place? That's so petty.

Some things I see and don't see; and some things, especially when I'm indirectly involved in it, I have to say something. People will walk over you just on the grounds that, "She's one of us, she's not going to say nothin'." —and that's not right. I didn't come here to gain any friends; if I have some, fine. If not, that's cool too. And, because of that attitude, sometimes I do find that I clash with some of these people. A lot of them I find are not necessarily...it falls under a lot of categories. They feel like life owes them something, and it really doesn't. You know, what you get out of life is what you put into it, and some people don't want to put in, they just want to get by.

I asked this girl one time, "How can you, with a clear conscience, pick your check up? How can you do that?" I said, "If I got away with the things that you did, I wouldn't be able to look in the mirror, let alone pick up my check—not with a clear conscience." She's one of the people that don't speak to me. [laughs] And I wasn't trying to be flip, I was being factual. I really wanted to know.

There are days here, far and few between now, that we literally get away without doing anything. That's because there's not that much work to be done. But you can't come in here every day and expect that—it's a blessing when it does come. Some days I come in here and work through and don't get a lunch, too much work to do. I know I'm going to have to do it, and I can't leave it for the next person without hearing about it. I do what I can, and after that I can't do anything else. But I will say, I can look in the mirror and feel good about what I've done each and every day, because it's an important job to me.

People just talk to the doctors any kind of way. As far as them having an attitude of superiority, in my opinion it's a defense mechanism, because they're already looked upon as though they don't know everything. They're not respected like they should be. Especially our new doctors—the residents, they come into a new environment, new surroundings, new attitudes and moods. They have to ask questions and you got nurses, clerks, and everybody getting smart with them unnecessarily. We have some major attitude problems here, so they have to adapt to that too.

They have to walk lightly, because they don't know what bridge they might burn that they might have to come back to. I understand that. But then again, a lot of them do have the attitude that they're better. I don't know why—your title doesn't make you a person. If you know how to treat people, then you don't have a problem. Forget whatever your attitude might be; if you know how to say "excuse me" and "thank you," that goes a long way here, it really does. I've seen progressively how they go from first year, all the way—their attitudes get different: they become meek and mild, then they become bossy. They feel their way, and they know who to be that way with, basically.

Have I ever gone out with anybody from the hospital? Oh, when we were out as a group we would dance together. I've had, um, I've seen somebody I would like to...But then judged from a distance what his attitude was like, and I had time to evaluate it, uh-unh. It don't take but a minute: if you look, you'll see. [laughs] My boyfriend is a nurse here. He's been here quite a while. I figured him out: he's kind of complex, but he's not as complex as he wants to make out. But I'll be the dummy, if he wants. [laughs] He's a great guy. Working with him, he doesn't play—it's all or nothing. He's as close to professionalism as I've seen, and he takes this job real serious. He carries the stress level with him. When we get together after work it takes a while for both of us to relax and just unwind from the day. It's a very stressful job.

I've been in a lot of trouble for doing a lot of things that aren't my job. Like, if our Transportation Department is running slow, and they don't consider: here's a patient who's been in the hospital trying to get this one test that has been canceled and rescheduled, canceled and rescheduled. And all the while he's here he's either having a light something to eat, or nothing to eat, waiting on this test, back and forth. If I see that everything is set as far as the test is concerned—everything except the transportation—if the patient's a wheelchair patient, a lot of times I'll take them to the test. Think about the legal repercussions if something happens to that patient; by me not being a transporter, I can get in trouble. But I don't think about that.

I've even had instances where somebody is seriously sick, and, say, they don't allow children on the ward, and some parents want to see their children—they're heartsick and all that. Things don't happen fast around here, so I take it on myself to maybe sneak the patient's kids up or sneak the patient downstairs, little things like that. And I've gotten in trouble for quite a few of them, but my conscience is clear. Maybe I didn't do just what I was supposed to, or maybe it wasn't in my job—but sometimes you have to go a little extra in situations like this, because this is not a grocery store, this is a hospital. These are real people. I have never been written up about anything—I've been reprimanded, but I haven't been written up or suspended or anything, because they know what my intentions are.

I talk to the patients some. I draw a line with IV drug abusers. I mean, somebody I feel is going to try to be slick or manipulate me. If they see you, for some reason, it's like they can smell somebody—they'll try. I'm kind of apprehensive about trying to help people. It could be somebody that sincerely needs help or sincerely needs something a little extra. I won't put myself out.

I've seen what people can do—people in my family even. It's not them doing it, they say. But I still have a hard time not feeling mercy or not feeling sorry for them…but trying to go that little extra for them, something stops me. It's not fair, I know, but it just happens that way. I've always tried to understand…That was the only blessing in coming in contact with certain kinds of people is that I got a kind of insight now. It's something in the way they move. That might sound corny, but it's really true. Something in their body language, their eyes—especially the females. They'll ask a doctor or someone for money—they'll say, for phone calls, or to go buy them some candy or whatever—and then they'll accumulate…I see them here trying to manipulate the employees and the doctors, and they accomplish what they're out for until somebody wises that person up as to what they're doing. And then there's a sudden change, *then* they want to sign out of the hospital. Some of the patients get high here. Some of them even steal things from other patients that are unable to stick up for themselves. It's like being a secretary *and* the police: you got to watch out for your ward, and watch out for the people as far as your job lets you.

The morale of the staff, on the higher and lower levels—even in-between—it's bad. People don't know what to expect with their jobs. You got the inspectors, and the people being inspected *really* catch it. That's just another ingredient in the low morale around here: we got the in-staff inspectors inspecting, and if the people's work on the ward isn't satisfactory, then the supervisor of the person doing the work has to go and ride this person. And in all fairness, if they're inspecting the day people, it's the night people that, say, left urine back there or something. So they're not getting the people that are actually causing the problem, and that makes it even worse for the person that's catching the brunt of it. I think it's each individual person's responsibility to do something to boost their own morale or help the situation here, because I can't see it getting any better. I wish I did have an answer for making things better.

My mother, my family always accuses me of wanting to save the world—and I've done some crazy things in my time to *really* give them those impressions. I'll never forget one time when I was about fourteen—there was nine of us kids, and my father was not in the home, and my mother was at work. I took the food stamps and fried up chicken wings.

Me and my girlfriend had sandwich bags and we took slices of bread and some chicken and came down here on Madison Street, skid row, and handed out the food. I was so happy! I felt like I was doing something...Did I think about whether I had food at home? I was so happy, because I saw people smiling, and I was able to give them something.

I think we were down there for about forty-five minutes, and we ran out. Those men started chasing us—they wanted more food. We didn't have carfare to get home. And then when I got home it was close to time for my mother to come home, and there was no food in the house—and I'm one of the oldest kids. I got my butt whupped.

Another time, I kidnaped this kid; he must have been about four. We used to call him a "trick baby," because he'd always be in front of the grocery store, begging. He looked White, but his mother was Black, and we knew she was a prostitute. We took that little boy and kept him downstairs in my girlfriend's basement. We got clothes for him, played with him, we treated him real good. I got a whuppin' for that too. I must have been about the same age. [laughing] That was a trying time in my life. But I loved that little boy—he didn't want to leave us. The pimp called the police. Somebody told my mother that me and my girlfriend had got the little boy. I got a whuppin', my girlfriend got a whuppin', and then my mother sent us to my girlfriend's house—we *both* got two whuppins'. [laughs] They didn't press charges, they just wanted to know where the little boy was. And the next day he was standing in front of the store again, begging for candy and money. It was really sad.

And here there's patients that can't get up and do for themselves. I don't necessarily think they get the care that they need all the time. There might be a nurse with four or five patients like that particular one. It might seem to be easy, but it's not. Sometimes the nursing staff, everybody might be— I won't say "burned-out," but maybe "overworked," because they're trying to get all this overtime to make their pocket look good, and their priorities aren't placed in the right slot. And then that person that could have got an ice bucket or an ice pitcher doesn't get it, because the nurse is way down *there,* and she's not going to come back down *here* again.

Most days, I love this place. And it really can work if we work it. I heard this clerk say...well, the doctor wasn't very nice about it: he came and said something. She said, "Don't ask me, I'm just a clerk." I said, "You're *just* a clerk? Oh, no—no, that's the wrong attitude to have. You are *the* clerk. That's a *very* important job." Then I said, "Are you using 'I'm just a clerk' so the responsibility or whatever he wants falls off you? Say that then. But your job is very important, and you should look at it like that." She was cool—she understood where I was coming from. Some people you can talk to; some people I just don't bother. [laughs] You got to know when to hold and when to fold. I just try to fill the water.

Dr. Michael McDermott

DIRECTOR OF ADULT *Emergency Services. He has a sixties aura: shaggy hair, a beard, a lanky frame that seems secretly dressed in jeans and a T-shirt. Loping past me in the vicinity of the ER, he mutters, "Madness, all kinds of madness," by way of a greeting.*

NOBODY IN MY FAMILY EVEN FINISHED COLLEGE. MY PARENTS were working-class people. For some reason I just had it in my mind to be a physician. I don't know why.

I worked at Lincoln Hospital in the South Bronx for eight years. I worked part-time, and my main interest and avocation was as an organizer. I was a Maoist, I was in the Revolutionary Communist Party. We started an organization here—it was called the Revolutionary Workers Headquarters—and I came to Chicago to work on that in 1978.

I came to Cook County because it was the obvious place to come work, for me. I found County to be overall not unlike Lincoln. I found that the patients here were a little quieter, they didn't complain as much. That was actually one of the striking things when I first got here. I don't know whether it's that they—especially the older generation of people that came here—had been successfully quote-unquote socialized to be more accepting of the level of services. Something I've found at County, over the many years I've been here, is that many patients have had a long-time relationship with County: they've been coming here many, many years. Many times it's a multigenerational experience: they may have been born here, their parents came here, perhaps even their grandparents came here. So I think that's on the positive side, in terms of just having faith in the institution and knowing what to expect. Feeling that it was their institution, and ultimately things would be OK.

For the first five, eight years, the social status of the patients was quite a bit different than it was at Lincoln, or than it is now, in the sense that it reflected the employment patterns, opportunities that existed for the African American community in Chicago. A lot of people worked in the steel plants, the auto plants, people worked at Sears, Montgomery Ward. All of which, without exception, are all gone. And so we had a lot of patients who were thirty or forty or fifty who were holding at that time $20,000- to $25,000-a-year jobs with insurance, who continued to choose to come to County. They had always come to County, and even though they had the economic access to other institutions, they felt that the doctors here had a more personal relationship with them. They always would say, "The best doctors are at County."

I tried to interpret that…I think there are excellently qualified people here, from any standard, whether it be research, teaching, or depth of knowledge. I think that probably, by some conventional standards, there are more of those at other institutions. So the conclusion I would draw is that the doctors here would actually focus more on the patients' problems, would treat them more respectfully, and would actually help them out with what they needed. I remember stories of people going to other institutions and telling me, "Well, I had this test and that test and the other test, but the doctor never talked to me." Some things never change in medicine. [laughs] And I'm sure that's not restricted to the African American population, as far as the complaint.

I think there has always been a premium here on the behavioral aspects of medicine, whether it's the patients or the physicians—trying to talk to people, trying to be respectful, trying to educate people. As well as probably some advantages in a funny way—of not having immediate access to tremendous amounts of technology and tests; of having to rely a little more on one's old-fashioned clinical judgment and not shunting people off to fifteen specialists—and maybe asking them more questions. I think that there's a lot of things that, even after the tests, not only don't you know any more, but there's not any more you're gonna do. So there's still plenty of room for compassion and hand-holding, and asking how the husband and kids are that's nice, and even therapeutic and healing.

What I always tell people is the quality of medicine at County is very good. The amenities are a little rough. And if you can't put up with that, then you might be better off, if you have a choice, doing something else. If you're going to be thrown off by all the uglinesses: the way that the pharmacy…the non-air-conditioned open wards, the appointments that aren't for ten-thirty but are for the whole half day. And if that's too much, and I could *easily* see how not only is it too much—but it ought to be too much—then if you have a choice, it might not be the best place for you. We're trying to change all that now, but it's a long, uphill struggle.

I'm the cochair with [Hospital Director] Ruth Rothstein of what's called the Medical Staff Advisory Committee, and we're working on three tasks: designing features of a new hospital, a medical school affiliation, and a whole ambulatory-care network that would have two outstanding features. One would be a decentralized, community-based clinic system. Another would be a different style of practicing medicine, with all of the things that are supposed to be there: emphasis on primary care, on prevention (you'd see the same physician all the time); timed appointments; a little less surliness from the clerks. But sometimes, in the back of your mind, you wonder what you give up to have that. Everything becomes more businesslike.

I think it's interesting that when you look at general health indices, like mortality within the hospital, we do as well or better than most places. I guess the way I would put it is, once people get plugged into the system, they've navigated the first few difficult places—getting to the clinic, to the emergency room, getting a physician you can relate to, either by luck or by skills of the patient—things work out reasonably well for that patient. But I think that there's a lot of people who won't go through that. For those with no option, if they don't go through that here, they don't go anywhere.

We unfortunately live off of, as a training program, among other things, advanced pathology. I don't endorse that; it's a terrible situation. But if it wasn't for the shortcomings of the health care system, we wouldn't see the advanced disease that we use to train physicians. So we become almost parasitical. We almost require—I hope this comes out in the text, with the same inflections, sarcasm intended—we almost *require* underserved populations.

In the Emergency Room what we've tried to do is develop innovative treatment strategies and innovative educational strategies that adapt to this. We make a big push on educating people who come to the Emergency Room about the use of inhaled steroids. Normally that wouldn't be a major effort in the Emergency Room; normally you'd treat the immediate situation, you'd refer the person down to their doc. From surveys that we have done, in some age groups—the younger age groups—80 percent of our patients don't have a regular doc. So we end up, within the limits of our expertise and energy and resources, trying to provide primary care service out of the Emergency Room so they aren't continually coming back. For example, we have little pamphlets that we've written on the importance of using inhaled steroids. We try to encourage residents to talk to patients about that. And on a more advanced level, people can interrupt developing attacks by the self-administration of more powerful steroids, like Prednisone. We have patients who, from talking to other patients in the ER while they were waiting, or hearing us talk, learned to dose themselves on Prednisone and interrupt their developing attacks—a very sophisticated operation—without ever having been to clinic. Is that good or bad? I think from a drawn-out point of view of what gets done where, it's bad. From the point of view of the needs of the patient, it's good. So I think that we've adapted to all kinds of things that actually lead to some innovative treatments, innovative diagnostic programs.

We have in the Trauma Unit, for example. If you go back years and years, they used to operate on everybody who had stab wounds. Well, at County it was physically impossible to operate on everybody who had a stab wound, so they were forced to develop stratagems like abdominal lavage to sort out people who really needed an operation from those who didn't. We were cost conscious long before private medicine feeding at the public trough ruined medical economy. Those years when people were being admitted for small problems and staying in the hospital for three weeks—we were never able to do that because the demand was simply greater than our ability to fill it. So we have been trying to shunt people to outpatient workups and triage diagnostic procedures for years, out of necessity. We've been cost conscious for years, coming from a completely different angle—coming from limited resources, trying to do the best job we can.

There's an impression that once health care reform takes place, and once people have financial access to care, there will no longer be a need for public hospitals. There's many, many arguments on the other side of that. Probably the one that I like the best is that we've learned to do some things very well, and given a little more resources, we would probably even do them better. It would be foolish to throw away the organization and expertise that exists now. Particularly the expertise that we have in dealing with problems that are common among the patient population we've served for so many years. Our expertise—whether it's in hypertension or diabetes trauma or asthma or low birth-weight babies—shouldn't just be dissipated.

Hospitals should be referral centers that are intimately connected with ambulatory care networks. More and more of the care is properly—not just to save money—but *properly* done, in the physician's office or at an ambulatory care center; less and less should be hospital based. So people don't become as sick, and they don't have to come to the hospital. Also, it's cheaper, so it's a better way to go. I think it's already begun: the County took over the Woodlawn Clinic from the city and they're expanding it. Prieto Clinic is tripling in size. There's Provident [a smaller, South Side hospital the County bought, renovated, and recently reopened]. The network is developing.

Within the limits of public hospitals in general, it's done as well or better than most other public sector hospitals. I think that the leadership of the hospital is properly committed to, I guess you might call it, a "mixed health economy": partnerships with community clinics that are church funded, government funded; partnerships with private institutions where we can establish a clinic that will ultimately, say, refer patients to a private hospital for certain reasons—surgery or…We may see people in neighborhood Y and the nearest hospital is a private hospital that's having difficulty filling its beds, and I think there's a mutual interest there that can be worked out. I think that we are willing to do that now. And these are *major* changes; these are flexibilities that would not have been conceivable fifteen years ago. I think that people are learning how to develop those partnerships.

Some people say Clinton's plan is going to allow everybody to go somewhere, so why should the taxpayer pay for County? It depends what people want. If people want to put up with—literally, it will come to check-points between the city and the suburbs, armed checkpoints—if that's what people want...I don't think you can walk away from the cities. If people want to live like some futuristic movie, where they drive in armored vehicles to the downtown area, then go back to the suburbs—and, basically, police are cruising the streets, and anybody with a beat-up car or a dark-skinned face can't enter the suburbs...If that's what they want for the future, that's what they'll get, if they walk away from the cities.

What I've seen happen in the city over the past fifteen years is really, really frightening. Talking mostly about the African American popula-tion, there has been a relatively small number of people who have done well, and they certainly deserve that. People have every right to the same opportunity as anybody else—every right to access the middle class, access the business class, professional class. There's been significant numbers of people who've done that, and that's fine. But a lot of them have left the city, along with everybody else.

What's left in the city? There are no more steel company jobs, there's no more Montgomery Wards, there's no more Sears. There's fast food, there's unemployment, and gangs, and nothing is being done to change that. Health care isn't going to change that—although [laughs] it can provide jobs. Somebody once said to me that the major impact that Med-icaid had on health care was that it expanded the health care industry and gave a lot more people jobs. It may be true. You know, these bloated structures may be serving a purpose that we're not even thinking about. It's much better for people to have jobs, income, health insurance, and everything else, than not. In the city, the results of lean and mean are pretty mean—and whether it's out of compassion or not wanting to see this civil war develop, I think it's in people's interest to have some reason-able health care system in the cities. I think we've developed the skills and the experience to make a major contribution. But that isn't going to change things unless action is taken from the top.

The American people have to make some decisions themselves. Do they want to spend 90 percent of their health care dollar on a disease process once 90 percent of the damage is done? You don't have to spend all that money at the end; you can have the same life expectancy—which is the situation in Europe, where you don't have all these cardiologists. In Europe they discovered eight years ago that the clot-breaking drug that costs $130 was as good as the clot-breaking drug that costs $1500. It took the United States eight years longer, and it's nothing but corruption of the cardiac research industry by the drug companies. Life expectancy in Europe is as good or better than in the United States, even for middle-class populations—leaving out the poor—without all the expenses.

So the American people have to wake up as well. They can have their cake and eat it too: you can live a long and healthy life, but you change a lot of things. You put your research money into how to prevent heart disease; you take serious dietary suggestions; you change the way you live. People want to smoke and eat meat every day and think that the cardiologist is going to bail them out and give them another two years of life—a pill or an operation—and they're willing to spend $200,000 for that, then this is what they're going to get.

I think the government will take action; they'll cut the number of training spots in these subspecialties. They'll stop providing education and stop providing money for these heroic interventions at the last stage. And that's not to cut people off or put them out in the ocean when they're fifty-five years old. You can have a long life without the end-stage high-tech intervention; you just have to start when you're twenty, or when you're forty, but you have to take it seriously.

I would like to see the day, in fifty years, when we look at daily meat eating like we look at smoking—and I think that will come. But in the meantime there's a lot of vested interests, not only the meat industry but the cardiac-bypass industry, that are not going to benefit from that. And the research money is not being put into that; it's *just* beginning—the way it should be. It's not going to be easy to change people's habits, but there's very little money being put into figuring out how to do that. If we want to see some changes in the next five to ten years, we will have to simply restrict the number of training opportunities, say, for invasive cardiology. Cut it by 30 percent, cut it by 40 percent.

My guess is that the government supports 60 to 70 percent of graduate medical education—a lot through Medicaid, some through research funding. Those priorities should change, they should change next year. There should be much less money given, there has to be a shift in priorities. Certainly, specialists are doing an important job—they're important as consultants—but the funding of graduate medical education is a major vehicle through which this could be changed.

People say folks won't enter medicine. I find it hard to believe that in a country as rich as this, as far as the people who go to medical school, that people are not going to go into a field to make *only* $100,000 year. I think they'll probably be able to find people, especially if they'd give more support for undergraduate medical education. It's a terrible problem now. People graduate from medical school with $60,000, $70,000, $80,000 in debt, and it's no wonder they feel they have to get a job right out of school where they'll make $130,000 or $140,000 a year. But really, I think people will take a job for $100,000. [laughs] I don't know how that'll come across. It's hard to believe that people wouldn't take a job for only $100,000 and work maybe forty-five, fifty-five hours a week. It's difficult. I mean, it isn't easy being a general care provider, but I think there will be people who will do it. It may not be the same people who did it before, but that might be a step forward.

Our residency program in Emergency Medicine is new; we've been at it for six years. It's hard to tell about the residents. To some extent, the people that are stereotypically the worst, quote-unquote, don't even apply to County—it would never cross their mind. I mean, what could be worse? Our selection process in Emergency Medicine definitely includes social screens—in other words, people who would be, say, overt, who would talk about "those" people in an obviously disparaging way, wouldn't make it past the first cut. We put a premium on residents who will understand the social conditions that our patients grow up in, live in.

We don't always get exactly what we want—it's kind of interesting. I always ask the people I'm interviewing for the residency how much of a cultural gap do they feel there is between themselves and the people that they'd be taking care of. And what I would characterize as the middle-of-the-road answer is, "I try to get along with everybody, I respect everybody." Which sort of avoids the question. I think the more enlightened answer is, "Huge!"—whether it's a White or African American applicant who comes from a middle-class or upper-middle-class family. I mean, people understand there's a huge gap, and that it's a major task to overcome it. I think the least desirable answer is "none," because it means they don't have any understanding of what's going on, or they're just flat-out liars. And that, in our selection process, counts against people: we want very talented people, and we've had some excellent residents who will go on and do great research and have big names and that kind of thing. But even in those people we always selected folks we thought could get along in the environment here, who could deal with the staff, the patients—at the very *least* could control whatever negative tendencies they had, and at the best had a real understanding, empathy, and willingness.

Whether people go out to the suburbs, or they go downstate, or they go to some hotshot academic institution, hopefully some of the lessons that we've tried to teach people here stay with them. Even if they take sort of an upper-class view—"Those were the grand old days of slumming with the poor"—even if that's *all* that happens, I think they're better off, their practice is better off, and their patients are better off for that experience. But, I think, most people do better than that: they have a better understanding of how to deal with people, of how to work with people that haven't had a lot of opportunity. I think the other side of the problem is there too, though.

One of the problems we face is that sometimes our patients don't have the expectations they might. I think even your skills, for example, on how to manipulate medications to avoid side effects, are difficult to develop at County, because it's hard to get people to complain—whether it's from low expectations, or being treated rudely, or just being raised in a social environment where people have had a lousy life and don't think much about themselves in that regard. Or, especially if they're dealing with institutions where they don't expect much, it actually harms people's medical development.

I work about twenty hours a week in the Emergency Room and, we're seeing a lot more unemployed—people who worked for many years and haven't worked now for years. We're seeing a lot of young people who've never worked, who are very angry, very bitter, and that's real scary. I don't know what's going to happen. I don't think anyone has a strategy for what to do in areas that are maybe 80 percent unemployed. Except maybe wall them off. It's frightening from a social perspective. I mean, nobody wants to see violence increase. And it's certainly frightening if you have any kind of social consciousness or commitment, to see that happen. There's no question that things are worse now than when I came to Chicago fifteen years ago, significantly worse. We see the results of there not being any kind of a decent ambulatory care system out there. We see 110,000 patients a year in the adult Emergency Room; what we call the Ambulatory Screening Clinic—that's the least severe, needs medicine refills, headache for three months, that kind of stuff—also sees about 80,000 visits. [In the ER] we see everything more acute than that for the most part—whether it's a severe headache for two days, abdominal pain for two days, sprained ankle, shot in the muscle in the leg but doesn't need to go to the Trauma Unit, knife wound to an extremity, hit about the head but wasn't knocked unconscious, lots of asthma, lots of hypertension, lots of diabetes, lots of heart disease...All those problems that come from a patient population that doesn't have good access to care, that has a lot of dietary, environmental, and stress-related problems that come from living in a terrible environment and being squashed down for ten generations. It's depressing.

The only time I feel like walking away is when I feel ineffective. It's important for me to stay involved in my clinical practice, the asthma patients. Because as good as the ideas seem, I have to have that day to day contact with helping individuals. You can't just be a policy person or a planner—I can't. And I've done that too long. I went through a whole round in my life where I thought we were going to remake the world with grand schemes, and that didn't work out, quite. And even though I think the grand schemes now are a little more based, they may not work out either—so you're left with your individual relationships. That's important. [Long silence, big sigh. His face contorts; he begins to cry.] Stress. Um...[He continues, with difficulty.]

I think that...Well, how do you keep doing it? I think you have to be real rooted in values both for what you do and for yourself. A lot of my adult life was spent within very formal ideologies on the Left, and I think a lot of that turned out to be limited. Not completely bankrupt at all, but I just think we have to find new ways. In the meantime, we have to find other ways of sustaining ourselves and sustaining our communities. I've become much more involved in environmental causes. I think it's real important to maintain a community. That's one of the good things about

County, there is a core of people—some of us have known each other for many, many years, some not so many years—that share some of those values. Whether it's my own core values, whether it's politics, or whether it's certain forms of relation to nature. That's nice—but I think the community is broader than that, and I think that community is what will sustain us for what I see as even more difficult years than we've had before.

It's a very hard place to work. There's a lot of demands put on it. There's been a lot of political corruption at, most problematically, mid- and higher-level management. But I think that's very different for high-level management now, professional people are there. I think it's still true of some ranks of midlevel management and that has impeded the development of an effective managerial system. People are in it because it's a patronage job—they're protected, nothing can go wrong. Given that, I think there develops a lot of inertia from top to bottom.

It's interesting, because I think that most employees here have a commitment to their task. They may not know what it means. They may not have had the experience with an efficient operation, so it may appear that they don't really want to do a good job. But I think that people actually do. And I think if you set up systems, once people kind of get out of the habit of not doing things, they would just as soon do things well. There's a lot of commitment on the part of all levels of the staff. There's a real feeling that we're here to do a good job, we're here for the patients.

Darlene Green

HER EXUBERANCE MAKES *her seem younger than her forty-four years. Her smile is warm, and she offers it often. She is an LPN [Licensed Practical Nurse]. "I don't work no overtime. All of my extra time I spend in the nursing home where my mother is. If I get a little extra money, I buy goodies for the whole floor for the holiday. I think in the back of my mind I'm thinking about my grandmother when I'm doing that. That's the person that most influenced me in life, and when I see these older people it's really who it reminds me of. Yeah."*

I GREW UP ON THE WEST SIDE. I WAS RAISED ON RACINE AND Taylor—it's a three-story project called Jane Addams. I have two brothers and one sister, and nobody graduated from high school but me. I don't know why I'm different from the others. I keep thinking maybe it had to do with looking at my grandma when I was a little girl. She was the person that I looked up to. I never saw her argue or get angry, but she always got the respect. She'd just look at you and you'd know to straighten up.

My grandmother had a brain stroke and she was on the third floor at County. I was thirteen and you had to be sixteen to visit, so I snuck up the stairs and I saw my grandmother. She was in restraints and her face was all swollen. She died at County.

I got married when I was twenty, and I had a son. My husband—well, I liked this boy since I was in grammar school, but he was an alcoholic, so I raised my son by myself, but I done OK. He turned out to be a responsible young man.

I worked at Wards for thirteen years, 'til they closed; I took my severance pay money and went to Dawson Skill Center and became an LPN, because I needed a job that would never go out of demand.

My mother, she has Alzheimer's, and I tried keeping her, because she kept getting away—she'd wander off. People from the projects would call and tell me and I'd have to go get her. I tried to keep her here, but one day she wanted a glass of water, and she picked up the pot of boiling water off the stove. You *know* they would have locked me up, they would have sworn I scalded her. You know that. It's not, You might get in trouble. You *will* get in trouble. One time my son was in the bleach as a little boy—he spilled mop water—and I took him to the hospital to make sure he hadn't drunk any, and the police were all around me. I'm like,

"Children do things like that, they climb in the cabinet." The police were right there questioning me.

I don't know, there's good and bad in everything and everybody. That's the way I see the world. You can't just go by one set of people. I work with the LPN union. I think most foreign nurses are terrible: they don't care about the patients, they're very rude to the staff, and if you're not involved in their little group, you don't agree with things they say, you're a troublemaker.

The policy says you shouldn't speak in any language but English while you're there, but all day long they just sit there and talk in their language. I'm like, if this was us doing something like that they'd be suspending us, writing us up. They play too much favoritism. They know I'm going to do good patient care, so that's why they tolerate me. They know they can't say I don't do my work. And the union saves me.

I'm on Ward 33, Ortho. The charge nurse gives you a certain amount of patients, and you write down the names, medications they need, go see the patient, see what they need: dressings, medicine, IV, whatever. You're in charge of those patients, you're responsible for all your patients, all his needs. I like total nursing care. I work the three-to-eleven shift. On Ortho we have gunshots, stab wounds, occasionally we get…Our ward has two isolation rooms, for the TB strain that's so hard to cure now. We get AIDS patients occasionally. We got a patient with multiple gunshot wounds right now. They come from Trauma.

I have a good rapport with the patients, I guess. Since I'm from the projects, I understand them. Everybody should be treated equal. Patients are patients—don't look at color, don't look at what they do, just treat them all the same. So they respect me, and they'll say, "I gotta do better, I gotta change my life." They'll make statements like that. Sometimes they'll come back and visit and show you that they straightened up.

I remember going to County as a little girl. I was anemic. I remember older, military-like nurses—they were very stern, but they were OK. Cabrini Hospital was near where I lived, but they didn't take Black patients. Everybody asked me when I graduated how come I didn't go to Cabrini, and I told them I remembered when they didn't take us, so why should I work there? We went to the doctor on the corner, or to County. I remembered going there as a little girl, and I said when I graduated, "I really want to work at County to help poor people." I thought about when I was poor, they was nice to me, and so now it's my turn. I applied and they called me! It's like wishes do come true.

They put me in Ortho right away. I like it, I like the patients. I feel they need more than medical attention—they need to be talked to. It's an all-male ward, and since I have a son I'm partial to males. I'll tell them my name is Darlene Green and I have a son, we was raised over there in the projects, and they're like, "I know Charles—he's nice. You his mother?!"

These boys need to be reassured that they're of some value to somebody. I tell them we're only here for a short while—they say I preach to them—and we have to make a mark in life. "How could you say that you have two children? When was the last time that you seen these two children?" They just look at me like, boy...but at least she's real, she don't put on airs. They call me "Real."

And I'm serious about dressing changes too. It is the nurses' job to change dressings and see how the wound is doing—but it's the patient's job too, to learn how to change the dressing, because they're going home with it. They have external pins they put in broken legs. It's like hardware, like Frankenstein movies, right? We teach them how to wrap it around, and they like this. They go home and they want everybody to see, like they just got out the war. Patients like being taught. And sometimes they'll say, "Maybe I should go into medicine. Where's personnel?" I tell them, "Right down there on Winchester." They ask you things like that. It gives them hope, I guess, because you take a little time with them.

I'll talk to the people on the job, we have people on the job, some of the males working Transportation, they come to work drinking. [sternly] You just don't come to work drinking. I'll be like, "You got a job, they fire you, you think they done wrong—and you're smelling like a tavern?" At first they can be angry with you, but later on they'll come back and say you were right, and they'll stop.

Some days I just let people do anything they want, I don't say nothing. They'll be like, "She sure is quiet today, is she all right?" They'll say, "You take this admission, you do this," and I'll just do it. The next day I'll be, "I'm so tired of this unfairness—I'm not doing anything until the supervisor comes and straightens it out." Unfairnesses like assignments and stuff. There's only two TB patients per ward and Team 2 gets them. I been having Team 2 for two months. I told them, "I'm not taking those patients today." The hospital does not screen all their staff for TB, hepatitis, or nothing. I've been upstairs to tell the coordinators that I feel that they should. They just look at me because they know I'm known to run off at the mouth. If you never say nothing, they'll think that you're happy. Even if they don't change it, they'll at least know how you feel. [laughs]

Everybody feels they're not appreciated. One person blames the other for whatever the problem is. Like the doctors—I hear them talk all the time about the attending [physician] makes me do *this,* and So-and-so didn't do *this,* and we didn't have any of *these.* Or I'll see some of the nurses get together and talk about a patient with a doctor. [incensed] Nurses should not discuss patients negative with the doctor! The doctor is there to treat the patient, he's not there to say, "Well, discharge So-and-so today, he's a behavior problem." And then the supervisor, no matter how much you do, it's never enough. So you never get thanks, you've never done a good job—you're short, you worked the ward, nothing is said.

I guess people just want to feel like they've done something worthwhile—but if they just spend more time with the patient they'll get that. The patients will notice the little things you do. I'll stop at the store on my way to work. I don't bring cigarettes because it's a no-smoking policy in the hospital, but I'll bring food, pop, whatever. Little things like that is important to patients, especially ones that don't have visitors.

I remember this patient, he was in his sixties. He had both legs amputated, he was just laying in the bed. He said, "You know, I should just die." I said, "Why? If they didn't cut off your legs you *was* gonna die, because you had gangrene." He said, "Yeah." I said, "Did you just become a diabetic?" He said, "No." I said, "Did you take good care of yourself?" He said, "No." I said, "Well, then who do you have to blame?" He looked at me and he thought about it. He had been refusing to go to physical therapy. I said, "You might as well get out the bed, they gonna send you home whether you can walk or not, so you better learn to do for yourself." He got up and went to PT [Physical Therapy], he got two artificial legs, and he's been walking ever since. And I like that. I like when he comes to the clinic, because he comes to visit me. He'll say, "I'm up here, I know you think I'm begging but I don't have bus fare." And I'm like, "I'll give it to you. Anything to get you off the floor." I know he has bus fare, he just want to see will you still do things for him. [laughs]

On the ward it's noisy, the patients play cards, they have girlfriends and children up there on the ward. We've found liquor bottles in the garbage can. And the patients sneak outside. You shouldn't accept the ward if you can't give account of all the patients. The patient might appear at eight o'clock and you accept the ward at three. And sometimes they'll be outside! They try not to give them to me because I hurry up and tell them, "You know, So-and-so is not here and I'm charting it, I'm calling the supervisor and letting her know he hasn't been seen on this shift. "Oh, give him a few more minutes." I told them, "No. I told you whenever you've got a missing patient, never give him to me, because I'm going to chart it. What if they go out and do something wrong? They're going to play like they were at Cook County Hospital in the bed. And me and you both know they weren't." Yeah. We need better security.

One time a Hispanic male came there with a stab wound to the thigh. The next Sunday afternoon a little Hispanic lady came up there, she had a butcher knife and she cut his leg very badly. She said the reason she done it was because he raped her daughter, so she came up there to finish him off. Right on the ward.

I get mad at the policemen too, because they're rough with the homeless when they be begging for food, and that's not nice. Dietary, when they get through serving breakfast, lunch, and dinner, they throw away the leftover food. Some of them are nice, they give it to the homeless, but then the officers be mad with them; they throw the people out, throw the food away. It's mean to throw away food when you see people that need it. Sometimes they throw them out into the cold, they throw their little bags out. I say, "You know you really shouldn't do that because one day this job might be gone and then what are you gonna do?" They look at you like, "I'll be here forever." That's the look they give you. Nobody be's nowhere forever.

County is a learning experience. I like it, so I can't really talk bad about it. I'm really not there for the staff, I'm there for the patients. Though the staff do care about each other: don't let it be nobody's child sick that's working at County but *everybody* knows that's So-and-so's son, *everybody* goes to see. No matter how you do and don't get along, if something happens, everybody is there. It's like a little melting pot.

People stay with their own kind, I guess, because you have more in common. But you get along with some others. We got a White nurse, and I know for a fact she's never been exposed to Blacks until she came to County. She'll tell you, "I'm really doing my best." I say, "You're doing just fine." We all got our own little...I wouldn't know how to act in an all-White hospital.

I'm happy being an LPN. Everybody say, "You should go back to school because you care about people and you'll be good—and all these things that you're finding fault with, maybe you could make a difference." I say, "Be happy with what you got and make the best of it." I'm never bored, I don't get tired, and sometimes I feel like I've done something worthwhile. That's what makes me, I guess, a good LPN. I always tell people, "There's no sense in discussing it, because I know I'm good at what I do, and it's a shame you can't say that about yourself." [laughs] They say, "I don't know about you, Green." To myself I say, Thank God.

Dr. Roger Benson

Attending physician at Cermak Health Services, the County Hospital arm of the jail. He is a very tall, large-boned man who seems to wish he were slightly more diminutive. Fifty-three years ago he was born in his grandmother's house, in a small farm town in McHenry County, Illinois. "Where I grew up nobody thought about being a doctor; we just didn't come from that background." He came to County as an intern in 1966.

As medical students, we were right across the street from the County Hospital. I had heard a lot about County Hospital, and it was such a huge place in terms of its image. In '66, County was still considered to be a very good place to train. I think our only *real* exposure during medical school came from friends, medical students who had trained there and told a lot of amazing stories about their experiences.

We did our autopsy course, our pathology course, at the County morgue. That was one of my first exposures to the almost brutal aspects of medicine. You would see these kind of cases because they were County Hospital cases that would get autopsied there. They were good teaching materials, in a sense, because they were in such bad shape, they were such complicated cases, and they were available for autopsies.

My first day on the job was in the summer, and I came to work with a tie. County didn't have air conditioning, and on the first day I got embroiled—even as an Ear, Nose and Throat intern—in resuscitating somebody. I went to the bedside—I was supposed to do a tracheostomy—and the patient had a cardiac arrest. This is the first day! I'd done this in medical school but, you know, now you're really the doctor in charge. The medical training takes over, and there's other people coming in to help out...But I remember just getting saturated with sweat. I took my tie off, and I don't think I wore a tie for the remainder of my internship, because it was just all-out work and the niceties weren't important after a while.

The thing that was disappointing to me about being on a surgery service was, being a physician, I liked to know who patients were and know them by name and know them as people. And the surgeons didn't like that. They actually got quite upset if you spent too much time talking to patients. They said, "Is the patient ready for surgery? Get the patient ready for surgery! Get the blood upstairs to the blood bank!" That's all they wanted. They didn't even know who the patients were—they just knew them by a disease.

That was my first and second months, and I was totally appalled. The only people that impressed me as being concerned about what's going on with this patient were the medical residents, who would come around and say, "Gee, what's wrong with this patient? What are you doing for this person?"

I think we were much more naive in those days, because our exposure in medical schools was different. You didn't question things, the way they were done. It wasn't like later, when students questioned ethics and the morality—the way women were treated, the way anybody was treated racially. Those things were not questioned in my early years in medical school; you didn't question anything.

There was a rule on the surgery service—this was later in the year, when I was seasoned and I knew my job and what was expected of me— that anybody admitted to surgery with gastrointestinal bleeding had to have a certain timed test performed. The patient would come in, we'd start an IV, shoot this dye into their body and, in forty-five minutes, draw all the blood for their blood tests, then race it over to the lab. The next morning, the attending surgeon would want to know what this test showed. I'd been doing this for weeks and weeks.

This one night we had a bunch of GI [gastrointestinal] bleeders, and I did the tests. I was up all night, no sleep: I injected the stuff about five-thirty in the morning and I ran over to the lab. In those days you had nobody to transport blood or anything, you had to do all that yourself. The lab tech[nician] was sleeping, so I knocked on the counter and woke him up. I said, "I've got the lab tests here, we need the results right away." He said, "I'm not doing them." I said, "This is an emergency." He said, "I don't give a damn, I'm not doing them." I said, "You have to—it's an emergency." He said, "No, I don't have to do anything you want, intern"—they always called you "intern." He said, "I don't have to do it because you say so." I said, "Wait a minute—I work for the resident. I got to call the resident." All I can think of is, I'm following the rules.

So I pick up the phone on the counter, and he said, "You can't use the phone." I said, "Wait a minute, man. I'm an intern here. I'm supposed to get this test done, and I want to find out from the resident what I'm sup-posed to do." I'd been up all night, no sleep—I was yelling at this point. I dialed the ward, I got the nurse, and I said, "I want to speak to—" and he disconnected it. Then he starts pulling on the cord. So I took the phone— I had absolutely had it. I wasn't usually argumentative, but under those conditions…I wound up and I threw the receiver at him, and I thought we were going to have a fight. He ran over to his coat, and I was thinking, What the hell is he doing? And all of a sudden he had a gun pointed right at my head.

I was so out of sorts and angry I kept saying, "This doesn't make any sense—I've got to call my resident!" I walked out of the room, saying, "I've got to call my resident," and found a hall phone. He came up to me and said, "You put that phone down"—he's *still* got the gun pointing at me. I could see the bullets in the chamber, he had it that close to my head. There were a couple of people standing in the hallway, and I said, "Can you *believe* this guy?! *He's pulled a gun on me!* All I am is an intern, I came over to get a lab test done!" I was really mad. I walked down the hall to the stairwell, and I went over to the ward and finally found a resident, and by that time I'd started shaking. I told my resident, and he called somebody over there and he said, "We want that test done immediately."

So the next morning, after rounds, the resident said, "You really have to report this." We had a hearing with the medical director, the head of the lab, myself, the guy who pulled the gun, and a bunch of other people. The medical director—he was in charge of all the interns—was sitting at this meeting and he said, "You know, we can't have this happen to our interns."

So the director said, "I still remember the day poor Bruno died.* We just can't have this happening." The guy denied everything, denied having a gun, he said I made up the whole story. They fired him because he refused to do the lab test, which he admitted. But County was such an awesome experience, you had so much to do all the time, that something like that disappeared, just faded into the background. So many outrageous experiences—that was just another one.

That was in '67 and '68, and it was a very tough year, extremely busy. This was right at the beginning, before Medicare had really come into being, and the hospital was really packed at all times. In most of those years the census in the hospital hovered around two thousand to twenty-five hundred. And in the winter it was much worse, because of people coming off the streets, needing a place to stay. Homelessness wasn't as great then as it is now, but it existed, particularly in the skid row areas. So people who lived in flophouses would get sick, they'd get TB, all of the consequences of alcoholism. A lot of diseases, a lot of pneumonia.

We were extremely busy, with shortages of everything. We never had enough supplies to go around—simple things, like IVs, needles, tubing. A lot of it was antiquated equipment, and they didn't buy the newer equipment. We didn't have things like blood culture bottles; test tubes were always in short supply. Most interns, including myself, kept a box in our rooms with a small cache of extra equipment: needles that worked, clean syringes, and blood culture bottles. We would requisition them when we were off call, so when you were on call you had all the items. You would bring this with you, because they might not have it available. You had to do virtually all your own initial laboratory tests yourself, the specialized tests. And you had to do your own EKGs, your own lumbar punctures.

* In 1956 an intern by the name of Bruno Epstein had been stabbed to death by a patient. They had a plaque to Bruno up there that said, DIED WHILE SERVING THE SICK ON WARD 24. I used to cover Ward 24 and I used to think, poor Bruno. And he hadn't even taken care of the guy who stabbed him.

I think one of the downsides of the County training was the fact that you were *always* doing things and taking care of patients—there wasn't enough time to keep up on the newest literature, you just didn't have time to get to it. We had, sometimes, twenty to thirty extremely sick patients, we were on call every third day, patients would keep coming in, and you'd have to evaluate them, get tests done.

We would actually put bogus names on the list—my resident taught me this—so that when you needed a test done...You'd keep a record of this, so that you knew the bogus names, and then you would erase that one and write in your patient's name, so you could get the test done faster. Even if you wanted any tests done as an emergency, you had to be able to justify it. We did crazy things. Like you would take a patient downstairs and put a bandage around their head and say, "I need this X-ray done now!" Sometimes we overdid it, because it was a game. I remember one time putting a bandage around somebody's head, and taking some blood from his vein and squirting it onto the bandage in order to get an X-ray of his head. That might have been an exaggerated response on our part—but we got the X-ray done. Sometimes these were people who had fallen out of bed, for example, who were a little out of it. Many times they had no idea what was going on anyway. Sometimes you could get away with stuff like that. Obviously not, hopefully, to the detriment of the patient, but to help them.

A couple of my classmates from medical school hated medicine once they got into it. In those days a very common admission would be a "John Doe," meaning that the person was mentally out of it, didn't know who they were, would be brought to the hospital either semiconscious or unconscious, and would get admitted as a John Doe. These guys hated those kind of cases, because they were tough: you know, treat the person based on what you could figure out from their blood tests, and hopefully bring them around to consciousness. But whenever these guys would get that kind of patient, they would cut all the identifying bands off, take off the hospital gown, wrap them in a sheet, and take them to the back door. Then those patients would be found by security and they would get re-admitted to somebody else.

There were other people who would actually pay the admitting clerk to give them credit for an admission even though they didn't get one. Every tenth admission would be your admission: no matter who it was you would get it. It was very cruel in those days, because some people would try and find ways of getting good cases. They would sneak down to the admitting area and try to scope out somebody who wasn't very sick, somebody who could give a history, or somebody who had an interesting illness.

Most of the residents, if we were single, lived at the hospital, so we lived there and worked there, and it was seven days a week, night and day—you really didn't have any time off. Once in a while we'd give our interns a day, because internships are very tough—and people did crack. There's no question there were times you'd just be so overwhelmed with fatigue and the amount of work, with the fact that nothing was getting done and you had to do everything yourself.

You'd go to the lab and they'd say, "We lost all the specimens—we can't give you lab results because all the specimens are gone. We don't have anything on your patient." And then you'd have to draw them all again. They had a lab tech school there, and students were actually supposed to draw their blood. In those days, most of the labor in hospitals was done by people in training; but many times the techs didn't have the same interest in taking care of the patient that we did.

In those days, County manufactured its own IV fluids, had its own bottling system, its own tubing and own needles, which they used to resharpen. We used to have to use County-sharpened needles, and they were often dull and had burrs in them. There were actually times—and it happened to me—when you could get a needle in but you couldn't get it out, because it was caught inside. Or it was so dull that you had to push so hard to get it into the skin that it would go right through the vein. We didn't have anything else. People who worked at other hospitals had more modern equipment—at that time, a lot more modern things to use for starting IVs, IV tubing, were being invented. We actually used to requisition things from other hospitals: you'd ask a friend at another hospital. They would, in all effect, just steal it and give it to us.

The racial attitudes then, well, I think that we never can fully know what it's like when you're on the other side of that racial thing. I think it wasn't so much a racial thing as it was a poverty thing—but I saw some racism. Not so much from doctors to patients; I saw it and heard it from other patients. I saw some absolute scumbag of a guy, once, a White guy: he was a down-and-out alcoholic off of skid row, probably an Appalachian. A Black nurse's aide tried to help him, and he said, "You Black motherfucker, get your hand off me." She was trying to restrain him, because he was trying to get off the cart. And I was so furious that this absolute scum guy, out of the gutter, would have it in him to make a racial slur, that I actually took his arm, twisted it, and threw him back on the cart. I said, "Don't ever say something like that again. Who do you think you are to make a statement like that?"

Now, granted, there was largely a White medical staff; there were very few Black physicians in those days. There was a lot of animosity between the Black people who worked there—support staff—and the White doctors. But I think it was much more of a class thing, because they saw doctors as being upper-class people who came here to practice on poor people, who happened to be mostly Black or Hispanic. Granted, there was a day when people started looking more critically at those differences and

the injustices and saying that it was a Black-White issue. To say that
that's not true would be ridiculous—I think there *was* racism there. But
to say that it was *all* racism, I don't think so. I had medical students in my
class who went to Selma, Alabama, in 1963, who were marching for civil
rights. Somebody was accused of being a racist and he said, "If you think
of it, if I were really a racist, why would I be here? I'd be someplace else."

In fact, the Black patients were many times more pleasant to deal with
than, let's say, a hostile, alcoholic White. A Black person might end up
there not because they were an alcoholic, but just because they were very
poor. And they felt more comfortable there: they felt like it was their hospital. That was a very common attitude, many of us had it, that Black
people saw this as their hospital—and I think most of us respected that.
Those were our patients.

I'm working at the jail now, and to me it captures the days under Quentin
Young [former chairman of Medicine]. When I first started working for
Quentin—it sounds kind of hokey—but there was this common purpose:
people all pulling in the same direction, an air of cooperation.

The whole correctional system now is really overloaded, with very,
very sick patients, particularly with AIDS and infectious disease. As is
going to happen in any system, the more entitlements that you give to
people, the more they actually do demand. Now, I think that could be a
problem in the society at large: once you make stuff available, there are
people there for it, because they need it. As the jail system has become
more responsive to their needs, I think it's engendered a better utility of
our services—and we certainly have some things they want.

They use medicines to barter—it's power. Within the jail system, medicines are used as currency in trading, so the prisoners manipulate us a little
bit. If I know it I try to avoid it, because it's not good medicine; but if they
manipulate you for something that's pretty benign, I say, "So what, give it
to them." It helps keep the peace a little bit. We're doctors, not guards, and
most of us go out of our way to meet their needs if it's within reasonable
standards of medical practice. There are a lot of what we call "somatic
complaints"—people who have a lot of headaches, stomach disorders,
muscle aches and pains, a lot of insomnia, hostility, feeling demoralized.

For people in the jail, a common attitude is, "You locked me up—take
care of me." They don't really say that, but that's my interpretation many
times: "I want my teeth cleaned...I want this, I want that." There's an
arrogance to it. On the outside they don't get any of this stuff done—for
one, because they don't have access. But on the outside they're free, they
can do anything they want: smoke, drink, use drugs, eat bad diets, whatever. When they're in there, though, it's, "I don't like this food, you're
going to change my diet." There's this attitude of, "You locked us up,
now take care of us"—it's resentment. And the system is far from perfect—the food, for example, is not great. It's a very bad place to be locked

up in. But, actually, I think people don't complain as much as they might. Part of the reason is acceptance. Acceptance in some ways could be depression, because they're accepting what's happened to them. Sometimes anger may be more healthy, because it's a way of fighting for psychological survival. But the ones who want to complain, complain. Most of us have a generally benign attitude toward it: if they say, "I don't like this, I don't like that," we try and see if there's something we can do.

I think their depression has a lot of ramifications. It's not out-and-out depression, where people are suicidal; it's more an acting-out, ongoing depression, being demoralized and yet blaming other people. In that sense, people would put it more in the area of characterological disorders. But even people with personality disorders can become very depressed, because they can't manipulate their environment. The severe stages are psychopathic people—borderline people are very common there, manipulators. These are pretty dishonest people. There are narcissistic disorders to beat the band.

Tremendous numbers of people are incarcerated largely because they didn't get their needs met when they were two months old. If you treat a kid badly, they're going to grow up never having their needs met: they'll never be happy, they'll always be manipulative at a very childish level. Put a manipulator in an atmosphere that's very difficult to manipulate, and they'll get depressed. The problem is, with such massive numbers of people, if you give something to someone, everybody wants it—and they find out about it *immediately.* He's a good guy, go down there, he'll give you a vitamin. I tried it when I first got there: I was really a good guy, I gave people vitamins, this and that, an extra mattress if they got back problems. So the next week half of the people want vitamins, mattresses—they *all* want to see me!

In terms of preventive medicine...As a society, we are really bathed in the idea that there should be preventive medicine, but nobody is *doing* it—it doesn't pay. *Sickness* pays. We are not a nation of people who take individual responsibility for our health. People think there's going to be some system that's going to take care of them when they get sick—but that system isn't interested in that. I mean, you're a commodity for them—whether it's the pharmaceutical industry, the insurance industry, or doctors themselves. Managed competition is a total sellout to the insurance industry, to the lawyers, the lobbyists, the pharmaceutical industry, to all the other high-tech businesses. People make a lot of money off of people being sick.

After Clinton was elected, the activist medical groups were trying to get a voice with him. They went down to Little Rock, and he was supposed to listen to them, but he just totally snubbed them. People who have done a lot of work with indigents, who are working in the front lines, who actually know the field, were brought to Washington to testify about these issues. There was some initial interest in it, getting the lay of the land; but it seems to me, unless I see anything different coming out, that it's going to be very watered down.

I think that places like County—public hospitals in general across the country—have been extremely important...Not just for training, but in terms of the social arena that people dealt with there, with that part of society—it planted a lot of very good things in people, made them better doctors. And not just in terms of the practice of medicine, but because doctors, in addition to learning their skills, rarely could go away unaffected by that experience, could never be quite the same.

Old Days

Dr. Quentin Young

HAS FOR YEARS *applied his diagnostic skills to individuals as well as to the body politic itself. Known nationally for his antiwar activism during the Vietnam War, he is currently focusing his progressive and prodigious energies on efforts for a single-payer health plan for the nation. In a perfect and equitable world, one suspects, he would go mad—nothing to fix, no one to finagle.*

MY FIRST ENCOUNTER WITH COUNTY HOSPITAL WAS IN THE forties. I went to med school at Northwestern from '44 to '47—three years, army-type training. I had some clerkships at County as an undergraduate, and there was an opportunity to go there for an internship in July of '47. The requirement was we'd have to agree to a two-year internship. The particularities were, after World War II, there was a huge influx of G.I. doctors who wanted to go into specialties.

County, at that time, was one of a handful of hospitals in the country, if not the world, that had a whole spectrum of speciality, simply because of its vastness and its history. It had over thirty-four hundred beds. But beds were different than now: now they have an official census which conforms to health rules and space rules. Then it was, you get another patient, you roll out another bed. It's still a very big hospital; but, understand, the number was large, for two or three obvious reasons. One is, I'd venture as much as a third of the patients there—maybe as many as one thousand—were kept there because they'd just recovered from an illness, and they were essentially in nursing home state. The other thing is, the average stay was much longer. I'd venture it was in the high twenties; today they probably have seven or eight days average stay.

The resources were such that a good deal of care was just bed care and support—and we had the space, but the space was horrible. There were rooms in what was called then the "Men's Building"—I think now it's called the "B Building." It was male medicine: it had eight floors, two wings on each, we would have sixty-five people on each wing. *Now* they have twenty beds on each wing, and they're not always filled. That means we had beds so close together you had to sidle through.

The stories are almost unbelievable. There would be two interns on a floor taking care of about 120 patients, and you'd get twenty admissions every night you were on call. Call was twenty-four hours on, and you were *on:* if you had time to sleep, you slept, but you were on duty. You didn't have a day off the next day, you worked twelve more hours. And there were serious consequences: there was a significant TB rate among the house staff—and occasional suicide. It was very trying. Very short-staffed, doctors as well as nurses.

I remember at night in that building with 120, 130 people on each of eight floors, there would be one nurse available for injections of morphine or what have you. The interns in that day and age did such elementary things as mixing penicillin: you'd spend the first half hour of the morning mixing penicillin and things of that sort. It was very common for interns to push the patients to the X-ray or the other places they had to go: so patients would be sent to X-ray, but by the end of the day there would be scores of patients waiting to be *returned*. Somebody would eventually go get them, but I want to give an idea of the very huge, almost battlefield conditions.

Now, County was started, as I recall, in the 1860s as a place for people who suffered from this or that epidemic. There was typhoid, cholera, and so on. It moved several times, but ended up at its present site, in the early part of this century. At all times, it was a very important, politically connected place. The head of the institution had the title Warden—which conveys its ancient quality, its similarity to a penal institution. From the point of view of patronage and contracts, it was notorious. Certainly, all of the administrative personnel were beholden to the political system. By and large, jobs too were available on a patronage basis, as were a good deal of the never-ending contracts for building, repairing, and so on.

Of the doctors, two things can be said. It was a very competitive situation—a lot of people wanted to go there, and it was hard to get in. For quite a long time, you had to take an examination, which was atypical—interns in very few places in the country had to pass examinations. Also, even the attending physicians took an exam. Being an attending at County was a very valuable thing. It had no salary, none whatsoever, but an attending physician at County was worth a professorship in any of the five schools that used the place. It was like a feudal principality: the attending physician had control of his ward and his service, and therefore it could be used for teaching, for human experimentation, for patient care activities.

The political was more than just structural, it was in the persona of a particular person—Karl Meyer—who ran the hospital. He very cannily and successfully made the whole County Hospital and its environs his bailiwick, by an odd admixture of skills and personality. He was actually kind of a mean-spirited, almost embittered person, very few social skills. He was a surgeon—very arrogant and authoritative in the manner of surgeons of the day. Everybody concedes he was a highly skilled surgeon, but he was not a nice person.

He very craftily used the hospital's resources in relation to the political power structure to guarantee his own enormous power. There was a whole ward at County—which is supposed to be a public hospital—that was essentially set aside for VIPs: people in the community, politicians occasionally, people with social and professional power. People like that would come in for surgery under him or other major surgeons. There's no denying that the hospital, broadly speaking, prospered. He protected it from the predations of the political; they got theirs, but at the same time, he preserved certain prerogatives.

Another crucial point was his strategy, which I think was right, of never letting one school dominate County: there were always four or five schools competing, and by pitting them in competition, he could get concessions. The schools wanted to use County as a teaching ground, so they paid for the junior staff that had to come in and do things. It helped the schools, to be sure, but it maintained a certain kind of excellence at County that served it well for many decades. The schools, the big four, were Northwestern, Chicago Med, Illinois, and Loyola.

So you get a scene, by the time I got there, of a huge, sprawling place. County was always a place where the most recent poverty group was taken care of. When I was there the first time you had to have a smattering of street Polish. Black English helped, but it wasn't the big issue; County was still majority White, albeit the Blacks were rapidly moving up, for obvious reasons. I would say in the forties, when I was there, County was sixty/forty White. You'd see all kinds of people there, it's the old American story: the most recent immigrants were the ones who used the public facility. There were no Hispanics to speak of, but now it's substantially so.

Then, of course, from that point onward there was an ever-larger use of the hospital by the Blacks, who weren't allowed to go anywhere else. They were Jim Crowed out of everywhere except Provident and County. By the mid-sixties eighty percent of the Blacks born in the city were born at County; fifty percent of Black deaths were in that one hospital—of the whole city! Beyond Provident—which at that time was a very tiny hospital, maybe three hundred beds—County was the one that really absorbed the Blacks and made it possible for breathtaking racial exclusion to be practiced every day in Chicago hospitals. Doctors knew that if they were silly enough to admit Black patients, they would not see their appointments renewed—they *knew* it. It was just one of those unspoken truths, like most racial compacts. Granted, in the South they had "colored only" and those sorts of things; but Chicago was just as well segregated without any laws. That meant that not only poor Blacks, but Blacks of all social classes, more or less, had to go to County.

It took on a very ugly extortionate quality, because Blacks by and large were in the mass industries: packing, steel, auto, Pullman porters—all of which had these wonderful industrial union benefits. And they'd go to County: Blue Cross would pay County five dollars a day as a nonparticipating hospital. Today, per diems are seven, eight hundred dollars a day; then it might have been as much as eighty or ninety dollars. It was a naked subsidy of the White population by the Blacks in the work force: obviously, if you have a work force that's half Black and half White, and the Blacks can only go to a five-dollar-a-day hospital and the rest wherever they want, the rates are kept down. That was all dealt with in some civil rights complaints. During the forties, fifties, they had no place else to go. That was broken explicitly in 1955 by an ordinance that was passed in Chicago, the Harvey Campbell Ordinance, which outlawed— in Chicago, under Mayor Daley—discrimination on the basis of race. In '57 there was another ordinance passed which outlawed staff appointment denial on the basis of race.

The hospital, during the forties and fifties, and to a large extent even now—though not nearly like then—was run by the house staff. The house staff was there—and attendings came, they'd make rounds. Some would be very conscientious: they'd see a few patients and make important contributions with their vast skills to understanding and treating the patient. But many didn't actually see patients; they'd review cases in conferences and stuff. So it was the house staff that gave the care, and it was by and large very good.

It wasn't a culture of "treat the patients nice," but there was a drive to give the patients good care. Why? Because the people giving the care were people in training, who were judged by their peers and by themselves, by how well their patients did. When you think a minute, a surgeon doesn't feel very good if half his patients die—but he feels *very* good if he saves the difficult cases. And, more to the point, the immediate peer group—which I would say is not the supervising doctors, but the fellow residents—could be very, very cruel if your patients didn't do well.

So, out of this quality of care, patients forged a really great affection. More than affection: when I came back as chairman of Medicine in the seventies, my service had 450 beds. It was the largest one. The best thing I thought I could do was to go to the Medical Admitting Ward. We literally had a ward for admissions: patients didn't come from the ER to the hospital room or bed, they went to a *ward,* essentially an intensive care center, since the typical admission was so sick that we had to have all the support systems. It looked like any intensive care unit in any other hospital: there'd be twenty or thirty patients who had been admitted that day. They were supposed to be moved out in a day; occasionally, some would be kept another day because they just couldn't be moved. I'd go there, because that was the concentrated essence of what was happening and how the hospital was working. I would read the chart and make an effort to establish some rapport with the patient.

I tell this story a lot, about this very old man who was obviously in heart failure. I greeted him and introduced myself and asked how's he doing, how's he feeling? At a certain point I'd say, "Why do you come here?" And he said, "I always come here." I said, "Well, but you know, why do you come *here?*" He said, "I been coming here six years." "But why do you come *here?* You have to pass twenty hospitals to get here." He says, "I *always* come here—this is my hospital." And I like to make the point that that old man, who probably lived in a housing project, did not believe that housing project he lived in was his, and he was right; or that the school where his grandchildren went was theirs; or even that the little scratchy park that might have been outside their project was his park. But he'd come to believe—and, with him, most of the users of the hospital—that this was *their* hospital. That's an amazing thing.

In the fifties and sixties, there was this kind of steady decline in the size of the hospital's operation, in terms of numbers of people admitted. But in every other respect it increased. Those were the same years that every medical center was doing more—the age of antibiotics, of heart/lung preparation surgery. You could get much bolder—and you could be sure that most things were done at County.

Earlier in that period, like when I was there in the forties, human experimentation was really crass: all of the safeguards of informed consent and the patients feeling they could say no weren't in place. I did a master's degree there doing renal clearances on people with late-stage kidney disease. Renal clearances involve getting blood, you have a catheter in the bladder—it's a very carefully timed procedure. By and large, it would be annoying to the patient; occasionally, it could be quite grueling. My informed consent mainly was: "Here—sign here." I would try and explain it to them, but I can't honestly say that they really knew, for example, that they could say no. I just didn't say it in as many words.

If somebody was really resistant, I would probably say no for them, or tell them, "If you don't want to do this, you don't have to"—and give them the right. But I would never claim that this had any of the modern standards of informed consent. And what I was involved in was pretty benign; I don't think I ever put people at risk. But the drug and surgical stuff...I'm not condemning, it was the age. It was from that type of unacceptable arrangements that latter-day human experimentation protocols were developed. And, obviously, there's no question that the reason that went on there, rather than at St. Luke's, say, is because these were disempowered people. County could be looked at as a huge trough, a lot of people at the trough.

When I was oriented as an intern in '47, there were a hundred of us. Now there are many more. Our orientation was very brief. The then–medical director...It's not clear whether he ever finished medical school, he wasn't too hot—nobody had *any* respect for him as a doctor.

He was a paid political hack from the machine, and I'll prove it. At our orientation, we were told this is where the lockers, this and that, were, and he says, "I want to tell youse guys something. A lot of people will come into the Emergency Room, and they'll have a little slip of paper in their hand—from their precinct captain or ward committeeman, or even their congressman. Now, you and I know they don't need that slip of paper to get in, but there's no need to make a big thing about it—just tell them you know the congressman or you know the ward committeeman, and then do what you have to do." That was disingenuous, but the vast number of people who used the hospital—whether once in a lifetime or every week—came to believe that they had to have that slip. Whether they did or not makes no difference—they believed it. It was part of the patronage system: that was part of the service that the party gave then, whether it was fixing tickets, or getting the roads repaired, or getting them medical care. And it was a very important prop, because you were dealing with thirty-three thousand admissions a year.

The interns, we got very devil-may-care...The work conditions were so oppressive that it was a kind of a battlefront bravado. We would tell them, even though it was perilous, "We don't need the damn slip!" Or if they *did* have the slip..."Oh, what are we gonna do with Ma? We can't deal with her, she's been screaming all night." "Take her to County." So they'd bring her—or whoever—to County, but there was no medical thing wrong, so we'd say no. And, you could count on it, they'd go up to the second floor, where the warden's office was, and the slip would come down: "Admit per Warden." He didn't know what she had or nothing!

That's how it was under the political patronage system. And it worked: people believed that it was an entitlement, they *had* to get that sanction, and they'd better be nice, meaning vote right and do what they want. We lived with it, and by and large there was very little interference—none, really, with the work you did. There was this kind of symbiosis. But the politicians were at the trough for jobs, contracts, and appearing to be the benefactors for thousands of people.

The people who worked there were also at a trough. Many of them treated the jobs like patronage jobs: they either didn't show up or didn't do a full day's work, depending on their importance to the party, whether they were precinct captains or higher. There was every kind of job—all kinds of maintenance jobs, all kinds of service, food delivery, and so on. By and large the professionals didn't do that kind of thing, because the wages weren't so good that you couldn't do as well elsewhere. But we had enormously untrammeled—one might say "profligate"—access to patients, seeing them and all these diseases.

We worked very hard to help them—but the experimental stuff and so on were what was and is placed in the trough: the patients were the food in the trough. The patients traded off their bodies and their illnesses in exchange for care. And that's what the model was—it's a very pejorative version, but I think it's accurate. And that doesn't mean...I mean, if there were no County, there'd be a lot more people dead. And a lot of very good things happened there.

I used to say there was no room for any liberals at County. Only two world philosophies worked with what you saw before you, because you saw the wretched of the earth: alcoholics, drugusers, late-stage disease, people with wound infections with maggots in them—I mean, really *bad*. And so you could come up with one of two conclusions: One was a very conservative, judgmental, almost religious view, that these were people who consistently violated God's law with fornication and alcohol and thievery, and they were the dregs of the earth and this was their retribution. But, in my opinion, it didn't keep these doctors from working hard to take care of them. They felt their mission was to cure the ailing—and even though they had that terrible attitude toward their clients, they still worked hard. The other was obviously the one I—and many of us— embraced, that this was the distilled oppression of society. These were people on the bottom of the economic heap, of racial discrimination, who were born to lose, and their whole life is a testimony to privation and oppression, and what we're seeing is the physical expression of it. And that obviously implied a more compassionate concern for the patients before you. But, I'd say, on any given day you couldn't tell the difference between who adhered to which philosophy.

And I would argue—as I recall—that both groups worked very hard, because the prize was how well your patient was. These doctors were guys who were paying dear for three, five years of very hard work, under very unpleasant conditions, not a lot of support. It was only to be thought of as a rite of passage: at the end of the time, you came out with a lot of notches on your belt. You really felt very confident.

And by and large it turned out a lot of great doctors. And its impact on the doctors...I always summarize it like this: At conventions where County doctors are—and there are so many thousands of us—they tend to congregate. They don't talk about whatever the convention is about; usually, it's about the speciality you're in. The normal tendency of doctors would be to talk about the hernias they repaired or the diabetes they'd treated. Sure, there's some of that—but mostly they go back and reminisce about County.

Dr. Murray Franklin

HE IS A VETERAN *of World War II. A war hero. The* Croix de Guerre, *Purple Heart, and Silver Star are only some of the medals hanging framed on his office wall. Others have gone to his young grandchildren. Still more are housed in a file cabinet—kept in a crumpled white envelope with "Extra Medals" scrawled in pencil across the front. He was a resident and fellow at County from 1946 to 1949 and an attending physician from 1951 to 1954.*

I CAME TO COUNTY IN '46. IN THOSE DAYS, THEY WERE JUST BE-ginning to do liver function studies in this country, and Cook County Hospital was the center for it. I came here and got associated with Hans Popper. They gave me a fellowship, and I learned the whole business about liver biopsies. I still had seven months to finish my residency. At that time, the residents were passed on by the medical board—that is, the doctors on staff. They were all very good friends of mine, and I was rather shocked when they turned me down for a residency. They told me no one in County Hospital had ever been a resident who wasn't an intern here first. So Popper, who had an in with Karl Meyer, said, "Look, they turned Franklin down, and he can go to University of Minnesota if he wants, he can go to Cincinnati." So, next thing, Karl Meyer—an absolute dictator, what he said goes—said, "If he's good enough for them, he's good enough for me."

And I did get a residency. [chuckles] Except, I wasn't paid—there was no pay, I got nothing, not even a room, a place. I lived in a whorehouse—it's where the residents quarters are now for Presbyterian. Then, there was a bookie joint on the first floor and a whorehouse on the second floor, and in between I had a room. I paid seven dollars a week, and was allowed one meal a day at the hospital.

For many years, in the twenties and the thirties and before, County was a renowned institution for learning medicine. It meant something. This was the finest place for me to do hands-on medicine: I got to exam-ine patients and whatnot, and then the pathology, the autopsies and all that. I learned medicine. I got to examine patients and treat patients dif-ferent ways and see which were the best ways, and I got to see bodies, autopsy material—this is what I wanted.

I saw all my patients, and I hung around from seven in the morning sometimes until one in the morning, though they closed at nine, so I had to get special permission to stay on the wards. I had some side interests. I used to play around with tests, I invented tests. The first kidney biopsy needle in the world I invented here. I didn't play golf and I didn't play tennis—I was wounded in the war, I couldn't. So, to me, working in the laboratory at the end of the night, that was what I had.

I finished my residency and went to the University of Iowa. When I came back to Chicago, I was offered an associate professorship at the University of Illinois, and my job was to create a teaching program in medicine at County for the juniors in Internal Medicine.

I'll explain you the system, because the system was a very odd one. Cook County had, as I say, a great reputation, and on the staff they had a few men full-time, like the pathologist and whatnot. But the unpaid staff varied from poor, I would say, to some very good men. It was *something* to be on the attending staff at County Hospital; it was something to be desired. It was the prestige they got. Unfortunately, many of these guys, they never did what they were supposed to do, their teaching, supervising treatment of patients. Which was a good thing, for some of them—I wouldn't want to be taught by some of those guys. For instance, my first year as a resident on Ward 75, I never saw my attending man until the very last day. Never saw him. [chuckles] I saw this guy walking around and I said, "Who are you?" He said, "I'm the attending man here." The very last day! The problem with County Hospital was that they couldn't change attending men very much.

To me, the prestige didn't mean anything, but I'll tell you why it was important for the schools to have men on the staff here. Four schools used County for teaching their medical students. Depending on the number of attending men each school had here, they were allowed to send two students per attending man.

To show you what I mean by the prestige...For example, in Internal Medicine, for the boards all the oral examinations for applicants from all over the country were given at Cook County Hospital. *Now* there are no orals, but in the old days there was a written and an oral exam—if you passed the written, then you were allowed to take the oral. All the big wheels in medicine from all over the country would come, and they were called the senior examiners. The good attending men here were teamed with them, one would go with each examiner. Some of these examiners were bad. I know one guy from Georgia who used to openly brag that he would never pass a woman applicant. I got in trouble one day: we'd put these six charts out with the doctor's name, and I noticed he was scheduled to give the examination to a woman, so I just exchanged that chart and I got caught.

Karl Meyer was superintendent from 1928 to '68 or something like that. He was an absolute dictator: he ran a tight ship, and the tight ship worked. He didn't bother himself with the mundane stuff, the politics and whatnot. Meyer was an excellent surgeon and—another thing about him—he had a private practice, and he was a very generous man and did a lot of free work for people. There are many people who swear by him that he did surgery and didn't charge them. He was known for that.

When I came here, I found that I had my name on papers with Karl Meyer—and I *knew* he didn't know anything about the papers. He once asked me a question: he said, "You know, they've got this new thing, vitamin K." Vitamin K had been out for years, and here it was something new to him! [laughs] So I went to my boss, Popper, and I said, "This is funny—he asked me about vitamin K, and it's been used for years! He didn't know anything about it." He said, "Well, he's got a couple of papers on Vitamin K." I said, "Yeah, but he doesn't know anything about it." He says, "Karl Meyer is a very excellent surgeon and he has a very fine reputation in the city, but in the country he's not known, and therefore we put his name on all the papers." So Karl Meyer's name was on all these scientific papers that he had absolutely nothing…didn't write them, didn't read them! [laughs]

Meyer had as his chief assistant a doctor called Ole Nelson, an older guy who knew absolutely no medicine and didn't pretend to know medicine. It was said he got his degree from one of these mills where he paid thirty-odd bucks for it. That was in the teens, 1913 or something. His main claim to fame was that he went to fifty-two Kentucky Derbies, consecutively. As a matter of fact, if you ever went to his office, most of the people there had to do with the racetracks, with the gambling scene— it wasn't medicine. So Ole did the administrative work and, as I say, he wasn't a medical man at all. I'll give you an example, it happened on my ward. A young woman happened to get on the ward who had diphtheria—she was immediately put in quarantine, and *nobody* was to go near her. I came the next morning on the ward, and the poor nurse was crying. I said, "What's the problem?" I looked in the room, the woman's boyfriend was there. I said, "You have *no* business being here, this ward is quarantined." He said, "You know who I am?" I said, "I don't give a shit who you are"—he was some low political precinct captain—I threw him out bodily. [laughs] He went to Ole Nelson and said, "Franklin threw me out," so Ole calls me down and was going to give me hell. I said, "Dr. Nelson, that patient's got diphtheria." Ole looked at me and said, "Is diphtheria contagious?" [laughs] I looked at him and I said, "Yes, it is." He told me later he'd called up the Board of Health, and they'd verified what I said.

He was the liaison between the politicians, who had a lot to do with County—remember, at that time there were three thousand employees, aside from the professional people—the liaison between them and the precinct captains and politicians. Now, Ole didn't butt in too much in the medical activities, such as with the residents and whatnot—*that* was

George Blaha's job. He was a younger man. He wasn't a bad doctor; he knew a little medicine, but he didn't practice. His job was to control the interns and residents, their schedules. And again there were favorites played. For instance, every month one of the medical residents was assigned to X-ray, which meant that you didn't have any other duties; it was a good thing, something to be desired. [laughs] He would assign it to his friends.

One of the fine things about County Hospital was the cooperation between the Pathology Department and the Medicine Department. At the end of the day, all of the autopsies which were done—there were sometimes as many as fifteen, usually between six and ten—the organs were placed in the old amphitheater building and the residents and the interns were invited to come down and see their "mistakes," whether they were right or wrong on the wards. The cases were discussed by the interns, residents, and pathologist. And we learned medicine! Over the doorway in the old Coroner's building was an inscription—THIS IS THE PLACE WHERE THE DEAD TEACH THE LIVING—and it was true. I learned a tremendous amount. Whenever we had cases whose diagnosis we didn't know, we found the answer at the autopsy table. We all made efforts to get as many autopsies as we could. In fact, we each chipped in two bucks a month, and the medical resident that had the most autopsies at the end of the month got the money. Now...they're doing maybe one or two autopsies a week, maybe less. They're worried medically, legally: everybody sues. In my day, no one was being sued—and we were doing five to fifteen a day! And when you see that every day, you learn medicine.

In my time at County there was one EKG machine, a lousy old Sanborn, a portable. It was not a direct writer: you had to put in a whole roll, like film, and take one EKG after the other, and then at the end of the day you go and you have to develop it. And if you forgot to put the roll in, which happened from time to time, you had nothing—or if you made a mistake and opened the machine and let the light in...So then Harry Isaacs, who was an attending man at County, his son was a resident—he gave his son a present. Another EKG machine! [chuckles] So we had two machines. And they didn't have technicians going around—we ourselves went and did it.

Now, the entire thing has deteriorated. I hate to say this...I don't know what has happened. In the first place, there are far less patients there now—we had almost twice as many patients. I saw every one of my patients. We had residents who were willing to do that—there was no dehumanizing of patients. It doesn't make a difference whether a patient is in a private room or he's on the ward. We had patients here who were rich and wanted to come to County. I had a patient who was a millionaire and insisted on coming to my ward.

It is a big old dirty building, and some people want nice working conditions. [angrily] But that doesn't mean that if you give me a brand-new shiny building that good work would be done there. I once spoke to a Nobel Prize–winner in his laboratory and he said, "I got a Nobel Prize. You came into my lab and it was disorganized and dirty because work was being done...I got now a building that's white, it's clean, and it's sterile because nothing is done here." You could do goddamn good medicine at County.

It's a dirty old building and nobody likes it, but that doesn't mean you can't practice good medicine there. Sure, you could go to a small hospital and get a hell of a good salary, but when you came out you hadn't learned anything. It depends on what you want. You want the nice white halls and all that, fine...I got nothing here: I had to pay my own goddamn seven dollars a week rent, I ate salami and bread at home—that's all I ate, except for one meal at the cafeteria. But I never had a better time. I learned more damn medicine here than I could have learned anywhere.

Dr. Frank Milloy

HAS BEEN A CARDIOTHORACIC *surgeon at County Hospital since 1983, but he was a resident there during the forties. "There was an old German place called 'Sieben's Brewery.' It was near the corner of Ogden and North Avenue. You could get a mug of beer for ten cents and the biggest sandwich, liverwurst or ham, for fifteen cents. There was a little bulletin board that was stuck to the door, and one time there was this scrawled thing on the back of a ticket or something like that: 'If the County doctors don't stop speeding on Ogden Avenue, I'm going to start giving them tickets.' [laughs] You'd never get a ticket—especially if you were in whites—if you said, "I'm a doctor at County." Because the police knew they may come in there at some time in bad shape.*

MY DAD WAS A DOCTOR. IN FACT, IN MY CLASS IN MEDICAL school we had 118 men, two girls, and no minorities. Very few Blacks even went to college in those days. Maybe we had two Chinese fellas. And so we had almost all White American males. The common denominator in that whole group was their fathers being doctors. I came to Chicago in '44. At that time County Hospital was thirty-three hundred beds, and we had a hundred thousand admissions a year. I remember the smell of the place was a little bit different than now. It didn't smell like a hospital, it didn't have that clean hospital smell. The smell was cooking food—and I suppose three thousand bodies contributed to it—but it had quite a characteristic odor when you walked into the place.

The wards were built in the old style—it's called the "pavilion style"—and they're built like that because of contagious diseases, so people were kind of isolated. This main hallway is two blocks long, and then these four wings stick out. You'd walk out, and when you started in the ward there were smaller rooms on either side, and then the back end of the ward was all one enormous room with about forty or fifty beds in it, and one bed next to the other. The smaller rooms were kept on the wards, when I was here, for real sick patients, people who were dying. They didn't want people dying out on the wards, it kind of hurt the morale of the other patients. The nurses were very considerate of those practical things.

We were supposed to start internship July 1st, 1947. We got a letter that there would be a lunch June 30th for indoctrination. George Blaha was the assistant medical director, and after lunch he said, "You're not due to start until tomorrow, but you could go to your wards and find out where your ward is and maybe see what the other fellows have to say, maybe get some advice."

The day we came, we got a full schedule for the two years. So I looked at my schedule and I had OB. It was over here on the fifth floor of this building, so I sauntered over [laughs] and I went into the labor department. They were delivering, I think, twenty babies a day then. It was just a simple labor line—the complicated stuff went to other wards. So I went in and I met a resident. There was a guy there, he was delivering a baby or something, and he said, "My internship ends at four o'clock." So the resident looks at me and said, "Would you mind starting at four o'clock?" So I thought, What the heck, what can I say? I didn't want to start off on the wrong foot. I said, "Sure, I'll start." So he says, "Well, let's go in and deliver a baby." So he went in and delivered one, and then he said, "Well, go ahead, you deliver one." So I delivered the next one. By this time it was five or six in the evening. He says, "I think I'll go get some dinner. I'll be in my room if you need me." [laughs] He left me. By the next morning, I'd had about ten or twelve deliveries.

I had a month in anesthesia. When you took a month in anesthesia, then you got anesthesia privileges—and from then on you could take anesthesia call at night, or if an anesthetic had to be given on the ward then you could do it. And I had a month of orthopedic surgery. They didn't have a neurosurgery resident, so the general surgery residents rotated through neurosurgery. Ward 22, it was mostly trauma: the West Madison Street crowd that came in, they got hit on the head and robbed. They were unconscious so they'd bring 'em here, we had to admit them and keep them for a couple of days. And then, of course, there were a lot of broken bones, so they had these old beds with the big wood racks on them—the fracture beds. And then they had the slide rails on them because they all went into DTs [delirium tremens]. Neurosurgery was referred to as "the jungle."

There was a contagious hospital, it was a little hospital across the street from what's now the Karl Meyer Hall—there's a parking lot there now. When you went there you had to live there. They only had forty or fifty beds. If a patient came in with the mumps or chicken pox they would usually send them home—but if it was complicated, they would admit them. And so you were isolated there for a month. You had to eat your meals there and sleep there; you weren't supposed to mix with the other house staff. A lady came in with something or other, measles or mumps, and she was about to deliver a baby. I'd had a month of OB, so I was the hero.

The psychiatry hospital was over in the other corner, on Wood. An old, dark, four-story building. And in the center, between the psychiatric hospital and the TB hospital, was the morgue, a little two-story yellow-brick building. It was also the coroner's morgue—John Dillinger was brought there after he was shot. And then all of our patients that died went to the morgue, and we did our post mortems over there at the morgue. If we had an interesting case and they were going to do a post, we'd go over and watch it.

So if you stand at the back door of County and imagine, to the left, is the psych hospital and directly in front of you would be the morgue, then to the right would be the TB hospital. When we made rounds, we'd be talking, a resident and a couple of interns, making rounds, we didn't want to say, "Well, this guy has cancer and he'll probably die"—so we'd say, "Well, he's headed for center field." Or if we thought it was TB, we didn't want to say TB because it would frighten all the other patients, so we'd say "right field." Or if he was crazy, we'd say "headed for left field." The expression "somebody is out in left field" is pretty common, but I think that's where it started out.

You got room and board and laundry. You could go to The Greeks in those days and get a steak dinner for a dollar and a quarter, and beer or cokes were 15 cents, 25 cents a bottle. That was the only building in the park. You walked in the door and there were big long tables: the nurses would always be sitting there before they started work. And there was a big round soda fountain-type bar. Then you went through a little door back into a room with a bar and booths, which was called the "Monkey Room"—the wallpaper was monkeys climbing on palm trees. We didn't have pagers. They would call your room and the ward and The Greeks. [laughs] And Pete was at the bar—he'd pick up the phone, "Canal 3696." That was the phone number of The Greeks.

When we worked in the Emergency Room, there'd be two of us, one guy on the male side, one guy on the female side. I think we saw six hundred people a day. People would be brought by their family; there were no fire department ambulances. The Chicago police had what were called squadrols. They were little panel trucks, except you could stand up in the back of them. They would hold two stretchers, one on each side. And if Grandma got sick in the slums, they called the police and they would come and bring 'em—and then the two big old cops would be carrying this poor soul in, and we'd look at 'em and of course they wanted to leave them. And if we refused and said it's just an old lady that needs some food and water, there's nothing to do for her, she's not sick, then they'd have to take 'em back. [laughs] Then they made a rule the cops had to stay until we released the patient. They would be telling you, "She's a wonderful old lady, doc—son's a priest." [laughs]

Each patient would be assigned to an attending. If it was during the day, his intern would work the patient up and see what kind of treatment was going to go on. The intern would get upset if you sent the wrong...I hate to tell ethnic jokes, but on Oriental patients when I was in the ER I always put down possible jaundice. So this guy used to come down and say, "Well, this guy's Chinese. Why do you say jaundice?" I'd say, "Well, how do you know he's not jaundiced." [laughs] So that was the kind of stuff that went on with us. Friday and Saturday nights were gunshots, stab wounds. Monday was the biggest day for medicine, because they were home Saturday and Sunday and they didn't want to be bothered, but Monday they'd have to bring Grandma to the hospital.

County was surrounded by the University of Illinois on the south, on the west was Chicago Med and Loyola, and then Rush Medical College, of course, had been at the northeast corner. So the medical schools always depended on County to a great extent—you have to remember that the attending staff in those days were the leading doctors in Chicago, and they came here voluntarily.

The system was Karl Meyer's creation. He was a master politician and a master administrator. He was the type of person that was admired, and he kept the right relationships, so these guys came. He was only about five-foot, two and very quiet, absolutely no sense of humor—just all business. Very serious, taciturn, hardly ever said anything. Meyer kept a pretty tight rein on things. He had strict rules about who got to do what.

During the day, you couldn't start a case until your attending man stepped off the elevator. In those days, they wore street clothes up and down the corridor and in the operating room. Now you have to change. We used to do spinal anesthetics and the guy would be looking down the hall—especially in the GYN, because you never knew when they were going to show up—and the guy would step off the elevator: "He's here." And bang, they'd do their spinal, then go down and change clothes and, of course, then they'd do the surgery. But that way it kept people from doing things or starting early.

Meyer ran a tight ship. And he was the kind of guy you did *not* fool around with—he didn't actually kick people out, but boy, if he wanted to chew you out, you knew you'd had a few words said. They tell a story about one guy that did something Meyer didn't like, a case at night or something—I don't remember what he did. Meyer put him in the morgue his last three months: he said, "He can operate all he wants over there."

I'll tell you one thing: When Meyer ran this hospital, there would have never been any kind of a strike by a doctor. I'll tell you a story about him to give you an idea. At one point during the war, the food got terrible here—I wasn't here then—but the residents got together and there was a little skinny guy named Roy Tanoui, who was from Hawaii. He was a surgical resident and he weighed about eighty pounds. So they said, "You go in and tell Meyer that the food is so bad we're eating all our meals at The Greeks, and could he please do something about it?" So Tanoui goes in and tells him. Meyer says, "Why did you come to County? To learn surgery or to eat?"

Gertrude D'Anno

A NURSE, RECENTLY *retired. When we meet in the Nurses' Residence building, she mentions that rarely does she return to the hospital. "I spent thirty-three of my fifty-five years here, and it's time for me to move on and do other things—and if I keep coming back it's just going to remind me of things that I know I'm not going to be able to change. It's somebody else's time now...The hospital will go on. It will survive. It has to, because the people of Chicago have to have some place where they can come for care."*

I CAME IN MAY OF 1960. THE DEAL WAS, YOU CAME AS A REG-istered nurse, you had to have a license. What you did was, you came here and you worked for six months. They gave you a room here in the nurses' residence. On the wall as you come in there was a rack of cards, and that was your mealticket. And you punched it. You went and you got a meal, you didn't have to pay. And that was what you got for six months, there was no salary.

I worked in the OR [operating room] as a staff nurse, and then I became the coordinator in '81. It was a whole different atmosphere: I think that people were friendlier, I think people in general were more willing to teach you. It was truly a learning experience. And it was really exciting—if you showed just the least little bit of interest there were so many opportunities for you to learn. The doctors were helpful and they were willing. If you were a sponge, you could not help—the opportunities were there for you to learn. I'm not saying that that's not happening now, but I think now it's more technology. Medicine in general has changed so much, there are so many new kinds of techniques. When would we ever think, even in 1960, of being able to have your gall bladder removed through a little tube? When I started, everything was done by hand.

There was a lot more camaraderie, up and down at all levels. It seemed like everybody worked together for the benefit of the patient; now it seems we've kind of alienated ourselves into, "That's her job, not mine." At that time, there was more teamwork, and nobody refused an assignment. "I don't want to work with her," "I don't like her," "I don't get along"—you didn't *dare* to say that.

It's very, very difficult to get people who are poor performers out of this institution—you really have to work at it. Unfortunately, in the OR, when you're the manager—and at times I was *the* manager for the whole

OR—you can't watch more than a hundred people and be on their attendance and their performance and every single thing *every single minute*. You need other people to help you. Unfortunately, when it goes to grievance and when it goes to reprimand and those kinds of things, you're the one who's on the firing line: it's you against the employee. And, of course, then, they have union representation and you have nobody. Sometimes I'd think, "Oh, there's so much red tape." It seemed as if, if you didn't document every little single thing, even though you knew what happened, if it wasn't written down…To document, you just had to keep on it *all* the time. You'd get so frustrated. It's very time-consuming—you'd think, Is it worth it? And then you'd think, Where are the good nurses? Why don't they just give me good nurses, and then I won't have to worry about the bad ones—I won't have to worry about the paperwork.

When I started, the nurses residence was strictly for nurses—it wasn't for offices, like it is now. It was like a dormitory. The nursing school was still being run. The place was immaculate, very well kept. On the second floor was what they used to call the Blue Lounge, and it was blue: the walls were painted blue, and they had blue carpets on the floor and lovely settees and sofas and things, chairs where you could sit. You could go there with a date and entertain. They had a grand piano. There were little rooms on the first floor—they used to call them "date rooms"—and they had a sofa with a couple of chairs and a lamp and you could sit there and socialize. There were a whole stream of people behind the desk. They sold meal books there, they took your telephone messages, and if you got telegrams or flowers or anything like that, it was all taken care of right there.

The cafeteria was totally different: there were small tables for four, and some for two. They had those racks with the cards, because you didn't have to pay. If you were an RN and you needed to pay, they had coupon books. They served breakfast and lunch, and in the afternoon snacks and things were available, and then they opened again for supper. If you worked nights, you used to be able to come—I think lunches started at one in the morning—you could come at night and have a meal. This was all ladies. Karl Meyer Hall was a residence for the residents and the interns. And if you were lucky, if you scrubbed for one of the doctors they'd say, "Come on, I'll take you to Karl Meyer for lunch." The food there was better, but the food here was very, very good. They used to do all their own cooking: they had kitchens in the back, and they'd bring out these great big trays of food. And the food was good in the hospital, too, when I first came. They also had a bakery on the premises, and we used to get fresh-baked bread and butter. It was wonderful.

The central supply, we used to make our own IV fluids too. There were a lot of things that they did. They had all their own maintenance. We had a mattress shop that used to repair the mattresses. They used to make their own uniforms. Down in the basement of the nurses' residence, there was a laundry—you'd get a laundry card. We used to bring our white uniforms over, you'd hand in so many, they'd launder them free, and you'd go back in so many days and pick them up. They did all the laundry for the nurses' residence: you'd get clean sheets once a week, and, I think, you got clean towels every three days. Once a week the maid would come in and clean your room. You would never ever see peeling paint. The floors were shiny, tiles. This here [gesturing around the glass-walled room we sit in] was a beautiful sun porch. They had lawn furniture out there in the summer [points to outdoor roof terrace] and they had potted palms.

There was a lot of overcrowding on the wards, especially in the winter-time because there were so many homeless people that came in. They'd come in with some chronic disease and just kind of bed down for the winter. There were beds in the middle of the halls...But at the same time, I'd say the hospital probably was a little bit cleaner than what it is now.

Of course, at that time too there was a lot of patronage. The environmental service workers, most of them were patronage workers. It depended on your precinct captain whether or not you got a job, and of course when there was an election you'd see all new faces. So if there was somebody who was a bad worker they'd go, and if it was somebody who was really good, unfortunately they would go too—you had no control. But I would say the majority of the staff that were hired were competent.

Now they have affiliations at private hospitals, where they go out and learn how it is and how to talk to patients, how to treat patients. [lowers her voice conspiratorially] When patients are not paying, you have a tendency to say, "I'm the doctor, you will do what I say." When you have a patient who's paying they can tell you, "I'm not going to do that, I don't want that." They can say no. [normal voice] I think it's more well-rounded, I think it's better. There were always certain services, like the plastic surgeons and the orthopedic surgeons, that would come here and do a rotation. They might be from Northwestern or from the University of Illinois. Especially the ENT [ear, nose, throat] and plastic surgeons: "Oh, I can't wait to go back to Northwestern." Go! The patients that we would have here, there were a lot of fractured mandibles, a lot of trauma surgeries that they wouldn't see in private practice. Some of them didn't want to deal with those kinds of things, with the clientele.

One time I had a patient—I think it was at night—they had to put a tube in the nose and then in the mouth. They wanted to spray the patient's mouth and he wouldn't open his mouth. The anesthesiologist kept talking to him, but he had his mouth clenched. I went over and I took his hand and said, "What's the matter? Are you afraid? How can I help you? Just tell me why won't you open your mouth?" He said, "I've got five dollars in there." I said, "What?" He said, "I have five dollars." I said, "Is that all the money you have?" He said, "Yes." I said, "I'll get a paper towel and I want you to take the money out of your mouth and give it to me and I'll hold it. When you wake up I'll give it back to you." He had a brand-new five-dollar bill way in the back—his teeth were imprinted on it.

If you want a patient's cooperation, you have to talk to him.

Dr. Agnes Lattimer

MEDICAL DIRECTOR. *"I grew up in Memphis, Tennessee. Very early in my life, actually while I was still in grammar school, I decided to be a physician. My parents were supportive, but lots of other people looked at me like…"* Her face wrinkles skeptically. *"Because, at the time, it was kind of unlikely, they thought, especially in the South."*

I WENT TO CHICAGO MEDICAL SCHOOL, AND I WAS ONE OF THREE women in a class of seventy students. Two White women and the rest were guys—mostly Jewish, because at that time Chicago Medical School catered primarily to the Jewish community. And Jews, like Blacks, were not accepted readily into medical school then, so that was one of the reasons that Chicago Medical School really existed—very much like Meharry and Howard.

When I finished medical school in 1954 I applied for an internship at County. We had about four thousand beds then, and it was a very daunting experience to be an intern. The patients were being treated so terribly. At that time, medical care was not being monitored like it is now: patients died, often because they were not seen in a timely fashion. There was no accountability, there was very little supervision by attending physicians. We worked tirelessly, because you could never get through all the patients you had. They didn't have but a certain number of budgeted positions—for example, the Department of Pediatrics had seventeen residents. We have sixty now. And there were three to four times as many patients, so it was extremely difficult.

But what was very difficult for me in those two years—I was an intern, and also a resident in pediatrics for one year—is that there was no accountability: patients could get the best care in the world or the worst care in the world, and there was no one really checking. I've seen physicians mistreat patients in terrible ways. I remember this one episode, when I was a resident here at County, in 1955 or '56, we had a diarrhea ward, with thirty-six beds; the children that were admitted to that ward were terribly sick.

We had hundreds of patients coming into the Emergency Room. They were all very dehydrated; that is, they had lost all their fluids. You could tell they were dehydrated: their eyes were sunken and their little skin, if you pulled it up, would just stay standing up. We'd sometimes have to line up two or three children—because we had only one more bed—and decide who of these three sick patients was going to go home or who was going up to the ward. All those patients were very, very sick. Sometimes we made a mistake, and those patients didn't make it because they were really too sick to go home...But we didn't have enough beds.

But this particular night, I was called by a nurse because an intern had started doing a cutdown—that's an incision you make on the ankle where the saphenous vein comes in. When the patient is dehydrated all the veins collapse and you can't find a vein that's standing up, so that's where you get blood. If you don't do it right, you can cut the vein there. So the practice is to just go up a little higher and make another incision.

So the nurse called me, [voice lowered, intense] and this little three-month-old baby was laying in bed. This doctor had made *six* incisions *this* wide [measures much wider than inch] from front to back on this baby. [voice rises in anger] Both legs from ankle to knee and the left arm, and he was getting ready to start on the right arm. I was so angry. I could have killed him. [fists clenched, head shaking in rage]

Anyway, that kind of butchery was so apparent, and one of the reasons I made up my mind that I would have to get into a position where I could make a difference. That's been the guiding principle of my medical career. It was that kind of lack of accountability...That isn't even sensitivity—it's just brutal. Brutal. We put him out. That kind of thing was going on all the time. Not that bad, usually, but a complete disregard for the integrity of people.

For example, when you do an IV you put the person's arm or leg on a board, and it may be immobilized in the same position for hours or even days. If you don't pad the board right, the bony prominences will ulcerate. How many children I saw come into the clinic—somebody had put their leg on a board, and they went home with it actually—they'd come back with these big holes over the knee bone, it was eroded. Unnecessary.

I think that medical education has to change too. Doctors have traditionally been taught that they are the ones who are in charge, and that patients have no—not rights, but no decision-making capacities. Whatever the doctor thinks is it. And it's a big step to move from that situation to one of empowering patients to feel competent to make decisions about their own life and their own body.

Anyway, I was offered the chief residency in Pediatrics, but I decided not to take it, because I didn't think I would get support for what I thought was significant reform. So I went to Michael Reese [Hospital and Medical Center] for my second year in pediatrics, but I decided that I would come back to County when I could really do something about it. So, through the ensuing years, I really—without consciously being aware of it—prepared myself to come back. I came back in '71 to reorganize the Ambulatory Pediatric Component, the same thing I had done at Michael Reese.

When I came back, it wasn't quite as bad in terms of overcrowding, because at that time I think they were down to oh, maybe eighteen hundred beds. We've actually closed a lot of wards. One thing that I like about the hospital now is, we're getting away from these long lines of beds; we've converted most of the wards to two-bed cubicles. When you go out on the ward now, it doesn't look like a ward. It's not the same as rooms really, but it's a lot more conducive to patient privacy and a sense of dignity for the patients. That's much better.

But when I came back, there was still this idea that existed about six years before, when I went to Reese—that doctors in the outpatient department were inadequate to be in the inpatient, if they were really good enough, they'd be inpatient doctors. So, there was resistance to really building up the outpatient department; it was the kind of a place you deployed people when you wanted to get rid of them. To reenergize that whole area and give it credibility was a daunting task. [laughs] But it was one that I really enjoyed.

One thing that we did with the people we recruited is that we took inpatient services, which demonstrated that we were as good as everybody else. Every department in a hospital like this has what's called a Medical Service. When you have a teaching program, you have residents and interns assigned to it and an attending in charge of that service. Maybe you'll have ten to fifteen patients that are the responsibility of that team—and there has to be an attending. When I say I'm "taking a service," that means I'm volunteering to be an attending on that service, with the outpatients or the inpatients. So I would be on an inpatient service maybe two or three months a year, depending. And so when I was capable and my staff was capable of being the equivalent of everybody else...

It's doing things like that that gradually elevated the quality of ambulatory care. I'll admit that outpatient care didn't used to be so good, any more than inpatient care didn't used to be so good, until people started saying, "It's got to improve." Bringing continuity to outpatient care was very important, because, before, patients would go to the clinic without any guarantee—not even a likelihood—that they would see the same doctor.

Another issue that was very important to me was to change the attitude and behavior of the staff toward poor patients. Generally, the prevailing belief is that poor patients shouldn't be treated with courtesy and respect: "They're not paying for it, so we're entitled to treat them any kind of way." Even now, in many clinics, that's the way patients are treated. It's a reflection of the prevailing attitude in this country, which is, "If you're poor, there's something wrong with you, you're deficient—so you're not entitled to the same kind of humane treatment as people who are not deficient." In fact, you see this everywhere people who are deprived economically are seen. In unemployment compensation, in WIC, even in Medicare and those kinds of things. These people have already paid their dues, but they're now on the "receiving end."

What we established was team-building. I started having meetings with the physicians, the nurses, and the clerks, and helping everybody to see how important each person's role is—including the person who cleans the floor—and to show what we needed to do in order to facilitate the care. We had a lot of role-playing sessions. I'm an excellent mom, and so I would play the mom and have them play various different types of providers—nurses, doctors, whatever. In the course of interchange, it would come clear: "Why did you feel that way? Why did you say that?" I would say, "We shouldn't have these patients waiting so long," and they would say to me, "Dr. Lattimer, why not? They're not paying for it. Why should we worry about it?" So they came to the recognition of why they felt that way. And I pointed out to them that what they were saying wasn't true: these people are paying for this in the highest coin of the realm, which is their self-respect. You require them to put their self-respect down when they come in, so they *are* paying you. They're paying you in a coin they should not have to use.

Dr. Robert Freeark

PROFESSOR AND CHAIRMAN *of the Department of Surgery at Loyola. His residency was at County. "I always say we were so busy trying to keep ahead, trying to learn everything we felt that we needed to know, that we didn't have the time to stand back and say, 'Hey, this is lousy—we shouldn't be doing this to people.' It astounds me as I think back on it; it never occurred to us to question."*

I GREW UP IN CHICAGO, SOUTH SIDE, THE SON OF A PHYSICIAN who was a general practitioner. I went to Northwestern for med school, and graduated there in 1952. When I came to County as an intern, I wasn't shocked by the facilities or problems. It's always been fascinating to me that all of us who went over there were so overwhelmed by our responsibilities, in the sense that we had all these people we were supposed to take care of, with varying degrees of supervision and varying degrees of knowledge. It's almost an embarrassment, but it never occurred to us that the system was bad. It took a whole new generation of kids coming along, the sixties generation, coming into the hospital, to say, "Hey, this stinks."

The most vivid example that I can cite is…At that time, I think, it was the largest hospital in the world, certainly in this country: twenty-eight hundred beds, and the X-ray department closed at nine o'clock at night. And here it was, the largest, busiest hospital in the world, all kinds of emergencies, but if you wanted to do a blood count or a urinalysis, or get a chest X-ray, you did the blood count and urinalysis yourself. After nine P.M., you could take the patient to a very primitive fluoroscopic unit up in the orthopedic ward: you pushed the patient yourself, you put them under the screen…God knows how much irradiation I got from that.

I would say that a doctor that came there for largely altruistic reasons was the exception—certainly, in surgery. The competition for the surgical residency was very intense, and almost everybody was doing it for what they could get out of it. I don't think there was a great deal of sensitivity to the patients. On the other hand, the patients—who subsequently were urged by the house staff to also rebel against the system—were incredibly loyal to their physicians. Until somebody came along and told them, "You're entitled to a private room or more privacy than this," it never occurred to them to complain either. They had great respect and admiration for the hospital—it had been their hospital—but they also had it for the doctors. You inherited a kind of esteem just because you were there.

There was a degree of disregard, on the part of some staff, for the patients' welfare. They would do an operation on this patient even though it might not be absolutely necessary, even though it might be riskier than was necessary. There were definite patterns of exploiting patients for that. I hesitate to emphasize that, because I think it was exceptional. It was one of the things that subsequent critiques by the Black community seemed to want to exploit—the idea that the medical schools were coming in there and taking advantage of the poor people, using them as cannon fodder to train residents, to do research, did not adequately protect their welfare...So that, I thought, got overstated. But it did exist to a modest degree.

But I think that the payoff, of course, was when you looked at what alternatives were available to these patients who were indigent, if they went to any...[lowers voice] For the most part, if they went to any of the local Black hospitals, they were likely to fall under the care of a private physician who wasn't near the doctor, or was not nearly able to give the kind of direction that they got at County Hospital. And they had pretty much figured that out. At other hospitals they were either turned away, or if they did get in, [near whisper] they were often under the care of a very mediocre doctor, and he was all by himself; nobody checked on him like we checked on the residents. So I think it was a reasonable trade-off, to make it an educational environment, maybe on occasion at the expense of some aspects of patient care. The payoff was clearly in the direction of the return far exceeding the...as long as there was not a better alternative. And, for the most part, there still isn't a good alternative for many of those indigent people.

There was another building to which all the male patients went, and they would admit the first patient that needed to be admitted to the first floor, onto Ward 15; the second on Ward 25; on up to the top of seven floors. Those floors were designed to have something like sixty beds on two sides. There was an "up ward" and a "down ward." There was one bath, no shower—one bathtub for the entire sixty-bed ward. Most shifts, there was one nurse for the whole floor, and she may or may not have a practical nurse or aide; sometimes, we only had a practical nurse that couldn't pass anything but a certain level of medications.

As an intern, you were on call every third night to cover that floor. So you had sixty patients. And in some respects, they were real sick; but there were a lot of things that we don't hospitalize for nowadays, but because these people were indigent and the like...It was kind of a mixture of critical and almost ambulatory patients. The patients were very good about looking after one another: they'd empty each other's bedpan. If a guy had a stroke, why, the guy in the next bed would get out and feed him. When it got busy and the census would get high, they would develop some middle rows, so instead of having the fifteen beds on one side and fifteen beds on the other side of a ward, they would fill up the center. At really peak times, you would have as many as 110 patients on that floor—with one nurse, one intern on call. Now he could, if he was lucky, get a resident to give him a hand.

I'll never forget the first night I was there. I came, green as grass, and the other two interns who were on the service with me had both made plans for that night, so I said, "I'll take call." I received that night eight new admissions—six of whom were dead the next morning. I almost jumped off the top of the roof! Everything I did went bad: I'd put a tube down somebody's stomach and he'd throw up all over me. And I had to run around to find the EKG machine, because I had to do my own EKGs. To this day, I don't know how I did it. I was terrified and also overwhelmed. I thought, Jesus, this is unbelievable. You either got overwhelmed and bolted—and several interns did—or...One intern took his life, committed suicide. One of them went crazy.

Our busy days were Wednesday and Saturday, the days that all the patients' families would come and visit. One of the intern's assignments was to get blood from families to keep the blood bank supplied, because it was entirely voluntary. And the only way you got blood to meet the needs of the patients who were bleeding was if you went out and bought it from the drunks on West Madison Street, or you got the families to donate. Obviously, some patients didn't have families. So you were constantly, as an intern, checking families. You're also under the gun because your resident said, "If you want to do surgery on this service you're going to have to get your blood bank built up." That was your job too. I'll never forget this one intern: the whole room was filled with patients and families, and he gets up on a chair in front of the room, [strangled yelling] "You goddamn people better bring in some blood." He went absolutely crazy! It just drove him right over...They carted him away. I don't know what happened to him. It was a zoo—that's the best description.

Now, there were five separate buildings with patients, but there was only one central X-ray Department. If you wanted an X-ray on one of your new admissions, you had to push him down to X-ray yourself: down the elevators, which were variously available, through the underground, miserable subway tunnel system—dirty and steamy and all that—then back up the elevators in the main building to the X-ray Department...and wait until the technician decided that you were next. And then the same thing on the return trip.

In the meantime, they're admitting patients that you're supposed to take care of. You used to hope for a patient with a stroke who couldn't talk, because you wouldn't have to take a history. [laughs] There were two kinds of good admission: one that you didn't have to take a history on, you just had to do a physical; and the other, of course, was a challenging one that had some unusual problem. What they would do is, the intern who was in the emergency room, who was having to make these life-threatening decisions, was also overwhelmed with the social consequences of the decisions. So he'd see a patient down there: if he wasn't sure what was wrong with this patient, he had the choice of telling the patient to go home—in the hopes that he'd get well on whatever medication he might order—or would come back, if it was more serious than he'd thought.

The other side of this coin was, if he admitted him to the hospital, then his buddy on the floor that he admitted him to would be on the phone: [nastily] "Goddamn you! What are you sending this crap up here for us to take care of?! I'm up to my ears with really sick people, and you send up this goofy guy that you think has lupus!" So if you wanted to be clever and thoughtful and intuitive about what's wrong with this patient, the environment wasn't conducive to that. So it was a challenge. And, of course, the societal implications of what you did were awesome: you'd send a kid home, but you couldn't count on a mother to use reasonable judgment.

And, at that time, one of the big newspaper scandals at the hospital was the Emergency Room. People were documented to be waiting upwards of twenty hours there. There was no triage system sorting out patients, so you'd see people who had waited down there on these miserable benches, people who had been down there twelve hours. When they finally got to see the doctor…What are you here for? "I think I'm pregnant." Twelve hours! There was no way of sorting those things out.

The system was bad, and there was nobody really looking after those aspects of the hospital. Karl Meyer didn't—he cared about the surgery. This was one way of keeping the hospital census down—because if we gave *good* service, there'd be a hundred thousand more! And there's no question about it, it was a deterrent. But, because of that, there was also no possibility of follow-up. Nowadays, we don't admit a lot of those people in the hospital; we put them on some medication and then somebody follows them on the medication, but there were no arrangements for follow-up. You could admit them, but in general you didn't. If you thought that they would get home all right, you'd tell them what they needed to do: "Find yourself a doctor and come back to the clinic." And the clinic, they'd give you an appointment in about three months. It was just awful, when I think back on it.

After my residency, I became the first salaried teacher of surgery there. Meyer's concept of this job—which was titled "director of Surgical Education"—was that I should take it for a year or two, make a reputation, and then go into practice. The whole orientation there was to prepare yourself to go into private practice—*no one* planned an academic career.

As I think back about it, I was admiring of Karl Meyer. He had some qualities that you couldn't help but admire. My wife despised him—he was very much a bigot and a chauvinist. He was very much an autocrat—but he set a tone there which insisted on you being a good doctor. He did not see himself as the savior of all these poor people; I think he saw them as people that were his responsibility, but I don't think he felt a great social conscience about them. He had been at that job long enough so that he knew the political overtones and he saw the things developing. I think he was as much of an anti-Black as I can think of, in the setting there; he had no sensitivity to the needs of the Black patient.

And I saw it in other ways too. While he had worked very effectively with a large Jewish component of the staff, I think that in truth there was an element of anti-Semitism in his behavior, in the way he talked about them. At the time, if you were Jewish and a doctor, your chances of entering a medical school faculty were almost zero. So the Jewish doctors, many of whom were the really bright people at the hospital, found that the one way that they could get onto a medical school staff was to take the Cook County exam. If they passed that exam—and I think Meyer kind of graded it the way he wanted to—they would become an attending at Cook County, and then the medical schools would give them an appointment.

I was director of Surgical Education for about three years; during that time my title changed to chairman of Surgery. The students that came in in the late sixties and seventies had a kind of a mixed agenda: on the one hand, they were smart enough to cloak their demands in what's best for the patient—but at the same time, they were very much interested in what was better for them. It was an interesting mix of, "We want to get paid more," "We want to have somebody else do these blood counts," "We want to have more laboratory"—but they quite properly blew the whistle on what was then an obsolete system.

I became the darling of this group of people, kind of. They focused much of their resentment on the County Board and the president of the County Board, who was at that time Dick Ogilvie. He thought that his problems would be solved if he could get rid of Karl Meyer, so he finally forced Meyer to resign—and then he asked *me* if I would take the position of hospital director. So all of a sudden I've got to run the laundry, I've got to run the dietary, the pharmacy—and I had no training for any of this. But I am the CEO for this big hospital, with all this money going in and out and everybody ripping it off. Ogilvie figured that if he could get me to take this position, he could get these kids off his back.

My deal with Ogilvie was an interesting one. I told him that I would be willing to assume that position under two circumstances: one, if I didn't like it, I could go back to being the chief of Surgery; and two, that if he were to be elected governor, that he would be willing to work to change the governance of the County Hospital legislatively. See, our biggest frustration was that by the time we educated a new president of the County Board to the needs of the hospital they'd run for something else. So we decided that if this thing was ever going to get fixed, we'd have to get it out from under the County Board—which was kind of a naive idea. But, sure enough, when Ogilvie was elected governor, one of his younger associates came over, and he and I wrote the first legislation that changed the governance of the hospital. We didn't know beans. When they finally passed it—it went through at the state legislature pretty well—the problem was it had no teeth, because it did not identify the control of the budget.

But it did call for a citizens' commission for Cook County Hospital, and it enabled a number of Black leaders who were so motivated to come in and begin to look at this operation. When they began to look at it and try to do something about it, it turns out they had no power to change it. So we made a second try at legislation a year later—and *that* piece of legislation gave a lot of control to this commission in terms of the money: they had to approve the budget, they had control over the contracts.

One of the premises that we all operated under was that the County Commissioners who were able to work the system would spin the contracts to their buddies—and ultimately get kickbacks in the form of campaign contributions and God knows what else. But that was the presumption: "It's all patronage, it's all on the QT and so on." So in the second legislation the governing commission was given that kind of power. Now, *that* one, not surprisingly, the Democratic politicians fought tooth and nail. And as that thing wound down, the fight became very dirty: the docs were busy going to the newspapers to tell stories about the county commissioners. And the commissioner in turn retaliated, using some inside people there to try and besmirch the doctors. This was '68, '69.

I ended up with a couple of real fiascos that occurred in the hospital. A little kid with appendicitis, a young Black girl ten years old, was sent home with a diagnosis of pelvic inflammatory disease; the presumption was that she had gonorrhea. And she goes home to die of a ruptured appendix, so it had all the overtones of misdiagnosis. Now, at that time there were three hundred thousand Emergency Room visits, so a thousand people a day came to the Emergency Room. The only persons that saw them down there were interns—the greenest, least experienced person in the world was all they had. So it was not surprising that that happened once in a while. And when that happened at County, in those days, it got in the newspapers.

Then there was the first guy that ever had a heart transplant in Chicago. The donor for that was a guy who came to the County Hospital after being hit over the head with a pool cue. It cracked his skull, and the guys, for whatever reason, told him that he was doing fine; he had a skull fracture, but it was not serious, and they sent him home. To make a long story short, he shows up two or three days later at another hospital, he dies, and they take his heart and give it as the first heart transplant. So the newspapers wanted to know, "Where'd the donor come from?" "Well, he got hit with a pool cue." "Why did he die?" "Well, County sent him home." So then it's in the newspapers and on the ten o'clock news.

So as the house staff is slinging all this mud and pointing their fingers at all the failings of the place, well, I end up having to respond to this. I walked a very fine line, trying to represent the needs of the hospital to the County Board, trying to keep this rebellious house staff off my back and off the board's back, and making sure the interns and residents were staying with their patients and doing their job. And the legislation appeared to be doomed. Somewhere along the way, this new governing commission decided that they were going to go out and look for an executive director who would be in charge of all County institutions. That was [James] Haughton.

Then the House Staff decided that they were all going to quit; and then the nurses—everybody had their own camp, but they were really coordinated—decided *they* were going to quit. They all went down to Springfield in caravans to see if they could get the legislature to pass the second governing commission bill. So, with this legislation still on the table, it appeared to me that the issues were dead and there was no way they were going to pass it. I knew by this time that not only was the County Board gunning for me, but now so was the governing commission, figuring that there's no reason we should have a surgeon running the world's biggest hospital. And they were right, of course. [laughs]

Finally, in a fit of pique—though I like to think it was somewhat calculated—I submitted my resignation, and *that* polarized the entire medical and nursing staff. They viewed me as their leader, as the one person who was a spokesman for what they felt the hospital should be. And by God, they then took it out on the mayor and the county commissioners: they said, "We're going to close this hospital!" So, Mayor Daley called down to Springfield and said, "Pass that goddamn bill—I'm not going to let this hospital close!" They'd already closed it on a couple of nights when they thought they were overwhelmed, just to kind of make a point, I suspect. And I had to defend them, because there was no question that they were overwhelmed.

I have not set one foot in that hospital since that time. My wife sees me driving down the Eisenhower and she says, "You don't look the same when you go past the hospital." I dunno. She thinks that I've never really gotten over that. [softly] I just...I don't want to go through it, to relive all those memories. I don't know whether I had in my mind's eye some kind of idea of being the second Karl Meyer, someone who'd run the thing for fifty years. I don't think so, but I just decided that's a part of my life I'm finished with. I'm not going to come back and recapture it in any...I don't mind talking about it. And I do get together for all of the reunions they have in other settings, but I've not walked back in the hospital since.

Dr. Rolf Gunnar

Director of Medical *Affairs at MacNeal Hospital in Berwyn, Illinois. He trained at County and was the chairman of Medicine for a time. "Measure it in months—eighteen months."*

In july of '48, i started at county as an intern. i trained there, and then in '51 I went on a camping trip for Harry Truman in the hills of Korea. I came back in '53 and was there as a resident. Then, from '54 till '63, I was a voluntary attending in General Medicine; then in '63 I became chief of the University of Illinois Division at Cook County Hospital and worked full-time in Adult Cardiology.

County was really used during that period of time. The attitude toward the patients wasn't sensitive at all, but that was societal more than just the physicians—they looked on it as teaching. And the patients actually got something out of it, they did get care—but there wasn't any feeling among the doctors that it should be any relationship like what you should give a private patient. I think the patient care got even worse during the early sixties because there were even fewer nurses. It got to a point where one time we had one nurse for seven hundred patients. As house officers, you would go out and deliver water to the patients because nobody was available to do it. Those conditions were just really bad.

But if you talk about house officers...I think it was in the beginning of the sixties: when patients came to the Fantus Clinic, they'd be given prescriptions and they'd go to the clinic pharmacy, where they'd be told the pharmacy was out and directed to the pharmacy across the street, next to The Greeks. So they'd go over there, where they would be asked how much money they had—and they were given as much drugs as their money would buy.

Well, two of the boys who worked in the pharmacy at County, it was reported to me, were seen taking drugs from County to the pharmacy. The house officers got the patient to bring back the scrips: they said, "If they say they're out of it, bring them back to us." They collected a whole bunch of these prescriptions and went down and forced them to open up the pharmacy. The drugs were in the outpatient pharmacy, so they were not out of the drugs. They then delivered this batch of prescriptions to Fred Hertwig, the hospital warden, who lost them. But they had made copies of them, so they gave me the copies; I turned them over to the *Chicago Tribune,* which turned them over to the state's attorney, who lost them.

The reporter at the *Tribune* told me he'd called up the guy who ran the pharmacy, who said, "Hey, this goes a lot further than me, and if you want to know who's involved, I'll tell you." The reporter was going to meet with him, but the guy closed the drugstore and left town before the meeting. There were those kind of shenanigans.

The governing commission was first created when the first bill was passed, and the state's attorney ruled that the commission was responsible for the hospital, but it didn't have control over the budget, personnel, finance...Apparently, to do this they took advantage of the fact that the legislation didn't state that the governing commission could sue or be sued, so how it stood as a governmental body was a question. We started organizing, and we went down and changed it: that's where I really got involved, because I thought it would be a simple change and there was serious opposition from all the politicians. This would have been about 1970; I was chief of Medicine at that time. We took two or three busloads of people down to Springfield to try to get this bill through. It was in committee, and we couldn't get a hearing; they let us sit around and, finally, they heard us at the end of the day, which was a real botch—it was an orchestrated botch. I had created a community advisory board for the Department of Medicine, and it started putting the pressure on Daley. Finally, on the last day of the legislature, Daley decided that he wanted the bill passed, so he sent word down and it went through both houses without a dissenting vote. That shows what his clout was. The first time I crossed the pols down in Springfield, both my father's *and* my income tax were investigated on a "random" audit, which was sort of interesting: same name, same family, same year. This happened shortly after I became chairman of Medicine.

Around this time—before, actually—there was a patient who had terminal cancer of the lung. She was in the hospital, unable to go home because they couldn't get her off the oxygen. Now, the resident apparently decided to see if he could wean her, and during one of these weaning periods, she died. The case came up at our four o'clock conference, where the case was presented—this was called the "organ recital." They would bring in organs from the autopsy and go over them, discuss the clinical. Her case came up, and the question involved the ethics of what the resident had done. It was a heated discussion, and one of the senior attendings said, "That was murder"—which was dutifully recorded. So, later, when they wanted my backside, I was sitting in my office one day and a guy comes in from the coroner's office and said, "You've been accused of murder." [laughs in disbelief] I said, "What?! How?"

Well, it turned out my involvement was I was chief of Medicine and, therefore, the resident was responsible to me, and if the resident committed murder then it was my murder. It was a serious case as far as the guy from the coroner's office was concerned; but when he found out that the incident occurred a week before I became chairman of Medicine, the case just disappeared. There were other threats. I mean, there are more subtle ways of telling you you're not in favor. When you step back from this distance it almost becomes amusing, it's all so...But that kind of thing was troubling.

Haughton, who was hired even though he'd never run a hospital before, started building up his own cadre of people. He made a major, major change, in that he would not allow County to be the hospital of last resort. He articulated the philosophy that "if we're full, we don't have to take you no matter how sick you are"—and he started implementing it. Haughton convinced people that all they had to do was send patients to another hospital, and County will pay for it. Fine. But on an operational level, the house officer in the Emergency Room faced with a patient who needed to be admitted said he'd call the other hospital, and they'd say they had a bed and would take them—"but you've got to send me the paper that says that the County is going to pick up the cost." But no such paper ever appeared, so the hospital would say, "No, we can't take them." So then they wanted the house officers to send the patient home.

The house officers then decided, "Well, if that's what you want to do, we're going to admit and keep every patient that needs to admitted—*and* we're going to keep them as long as they need to be in for." Well, that of course was essentially a Heal-in—when you fill the hospital up to the point where it bursts—but you couldn't prove it, because the patients were all sick. I got called by the president of the AMA, telling me that this was a Heal-in, and that I should clean the hospital out. I said, "Come over and make rounds with me, and we'll together see if there are any patients who can get discharged." He wouldn't come over.

The doctors were unified in pushing the administration for changes that had to do with patient care; it had nothing to do with money for themselves, anything self-serving. This was late '71. They fired five physicians, three of the residents and the two who were the leadership of the residents. I resigned, to be effective at the end of that next year. So they called me into a room—I forget his name, he was second in command—and said they'd like me to advance my resignation to immediate. But he didn't tell me that, at the same time, Haughton was holding a press conference saying that he'd fired these five and that I had resigned. So when I came out, I found out that I'd resigned and that they'd fired the five. It was a zoo.

I had planned on staying at County—it was my career. I really thought it was a wonderful place to get things done, and I welcomed the governing commission and welcomed Haughton. But it turned out to be that he was more interested in his image and control, and he created racial tensions that had never existed before. If we criticized him, he would have meetings where he'd put on a dashiki and call the African American workers in and imply that it was just a racial attack on him, that we attacked him because he was Black and not because he was incompetent. But he'd never run *anything* before, and he was surrounded by people who really were inept at their job. Of course, he had a differential policy for promoting African Americans—which would have been fine, except some of them really were promoted into positions they couldn't fulfill, they didn't have the training to do it. So it wasn't promote and educate, it was promote and drown, which caused a certain amount of tension.

Maybe with health care reform, they won't have a need for County. But then you have to open up some of the community hospitals. I'd recommend—nobody will listen to me, I'm sure—that each university be given a corridor of care. I think we should look at it as an integrated system: there's primary care, linked to a community hospital, linked to a university hospital. That way you could shake up the system. If we get health care reform, if these people are taken care of, then you could use the community hospitals that are closed or are underutilized—but you need to develop an integrated system, so that the primary care physician relates to the community hospitals and relates to the university hospitals.

There are sixty-five hundred physicians in training in a year in the city of Chicago—that's a *large* work force. But I sure wouldn't give the County hospital up until you have another system that's proven to work. You either have to fix it up or find a different system. I think it's an emotional thing when you say, "We can't close County, we cannot walk away from that job." By closing County you might force the system to take more responsibility. It's always easy to say, "Send it to County."

The Seventies

Dr. Quentin Young—Part 2

HE RETURNED TO COUNTY *as the chairman of Medicine from 1972 until 1981.*

WELL, THE ATMOSPHERE WHEN I CAME BACK IN 1972 WAS appalling. The only reason—certainly the required reason—for me being asked, was that the executive director of the Health and Hospitals Governing Commission, Jim Haughton, had fired the chairman of Medicine, Rolf Gunnar, and five other doctors, residents, and attendings in the County Medical Department. It was completely unwarranted and it was a rather dangerous, if not destructive, thing to do. The act was more than just losing some very dedicated and prestigious doctors. County is a very fragile place, and if you have an administration that does that to doctors...They're not used to that kind of reprisal for nothing—*nothing* had happened.

That event resulted in a huge and sudden exodus of attending physicians—particularly in the Department of Medicine—and house staff. Well, that hospital can't run without house staff and attendings. Haughton had recklessly created a condition which could have easily brought the hospital down—and that's not exaggerating. Haughton was influenced to consider me by the leader of the Medical house staff, Nick Rango, who ironically had been fired also—he'd been restored by a court order. Nick was a very charismatic guy, and he went into Haughton's office and said, "You've got to hire Quentin Young to be chairman of Medicine." Haughton said, "He's a communist, isn't he?" Nice way to respond. And Rango said, "I don't give a damn what he is, he's the only person who can save your ass." What he meant was that my work in the medical community for human rights, and in support of the student health organization, had given me some national exposure that would attract house staff who would be willing to overlook what had happened.

I didn't want to do it. It was the largest Department of Medicine, by far, in the Midwest, and one of the largest in the country. We had 480 beds in Medicine alone! Suffice it to say, County now is approved for 960 beds *total*. So the magnitude was awesome. We had about 150, 160 house officers—resident, interns, fellows—just a *vast* empire. I didn't feel it was overwhelming, but it wasn't what I wanted to do. I obviously felt strongly about the opportunity to shape the way care was given to a huge number of people. We also had clinics at Fantus, on the order of four hundred thousand outpatient visits a year, and at least half of them were to medicine. We also ran the Emergency Room, and there were nearly three hundred thousand visits. And the resources weren't there in terms of personnel—and they'd just messed up the work force! So I had to be persuaded.

It's very hard to summarize that decade there. There were some things that are very, very good—say, the creation of an Occupational Health Service, which, because it admitted four doctors every year, immediately became the largest occupational health program in America. Most schools of occupational health essentially trained company doctors; *we* stressed that this was a worker-oriented occupational health program. It wasn't an even-handed approach, and we ran into real opposition—not least from the County Board, who said, "Why do you want an occupational health program in a hospital where everybody is indigent. They're not working." Well, the answer to that we knew—and we went on to verify it. A huge fraction of people who use County have to rely on indigent services because of damage they've sustained in the workplace: they were injured, they were sickened, and they had to come to County. So it's been a resource ever since for evaluating occupational and environmental hazards, and for helping workers who deserve it to get the recompense that comes from workers compensation. So Occupational Health worked very well; it's been turning out doctors, at least four a year, for all these years. They've gone on to make their mark in OSHA [Occupational Safety and Health Administration] and NIOSH [National Institute of Occupational Safety and Health] and even in company medicine. Some went to work for unions.

And there's Jorge Prieto—he's an extraordinary human being and a dedicated doctor. We needed a Family Practice Chief, and I was chair of the search committee. He'd agreed to come, and then he said no—he called me about ten o'clock at night, which wasn't an odd time for me to be at my desk, and we talked for four hours. I wheedled and finagled and manipulated and held his hand. We were on the phone like two schoolboys. At the end, I convinced him he had to do it: it was a people's hospital, his people use it, he'd have much more influence...I used all the arguments I'd used on myself. And he came and fashioned a spectacular program: he insisted that everybody become bilingual, he established a community clinic and got the governing commission to buy it for the community, and then let the community buy it back, so they own their own clinic. He's moral and honest, and was a great influence over there.

And then there was the Jail Health Service. The circumstance was very "County": there was yet another scandal. This time, Mount Sinai Hospital was found—exposed by the Better Government Association—actually *trading off* a stay in the hospital among these prisoners, in that cesspool of a jail, if they agreed to have an unnecessary operation that they didn't need, for the training of the residents. They would do circumcisions! Herniographies! It was vivisection, but such was the prisoners' desperation that they would agree to such a thing. They'd get a nice week in the hospital with good food and sheets on the bed—out of that terrible jail, in exchange for having a hernia. But when *that* got exposed, it created an instant crisis that couldn't be fixed by *any* wallpaper.

They had this huge scandal, and Dunne [then President Cook County Board of Commissioners] calls up Haughton and says, "This is a health facility, it's run by the County, it's yours." Haughton comes to me, the bleeding heart among his chiefs, and says, "We've just been given this jail..." Well, it was ridiculous. It's a *huge* place: now they get about six thousand people in there, then it was about forty-eight hundred. Just huge. And the most adverse conditions: people didn't have enough beds and so on. And the thing people don't understand is that the jail—as opposed to the prison—is a detention place where people *can't* make bail. In a jail people are going in and out all the time. How many? Try fifty thousand a year. So, from a public health viewpoint, it was the concentration point for alcoholism, sexually transmitted disease, drug use and abuse, contagious diseases of all sorts. From that point of view, it was extremely interesting and attractive to a reformer.

I told Haughton I'd give it a try, and I had some of the doctors go to the jail to see what could be done, because the prisoners had to have health services, people were sick all the time. They told me what it would take, and I put the demand on Haughton for staffing it—and I got it. That started the Cook County Jail Health Service. Little did I know then that it would be historic in terms of penal medicine. The doctors there, Burt King, Jack Raba—a fantastic guy—and three or four others, became the reformers of health care in America's jails and prisons. There were some efforts at reform in other parts of the country, but I think it's safe to say that, because of these peculiar conditions, because we had the resources of the County Hospital, we were unique. We developed a very good service and started to move into the opportunities for early detection and prevention. But the other big legacy was that these doctors stood ready with the Prison Health Project of the ACLU and the Carter administration, and the Justice Department, to be expert witnesses on the conditions in the numerous jails and prisons in the country where lawsuits were brought. Literally scores of jails were forced under court order to clean up and provide certain levels of humane care.

In preventive health, we did far less than we wanted. My big push was for clinics—outpatient clinics—and I managed to get four of them established. But we ran into hard times with the governing commission, which had to do with the fact that we had a house staff union and a strike. Haughton was putting pressure on the Medical staff to press the house staff to settle. His logic was: "You are their teachers, and you should tell them to go back." The only flaw in this was that we could make them come back—but then we'd never get another house officer. The same thing that Nick had been telling him before. And the things they were demanding were things that even the governing commission didn't find that farfetched. They demanded that there be call bells at each patient's bedside; each patient should have a light so that when you brought a person into a forty-patient ward at two A.M. you wouldn't have to turn lights on and wake up everybody. They were acting to break the strike—and, it's conjecture on my part, but it's my view that Haughton was stimulated in this by the American Hospital Association, which at that time feared and had reason to fear a growth of house staff unionization.

Anyhow, as soon as the strike was settled—that was on a Thanksgiving weekend—I was called in and fired. They didn't give a reason; that was their mistake. They said that I was being fired because my position was so high: like a cabinet minister, I served at the pleasure of the governing commission. I argued that I'd done nothing to be fired, I didn't want to be fired, and I would stay at my post. They were like the gang that can't shoot straight. The first thing they did was to padlock my office—so the house staff took the door off. Then the press got interested. The house staff occupied my office during the night. I remember after this started, I got wakened at two A.M. by one of the radio stations: Could I tell them, was the vigil still on? I said, "What vigil?" They said, "The people in your office." I said, "Call the office. If they don't answer, it's off. I'm trying to sleep." Then they ordered my clerical staff, under pain of being fired, not to help me. And every time they'd do this, we'd go to the press—and they looked more and more stupid. Then the attending staff was ordered not to recognize me as the chief, but they couldn't get anybody to replace me as acting chief. Then I proceeded to make rounds with forty attendings as a show of solidarity. Finally, they took my parking place away; they blockaded it. I said, "Now *that* was serious!"

The problem we had was legal: the question was, who was going to sue who? Were they going to sue me to vacate, or was I going to sue to get my job back—and my parking space! We decided to go to federal court; we drew this guy, Bernard Decker, a Nixon appointee known for his terrible temper—very conservative, but a strict constructionist. We claimed that I had been fired without due process, and we were seeking a temporary restraining order so that I could resume my duties until this matter was resolved. We claimed that they'd violated the statute—and they *had*. The trouble was, the governing commission's lawyer kept referring to some statute that was operative, claiming it said I wasn't entitled to a hearing. And Decker kept getting angrier: he couldn't find it. My lawyer told me they had amended that law, and that the other lawyer was giving Decker the law before it was amended. I said, "Well, why don't you tell him?" He said, "I want Decker to get good and mad." So Decker goes back into his quarters and then he comes back and says, "Counsel, I cannot find it." And so my guy gets up and says, "Perhaps, your honor, I can help you: he's showing you the book before it was amended." Apparently, in the courtroom, to mislead a judge is like spitting at the king, whether you do it deliberately or stupidly. The judge got *real* angry, so he ordered that I be restored, and that we have a hearing, and that they give me charges and so on.

It took them six weeks to decide what the charges were. We had a hearing. They came up with six reasons: they found me not guilty of four of the serious charges and guilty of two. They said my conduct was such that my penalty should not exceed thirty days' suspension without pay. So *that* went to the governing commission. They had voted nine to nothing to fire me the first time; they voted six to three to fire me *again*.

So we went *back* to the court. Decker had also instructed them on how to fire me: they had to issue a resolution which indicated the reason for whatever they did; they'd written a resolution which made me responsible for everything from the Crucifixion to the Chicago Fire. The judge got really mad and he issued a statement saying, "This governing commission is incapable of judging this fairly, and I order them to reinstate Dr. Young or, if they wish, to give no penalty greater than thirty days." So, then, this time we went back again, and this same governing commission voted nine to nothing to restore me without penalty! [laughs] Is that pretty good?

Mind you, that was the middle of my decade. I stayed five more years. See, Haughton wasn't a bad guy—he was just so self-important. There was never any rancor. The son of a bitch fired me, held me up to public shame, but "Yeah, you're back—all right, let's go." As it turned out, the governing commission collapsed because of the underfunding and a deal made with Governor Thompson and Dunne: Haughton was humiliated and driven off, unnecessarily early. I stayed on—there was no way they could get me, the law protected me. But *Dunne* knew how to get me, he proceeded to do it the right way: he just stopped handling what I needed to have handled. If I had an empty attending position and I'd recruit somebody, somehow the paper never went through. Or this doctor who had come to the point where he was supposed to get a raise: I'd send the request for a raise and it would never happen. I don't argue they did nothing, but it was just enough to make me increasingly impotent in running my department. I knew I couldn't rouse public opinion about not raising a doctor's pay, and I knew that Dunne was entrenched and that he hated me—I reveled in it—so I resigned.

Dr. John Raba

DEPUTY DIRECTOR FOR *Ambulatory Services. He's got the build of a street-lot basketball player, but a presence so serene he'd look perfectly normal garbed in a friar's robe and tire-tread sandals.*

I'M A CHICAGOAN AND GREW UP ON THE SOUTH SIDE. THERE were farm fields when I grew up, though it was still in the city. I went to Catholic grammar school, Catholic high school. I was in the Catholic seminary for a while. As a junior and senior in high school, you had to do something one day a week that was considered a service project—whether it was visit the poor, or help the poor visit the sick, or tutor, or volunteer as a coach.

What I did was, I went to County Hospital. This would have been in '59, '60, and I was fourteen, fifteen. I have images of this place: the ward we visited was the same one I was eventually an intern at. We never had a chaperone, we just showed up and visited. It was very packed, very congested, you didn't see many nurses. It was a big open barracks—there used to be patients lining the corridors, like in a war. I forget about that image sometimes because it's changed a lot, but it's still in the same building, it's still the same ward, it's still the same facility that they said should have been closed down in 1930.

I remember the lights would all go on at once: all the lights for the whole ward were on one light switch. And when I was an intern, that was *still* the case. I just remember being overwhelmed by the crush of humanity. I knew this wasn't the way it is for people with money. Mainly, it was the crowds, the congestion. The lack of privacy was staggering. It was like a flophouse in some ways.

I started as a resident here in '74. At that time, house staff unions were starting to be formed throughout the country. I was elected president of the house staff in my second year. I hadn't been politically active in anything. I think they wanted me because I'd rotated around a lot and I knew everybody and didn't have a label, and I wasn't a member of a party. And there were members of parties here—Communist party, other parties.

At that time, the County Board funded the Health and Hospitals Governing Commission and they ran the hospital. The governing commission had appointees from the mayor and the governor and the medical school deans, and they really made the decisions about how the hospital was run. The contract had to be negotiated with them. We didn't want to strike and there were meetings upon meetings, but no action of any importance. We finally went on strike in October of '75, and we were on strike for seventeen or eighteen days.

It was very hard for the doctors to do anything like that. We made a decision that every patient that was in the hospital, we would continue to take care of—so if a patient was yours, you had to keep coming in. Everyone was working, but they were picketing. We were wimps: we didn't burn cars, we didn't turn violent. Some of our foreign-born staff said: "This is such a lightweight strike—no guns, no nothing." They wanted to blow up cars.

The nurses were very supportive. There was some anger from some of the attendings and the department heads who yelled and told the residents, "You go out and we fire you." It was an ethical issue: Do you really take good care from the poorest of the poor? We had huge ethical arguments about whether you could step back one step to move forward two. Do you deny care to people who have little choice? Yet the response of the house staff was overwhelming. Of the five hundred and some doctors, somewhere around four hundred and some were truly on strike. They did exactly what I did: they would go to work and say they were on strike. [sounding amused] And the newspapers said we were on strike, so we were on strike.

The support was wonderful. There were a couple of marches downtown in which there were three hundred doctors in white coats walking down the street. We all got to know each other. Never in the history of County Hospital did all the medical people know all the surgical people. So you had all these five hundred docs, four hundred of them now recognizing each other and shaking each other's hands, who decided it was something they should do.

For a couple of weeks, we were vilified in the press, which said, "These doctors are striking for money—irresponsible!" Finally, we went down to the press and said, "*Who* is talking to you?" We had these four very saintly type doctors with us, who told them, "One year from now I can start off at another job with fifty, sixty thousand a year. I'm not going to go on strike for an extra thousand a year. Are you crazy? Do you think we're stupid? Would we jeopardize our entire career to make fifteen thousand a year now?" And *boom!* everything changed—even the editorials changed, saying that there are issues that they want to correct: it's not an issue of money or hours, it's really service issues.

We had been given a court order to go back to work, but we didn't comply with the order. We had a court hearing—we settled the strike the night before that. But when we went to the hearing, the judge sentenced the leaders of the house staff to ten days in jail. We went back to the house staff meeting that night, and two or three of the leaders wanted to go on strike. But most of us decided that because we had accepted the contract, it was dishonorable to go back out on strike after we had agreed to settle. The house staff voted to accept the contract and we went to jail.

It wasn't a difficult time. We were on television; when we walked into the jail, the inmates were cheering. We had all worked at the jail as part of our rotation in medicine and family practice, so I knew the officers and they knew who I was; there wasn't a sense of antagonism. One night, the resident on duty in the jail's Emergency Room got sick and had to be sent home. They called over and wanted one of us to cover, so I volunteered and ran the Emergency Room for the night. I didn't sleep all night, I was really busy sewing up people—the police used to bring people there instead of going to private emergency rooms.

I was so tired...I was wearing the hospital greens which they gave me—it was nice, I didn't have to wear inmate clothes when I was seeing patients. And I walked right out the door. I just said good-bye, like I did every morning when I was on call on the weekend, and I walked out the door and got to the parking lot—and realized that I had escaped from jail! This was after Thanksgiving. I thought, I should just take a bus home, have some turkey and come on back—they'll never know I'm gone, they'll just think I'm still over working in the hospital. And then I thought it might cause myself some problems, and it might cause some others even greater problems—so I went back. All the way around to the other entrance of the jail: there was this huge metal door that had a little tiny door in the middle of it. It was a special entrance for inmates assigned to the unit I was in. So I'm banging on the door, and the guy opens it up and goes, "Holy Jesus Christ! Get in here!" He pulls me in, shuts the door: "Don't *ever* tell anybody this." It was really funny—my escape from jail...

Eventually, I became the medical director of the jail and the chairman of Jail Health Service at County Hospital. It's a dual role. I worked at a small, 110-bed hospital in Guatemala during a break from medical school and learned that you don't need doctors to take care of most people: you need community health workers, you need ancillary medical staff. In the jail, we had twelve or fifteen doctors, but what you had was seventy medics. Some had trained in Vietnam, some were paramedics trained by fire departments—and *they* were the ones that were most important in delivering care, because they were the ones that the inmates saw every day in the tiers. I started to realize, as the medics got better and better at what they did, that they were becoming health providers in the community, in their own home. They'd say, "Yeah, if somebody has a problem on my block, they call me first. And I walk down there and I say, 'No, don't go to the ER.'" So what we were doing, in a nice way, was starting to expand the equivalent of a barefoot doctor system, which is cheaper and more effective.

Now the jail is a little community: a little, tiny city of, at any one time, as many as nine to ten thousand men and women who are walled in. It's like a medieval fortress. And we had to do things to start to improve the health of that community. I used to get sad walking through the jail: brand-new buildings going up, solid, clean, with little gyms so people can exercise. The only thing that gave me hope was that if our society got a little smarter about what got people into jail—and what causes some of the problems that lead to incarceration—these clean, new, dormitorylike bedrooms, someday would be great for long-term drug treatment centers. Maybe instead of incarcerating nine thousand, we could incarcerate five thousand, and those with serious substance abuse, they'll live there, sleep there at night, work at something, but it's part of a drug treatment program. If I had to spend money on incarceration, I'd rather take twenty million of that and put it into substance abuse, because maybe that would be one way of starting to solve the problem. The buildings are there. It's worth a shot.

Most of the prevention work that we did was initially just in early screening—picking up illnesses that they had, treating them quickly. But then it became clear that's not enough. If people left there with some information about keeping themselves healthy, we'd be better off, because the patients that came to the jail were the patients that would most likely eventually end up at the doors of Cook County Hospital. The first jail in the country to be able to hire budgeted health educators was right here at Cook County Jail, and the disease that we focused on to begin with was HIV. Eventually they started to do pretest counseling, but the initial thing was simply to start talking about what it means to use a condom. The guys didn't know how to spell condom, they didn't know what it was. It wasn't for them. Women were much more receptive, as they are in any society, to protection. So I think major inroads started there with health education.

We also realized that you can't force people to travel great distances for care. Well, that's true in the community: the more barriers you put up to health care—distance, transportation problems, scheduling problems—that aren't convenient to the patient, you interfere with their ability to access care. We realized that we had to bring the clinics to the living areas. So we brought the docs to each building, five sessions a week—so all the men and women had to do was walk down the hall to get care. We then set up a system where the docs, once a week, had to make tier rounds. The word would be out that there'd be a doctor on the tier, and the patients who wanted to talk to the doc would line up. So it's just another way you bring health care to people.

And then, to come to County Hospital, it's the same thing. I've only been back here a year, just a little over, but we're trying to figure out how to force care back into the community. And, honestly, some day—I may not see it in my lifetime, and the AMA would *die* to think about it—but I really wonder if we should have clinics throughout the community staffed by nurse practitioners and physicians' assistants, with maybe one or two family docs or primary docs working with them to solve some complicated problems. Maybe a nurse practitioner would have a relationship with one corner of this community, and another one with another corner—someone who knew the stores, knew what was available, what other private docs were there, knew the health problems. Someone able to sense what the communities, needs were. Break it down, so there's a personal tie.

Now, this is not a socialist utopia we're talking about here, and it isn't going to happen for a long time in *this* society. But someday we should be looking toward it—so every three-, four-, five-block area will have access to a primary care provider at a basic level. Someone who would screen and triage out complaints, and respond to 80 percent of the complaints—at a lower price than it would cost for somebody who went to medical school for four years, a residency for three to six years, and now is out taking care of colds and runny noses and ear infections. My goodness. I can't tell you how it embarrasses me to make what I make at times when I'm taking care of very routine problems. I know that my mother and my father, if they were given the right to prescribe twelve drugs, could take care of 60 to 80 percent of what I do.

You can offer great health care, but wonderful health care doesn't mean you're healthy. Sure, I can control your blood pressure—but if you're unable to lose some weight, if you're unable to modify some of your dietary intake, I can't control everything. I may be able to sew up your wound, but at this moment I can't keep you from getting shot. I may be able to take care of your cancer, somewhat, but I probably can't change some of the pollutants in the air that caused your cancer. Many diseases are related to the lack of good housing, social problems in the community, the lack of access to proper food or proper knowledge or proper health care, in some phases.

Sometimes, people organize around health care and then realize, "We didn't need a doctor—we *really* needed to get rid of guns. What we needed to do was to get a foundation to help us clean up our houses, so children aren't falling out of windows, or they aren't tripping and falling and breaking legs...where their playground is a mattress surrounded by walls topped with nails and broken bottles." Certainly, a hospital can't do everything. It *can* do what it has to do well; and it can do it with respect and decency and kindness and accessibility.

County Hospital fits into this safety-net hospital system throughout the country, which they call the "public hospitals." For the people who fall through all other coverage—who, for a variety of reasons, aren't acceptable to be treated at private facilities: either because of their total inability to pay, or the severity of their illness, or because they're unacceptable for other reasons—which could be drugs, alcohol, abusive patients, tuberculoses, sexually transmitted diseases.... That isn't to say that private hospitals don't take care of indigent patients, because they do. Medicaid pays for a third of the bills at the University of Chicago Hospital. But only about 5 percent of their care is nonreimbursed or indigent. County *must* be 65 percent indigent care.

So County gets those that are identified as being people with no source of payment. And that's where they serve a real need. And the question with a national health program is whether County will continue to have that place or not. I'm not totally sure. If patients have a choice of where they want to go, we have to be able to provide a service that's a little more competitive in this world. I don't mean financially; I mean that we should be a little more sensitive to patients' needs. I think we should start respecting the fact that they've *chosen* to come see us. Right now, it's not unusual that we have done little to make patients comfortable here, to make them feel truly like we're serving them. Doctors and nurses, once they get that one-on-one contact, they *do*. But the whole scene—setting up before and afterward, coming in and going out—it's not just a drab, dreary physical plant...Not a lot of money has been placed in keeping it clean. We've had to battle to keep the patients' bathrooms clean—and you shouldn't have to walk into a hospital or a clinic and have filthy, dirty bathrooms. We do have some timed appointments, but there is a core of our clinics where you have to show up at eight, because it's first-come, first-serve. Well, there aren't many places that you do that anymore. Fire sales—you do it at Sears or something. But you don't do that in health care clinics.

We don't have an ingrained system where the same doctor sees the same patient repeatedly, except in a couple of our long-care clinics, General Medicine and Pediatrics. For most of the other ones, whoever the doctor is that day who sees you, and the doctors change—there's little continuity. Even the attendings who are the supervising docs don't always set up a system so that they can see the same patients. Some do, but they have to fight to do that. Now we're trying to make that the culture of the building—so you see the same doctor, you have a timed appointment, you're expected to be there, we have to see you on time.

We do have a facility, a physical plant, that's very difficult to keep accredited. It's a very uncomfortable building; it's so spread out that it's difficult to offer efficient care. It has no pneumatic tubes; you have to hand-deliver everything. There's some computer systems now, for lab and X-ray, but it's not totally available, though they are expanding it. There's no computerized appointment system, for instance, unless somebody has their own PC or they've worked one out on their own time. There isn't one where you can sit at one clinic and schedule a patient for another: it's got to be manual, it's got to be phone calls.

My feeling is that there is little pressure to change. We thought we were the field of dreams: you build your clinic and patients will come. That if you did set up a timed appointment system, these patients wouldn't show up on time anyway. I think there was a racist, elitist attitude, and some classism, that kept this happening. We served individuals who didn't pay up front, so therefore people didn't complain as much as maybe they should. Those that did were written off: "Why should you complain? You don't pay anyway." The individuals that choose County for service don't have a lot of political clout: they don't have a constituency base that can yell and scream at politicians. We don't serve a geographically limited community; we serve everyone in the city from all over, so people are disbursed out and don't have the ability to get together to organize.

I would make a rule that everybody here that made over $70,000 or $60,000 would have to use this hospital for their care, or they would have to pay for their own care somewhere else. Right now we all get insurance, we can go where we want. Doctors can choose where they want to go; very few choose to come here. Some employees do. Interestingly enough, many employees bring their parents who have lost their insurance, who are covered by Medicaid or Medicare. Some of the families have historically come here among the employee groups, especially clerks and techs. Their mothers and fathers have always come here, and would come here forever no matter what. They believe that this is the place that will never turn them away. It's theirs, they own it. They may not complain about it because, "Good or bad, it's mine."

So, jobs, safe homes, get rid of lead paint, living in a safe community. If you've read Alex Kotlowitz's, book, *There Are No Children Here*—he came out and talked with people at the jail. We thought it was very important for us to listen to him, because he saw the children before they got to the jail. And for us to understand the phenomenon of it, for those of us who don't live in a community like that—to understand what it's like to be afraid for your life every day, afraid for your mother's life every day. The stress…And I know, based on reading the newspapers, that every week somebody gets shot at, every day there's gunfire, every day there's an episode of violence of men against women, men against men, every day somebody is drunk or overdosed on your corner. Every day, every day, every day…That has nothing to do with health care, but it has a lot to do with health. So County has to think about this now. We want to talk about how health and County can become more a part of the overall solution.

What we feel is that if you want to keep people healthy, all your efforts should be on prevention and should be in the ambulatory setting. You should try to avoid putting people in situations where their health deteriorates to the point where they have to be in the hospital. So everything we do on the ambulatory side means better health for patients.

Dr. Linda Murray

MEDICAL DIRECTOR OF *the Winfield/Moody Health Center.*
*"My great-grandmother always had a clear notion of the world. She
used to say: 'You're Black and people are going to try and keep you
down, period. And the only question is whether you're just going to
lay down, or whether you're going to stand up and fight. And those
are your only two choices, so you might as well decide.' And so, it's
only one choice for me, and that is you have to fight. And you know,
it's not particularly pleasant."*

I NEVER HAD ANY INTENTION OF GOING INTO MEDICINE. I
wanted to be a political rabble-rouser. I was not a hippy. I was a Black
young child in the sixties, and, certainly, there was a consciousness that
as a people we didn't have lots of things that we needed, and that's why
we were out on picket lines et cetera. And one of the things we didn't
have were enough people with skills.

I started off at the University of Chicago, and I went to New York with
a friend for Thanksgiving. Her parents were doctors and her mother,
[chuckles] was horrified that I did not know exactly what I wanted to do.
She said, "Do you know how many Black doctors there are?" I said,
"Well...not enough." Actually there were worse than not enough and
she knew—to a person. Three thousand, whatever it was, it was very,
very small. And then she proceeded to tell me that it was disgusting that
someone like myself wasn't clear on what I wanted to do, and we didn't
have time to be mucking around. And frankly, that's why I decided to go
into medicine. I was shocked at the numbers. I said to myself, Well, now,
doctors have skills, and what they do doesn't appear to be very hard;
they sort of look in your throat and give you shots. I mean, my experience with doctors! I said, Well, I could probably do that.

I was a medical student during the County house staff strike. It was very
clear to me that the issues during that strike...What were they striking for?
They were striking for the ability to get a CBC [complete blood count], a
basic blood test. To be able to have that available to them twenty-four-
hours a day. Well, you know, every other hospital in the city you could get it
twenty-four-hours a day. And for a situation like ours, where you're taking
care of such sick patients, that's even more critical. What other kinds of
things did they want? Crash carts—what people see on TV, where there's a
cardiac arrest, you know. Not just two or three in the building—this is a

huge complex—but to actually have them on every ward. The ability to set up some kind of committee that would allow the house staff to work on these patient care questions. Now, the notion at the time for management was, Well, these are management prerogatives—it's not the prerogative of a bunch of young asshole doctors to tell us how to run the hospital.

These were physicians who came of age in the sixties, who had been against the Vietnam War. It was a natural thing for them, working in these public hospitals around the country and seeing the conditions that existed in the public hospitals, to say *no!* What we said was, "This is part of our working conditions: it's an inappropriate working condition for me as a physician to have to wait eighteen hours to get a CBC." But I don't want to minimize the self-interest; I mean, after all, we were physicians in training and it's very difficult to learn medicine if what you're doing is pushing patients around to X-ray and waiting days to get a test. I mean, that is not the way to learn medicine. So, this is an instance where the clear self-interest of physicians in training meshed with patient interests. I think, for most physicians—if we would just step away from monetary greed—I think this is true most of the time. It really is much more pleasant to take care of patients in a health care setting where things are working rationally.

There was a tradition that you would be house staff president in the second year of your residency, which was perceived to be—and it was—the easiest year; and that you would only serve for one year. I was the first Black and the first woman elected president of the union—and it was a difficult decision for me to run, to be honest with you, though I suspect many people won't believe that. I was much more comfortable being active in the Black Physicians' Association. Within the African American residents, there was a similar split: there were many people who were here, they wanted to get through here—they really didn't want to pay attention to too much stuff. Just to get out and go fulfill their dream of practicing medicine. And there were a number of others who really felt strongly that we had an obligation to the hospital and to our community, who felt strongly that we should be active in the union, even if all we did was function as a veto on—as we said—the crazy White folks [laughs] who would go away and leave us alone, stuck in our communities forever…There was a real feeling that there was an obligation.

It's really Terry Conway's fault that I ran the second year. He said to me, "You have to run a second time," and I said, "You're crazy." He felt that the hospital was in real danger of closing, which was our collective analysis of where things were. And we were correct, it really did almost close. He said that, politically, the only way we were going to keep it open was if we had support from the Black community, and that we couldn't risk having some nice young White boy as house staff president. We had a number of emergency meetings of the Black House Staff Association, and a decision was made that I would run, and then this other group of people would run from the Black house staff. It's very interesting that the surgeons and the more conservative elements of the house staff, their position was, "This makes sense to us—after all, it's Black patients and it's a Black community that we got to deal with, so yeah…" Everyone active in those days, they really thought hard and did what they thought was the best to keep the place open. And, clearly, we didn't agree all of the time; most of the time we didn't agree. [chuckles] But the place stayed open. We sort of struggled along.

I wasn't an attending at County. I was basically blacklisted and was not allowed to become an attending. I was blacklisted by our good friend, George Dunne. He didn't like me. [big laugh] He didn't like me. It's easy to say it was because of my union activity, but the reality is, for example, Dr. Raba, who led the strike and was a house staff president and was jailed, was asked to be an attending. Actually, I was the first house staff president that was not offered—could not get—an attending job even though I wanted one. I think it's clear that it was because of racism; it's not that no Blacks were being hired, it's just that I was a house staff president who was Black. It's one thing to be an uppity, arrogant, obnoxious, rabble-rousing doctor. But, you know, Blacks aren't allowed to be any of those things: doctors *or* uppity *or* rabble-rousing. [laughs]

I think it's unfortunate, because it sent a very bad signal to other Black house staff physicians. And in fact, one of the arguments for not becoming house staff president from Black staff—it had nothing to do with political leanings—was, "If you do this they will kill you: you will hurt your career, you will not be able to get a job." And, effectively, I wasn't able to get a job with the city or here. That's how it came to be that I left the city for five years.

It wasn't until Harold Washington was mayor that I officially became a volunteer here. In fact, for years the house staff here in Occupational Medicine used to call me the "underground attending." The real problem was that I could not get voluntary privileges here—that means working for free, in essence. I couldn't see patients of course, because I had no malpractice coverage because I wasn't on staff—but I *could* give lectures and things. A lot of my attitude was just one of arrogance. My attitude was, "Well, you assholes don't want to give me privileges? Tough shit: as far as I'm concerned this is *my* hospital as much as anybody else's, and this is *my* division as much as anybody else's."

For over a year I've been the medical director of the Winfield/Moody Health Center. It's a federally funded health center. It's twenty-five years old and has a long and interesting history. County house staff have been medical directors there—there were three before me [including Dr. Terry Conway]. It's in the Cabrini-Green area, and it has strong community support. My original goal was to go out to one of these community health centers, because they're a place where everything sort of meshes together.

Where you ought to have teaching going on, you ought to have research going on; you have day-to-day work in the trenches going on. The issue of clinical medical care really comes together with public health and preventive care in those settings—that's where you are forced to deal with the real world. That's one reason I like working in the city: there are lots of jobs in public health, and a lot of people don't like working in city health departments. But again, my attitude is, "Hey, if you can't get it done in the real world..." It doesn't matter if you sit up in CDC and say, "Here's a strategic plan for AIDS," if you're not able to sit down with four community groups in the city that are about to kill each other over these little pennies of aid. This is what you had to do, you had to try to make peace among community groups—at least a temporary truce.

My relationship with County has been official now for some time. I often speak in the name of County. My occupational and environmental professional career—which mostly right now is national committees and peer review groups and things like that—I really do out of County. And in my public health persona—I'm active in public health circles and in elected offices in a number of governmental and nongovernmental groups—I do that most often as a County person.

My thoughts on what's planned for national health care reform...Well, it's very frightening. First of all, there's no debate about health care reform. What *is* on the table is not health care reform: what they are arguing about is how to direct the money through the medical care system. That's very, very different than a discussion of health care reform, and we really do need health care reform in this country. But what we have is a very narrow discussion on, frankly, the least important part: it's what politicians are comfortable discussing, what the right wing is concerned about in terms of cost control. There's no *real* discussion.

You know, we have a public health infrastructure here that's in shambles. That's not being discussed at all. I don't even mean public hospitals. Cook County Hospital is part of the medical care system and, yes, it happens to be a public hospital. Medical care is when you go to your doctor, you get an X-ray. I'm talking about public *health*. That means, what's going on with air pollution, what's our water quality, what about the restaurants, what about antismoking campaigns on TV? What about violence? Now *that* is a public health issue. There's a whole range of other ones—teenage pregnancies, AIDS, tuberculosis. These are all public health issues, but they're not part of the public health care reform debate. Now, within that very narrow debate that is being discussed in the press—how do we finance medical care—I happen to be someone who believes that a single-payer system is the only obvious mild reform that we can tolerate. Anything less than that will fail totally. I would like to be wrong, but I personally don't think we're going to see any health care reform in this century.

Margaret Morris

NURSE PRACTITIONER. *"I grew up on the West Side. It's not the prettiest, but I love it. I went into nursing as just a job. And not only that, some of the nurses that I'd met...I'm like, 'Well, it couldn't be too difficult if this one is doing it.' [laughs] And I really liked it."*

I WAS AT PRES[BYTERIAN] ST. LUKE'S FOR SIX YEARS. THERE WAS more than one level of care there, and it was kind of discouraging and disgusting for me to see that. If there were two-bed rooms, and there were empty beds available, you still might find Black patients in the hallway beds because...there were actually patients who would say they didn't want a Black patient in the room with them. And that would be a bed available, but it would not be open to Black patients. And this was in OB/GYN! There was no ifs, ands...There was no, "you didn't hear it right." It was just a statement that was made—it was black and white. I got kind of fed up with that kind of standard of care. So I came to County, and I haven't really looked back.

When I came to County, I was an RN in OB/GYN, in the delivery room. Labor and delivery was pretty good—I did that for about a year, and then I transferred. When they opened the abortion unit—in 1974, I think—I decided to work with them. You didn't have the picketing. You had conscientious objectors that didn't want to work on the unit, like doctors that said, "I won't do abortions," and nurses that said, "I won't work with these patients." Fair enough.

At that time, that move was no big increase in pay—but there was a lot of knowledge to be had and a certain amount of freedom to do a job. It was autonomous, we worked on our own. We were working from a whole different aspect of medicine: as opposed to nursing we were kind of getting into assessment—a little bit more diagnosing, hands-on history, talking to the patient. And that appealed to me, because it was more fulfilling; it was more challenging than just service—making the bed, giving the bath, passing the meds—and not necessarily getting a chance to actually see enough of your patient, if you had a big patient-care load. Because it kind of gets left out when you're in a hurry and you're thinking about the next bed, the next patient, the next bath. To actually get to spend some time with people, without all the other stuff that goes with nursing: grabbing the phone, hanging the IV, a lot of the task-orientated stuff.

We got to follow the patient from admission to discharge—you got to build up a rapport with the patient. At first, we also assisted in surgery to a certain degree: they'd let us do suturing and stuff. Now we don't do that. I think one of the directors of the hospital was saying that a lot of the med students weren't getting as much experience as they could because the practitioners were doing some things that *they* could have done—so they kind of curtailed it. But now I notice that the physician assistants are being taught and allowed to do as much as what we were doing before. It was taken from us, now it's been given to them. And I think that kind of sucks. It's insulting.

In '77, I finished the nurse practitioner program and went to Oncology. From life to death. I was about twenty-eight and that was really a great experience in that you really start getting kind of a handle on life yourself. You're taking care of patients and they're like, "I wish I had, I always wanted to…" And they never did. I'm like, "My God, let me take some time to do some of those things that I always wanted to do before, because I don't know when my bell is going to be rung." It gave me a new attitude. I had the time to talk to them and really get a sense of their life. And you saw some lives that had been totally wasted: never went anywhere, never done anything, never lived life—just existed—and then you die. It's a sad situation.

I had one patient that was just…the fear…She was very terminal, it was the last days. And her eyes were just bugged. She was shaking with fear, and it was sad. I walked in the room and said, "Are you in pain?" She said, "I'm just scared, so scared." And just one thing: just holding her hand, and saying, "We know there's going to be some pain—we'll do what we can with that. But as far as the fear and scare, just have a little faith in your God." And she visibly, visibly relaxed. I could feel it. It helped her. And from there she didn't complain of any more pain; she just kind of closed her eyes and relaxed. She accepted it and she rested from then on. Later on that night she expired, but she did not expire the way…that pure panic that you saw in her eyes was not there anymore. It's little ways that you can be useful. But you've got to work with yourself first and realize that you're not going to be the savior. Once you accept that about yourself, then you realize you can help people just by being with them and being for them.

I was on Oncology up until '79. I decided, "That's it! I can't take it, it's time for me to get out of here." I quit for about a year. There were aspects of the hospital that were kind of ticking me off: you couldn't get things done when they needed to be done, there was a lot of red tape—you know, a phone call and no answer. It got frustrating to the point where I said, "I need a break or else…I'm going to strangle someone." [chuckles] And that's one thing that I notice in nursing: you'll see people you work with and you'll say, "Boy, does this lady need a long rest." You know? And they *don't* take it. They're obnoxious, they're hard to work with—

I'm sure the patients don't want to see them coming. I realized that when you get like that, you need to be alone. [laughs]

Then, after a year, I was ready to go back to work. But I didn't know that I wanted to go back to patient care, so I started in health services—I became administrative supervisor of Health Services. I was in Health Services from '79 to '86, and then I quit. [laughs] I worked a little while doing some political work, and at Lakeside VA for about three months, and then I came back here.

I have nothing against County. County is a great hospital—you're a little freer here, to a certain extent. I've been a patient at some of those nicer hospitals and it's nice, it's clean, it's pretty—but what's the level of care? This might not be fancy, it might not be cool as in *pretty*, but the patients do get taken care of. My nephew was supposed to have ear surgery when he was two years old because they couldn't clear up an infection. I'm like, "Before you let the baby go into surgery, why don't you bring him on over to County for a second opinion?" My sister brings him out, and they give him ear drops. She said, "Well, how come the other ones didn't heal it?" The doctor said, "They were giving him the wrong ear drops." Here's someone talking surgery for a two year old. I think that the volume of patients that the guys get here opens them up to being better diagnosticians. That sheer volume, some of everything from A to Z. It gives them a big edge on assessment and treatment. I come here; my grandmother, my kids, we come here.

Way back when I first started, there was a big sense of family in this hospital: as large as the hospital was, and as many employees—most people knew each other. But then, County was a very social place also. There used to be parties in Karl Meyer Hall and in the Nurses' Residence: routinely, people socialized together. That was before and after the strikes. Whoever was in charge of administration stopped the parties. It was where you got together—doctors, nurses, all the different employees. You'd hang out on a Friday night or something, and everybody would come through. You meet people that way, and you see them on another level; now you just don't know people the same way…And then, The Greeks was open across the way, and *that* was a social center there. People used to meet and have lunch or dinner, or sometimes we just howled at the moon over a few beers. [laughs] I think it burned to the ground in 1977 and I guess the medical center said thumbs-down on rebuilding.

Anyway, I came back I came to Trauma, and I've been here ever since. Right now, I'm basically working with the Trauma registry—that's the reports that we do for the state: the statistics, the coding. Sometimes I miss doing hands-on nursing, but it's not any gut-yearning, gotta go out and lay on hands. No, nuh-uh. [laughs]

I was the president of the local union at County during the nurses' strike in '76. There was talk of taking back sick days, which was kind of a key thing for people—docking folks for using their sick time. And also, the money was not right...a number of things. It was a big decision to strike. I don't think the house staff strike had anything to do with whether we struck or not, because their strike, to me, was like they really weren't out—they really didn't have a strike as far as I'm concerned. I was there and I was like, "There's more doctors here than I've ever seen in my life! Who is *this* one?" I didn't even know that these people existed. [laughs] The doctors would meet and say they were with us and for us and they were going to support us, and there was talk about not crossing the nurses' picket lines, but they never did it—they always wanted to keep in touch and be on top of what was happening. I ended up telling one of the guys, "Hey, you guys had your strike. Leave us alone and let us deal with ours." Everybody started getting on each other's nerves.

There were so many nurses that joined the union during that period of time. I was surprised. When we first started out, you really weren't getting a lot of people that were coming out for union meetings. They wanted someone to do it for them, but they didn't want to join. I said, "Wait a minute—I wonder if you people realize that *you're* the union. It's not me or her, it's *you*. You as a body whole: your numbers make you the union. So if you want the union to do something for you, get up and join hands." That was the first step. And then when the issues started coming out, then people started uniting behind the cause. When we took the vote, it was overwhelming—ninety-something percent.

We're dealing with the administration and then come to find out that our union, the INA [Illinois Nurses Association], is telling them, "They're not going to strike. Don't worry about it—we got it in hand." The union was dealing behind our backs! There was this sweetheart relationship taking place, and we were renegades, to the union. We went on strike, and the next day there was a court order telling us to go back to work. And we all said no. We went to court, and they told the union that for every day of the strike the union would be fined—and the INA said, "Hey listen, those people are autonomous. They do their own thing." [getting angrier] The next day, we got a call from downtown and the INA said, "We're dropping you guys. We're not going to support you because we don't want to be fined." I said, "All I'm asking you guys to do before you officially dump us is to allow us to go back to our membership and let them know that this is going to take place, so that they won't be surprised." They told us no and they announced it right away.

When we went to our membership that night, we had to tell them that INA is dropping us. There were tears everywhere. And the very next day, before we could get back to the office, they had been through there. They went through there that evening and moved everything out—they left a couple paper clips. They actually took paper, pencils, everything! It was so petty—they were out to hurt us. They were more punishing and vengeful than the administration ever was. They were spying on the office. It was really enlightening, because there were so many people that started sending money to support us—we weren't deserted by others. We got money from other unions, other nurses.

The strike lasted thirty-six days, the longest strike in the history of nursing. It was very traumatic: some people actually quit and went someplace else. I kind of just dropped out of the union after that. I'd had so much faith in the union, because my father and mother were union people. It was very disappointing. They didn't care about us, they only wanted their dues to keep rolling in—and never mind that County Hospital provided over half of the dues that were collected in the whole state. We weren't treated well by the union, not at all.

You know, every ten years, every five years there's a story that County's closing. This is it, this is the real thing. They used to have these little metal tags, circular, that had COOK COUNTY HOSPITAL engraved on them. That was the tag to let you know that something was hospital property. And all of a sudden, there was this hunt all over for people to get these tags. I was like, "Boy, would you look at these people, they're really obnoxious. County's not closing." And then I realized that they had taken the circle tags off everything, from wheelchairs to beds—and when I wanted one I couldn't get near one. I lost out—never saw another one around anywhere. And believe me, we looked. But they were like, "Get something from County, because it's not going to be here and we want to have part of it, a physical part of it." And all over this country, there's people who've passed through County Hospital out there with those little metal tags—and part of County is out there with them.

The Patients

Ida Milam

IS SIXTY-EIGHT, *and there is something both comforting and inspiring about her—you wouldn't ever want to let her down. She worked for the Board of Education for twenty-one years. "I taught preschool fifteen years, and I hear the children are going on to higher education, most of them." Of course.*

I WAS BORN IN ALABAMA, BUT I GREW UP HERE. BETWEEN MY husband and I—with his children, I didn't birth them—we still have twelve children between the two of us.

I started going to the County around '49. A lot of people, we didn't have too much other choice but to go to the County at that particular time. We had two hospitals: the County and Provident. I knew better than to go to another hospital, and so I always went to the County.

The first time was with my having children. We had some insurance then. I don't care what sort of insurance I had, I always went there. Once upon a time, between my first marriage and some separation time, if I had to go with my children I went when I didn't have insurance, and I got the same treatment. They don't look at you because you got insurance, you know? As my mother always used to tell us, "You don't bite the hand that feeds you"—so I feel why not give it to them when you have insurance. Help them to help other people, like they helped me.

Now, me, I haven't had no real bad experience, like I have heard some people say, "I'm always sitting there, waiting." I really truly can't even say I ever really run into no real nasty person there. I've seen it happen now, please believe me, maybe to other people; but I also feel, looking at things on both sides, it was a two-way street. Those other people maybe could have caused some of it: they both was agitating each other. Maybe that's not the way the professionals should have handled it, but you're a human being, you know? You deal with a lot of people there. Like sometimes I go in there, I talk to Dr. Hoffman—I say, "Are you tired? How *you* feel?" You know? I say, "All work and no play, it's not good for you." There's too much pressure. They're human beings.

One day Dr. Hoffman passed me, he said, "Mrs. Milam, you know everybody, don't you?" I said, "Well, Dr. Hoffman, I stay here enough, I should." [laughs] My son-in-law told me, one time, "Mom, please don't talk to strangers." Before he could get it out of his mouth I'm standing up there talking to another lady. He said, "Lord have mercy. I told her don't talk to strangers and here she is running her mouth." I just like to talk.

Things have changed over the years. For one thing, the upkeep of the County, its cleanness. We ourselves have to help. We shouldn't let our children just go in there and throw things around. But once upon a time, if you'd go in one of those bathrooms, it was terrible—I've seen a lot of clean-up done around that hospital. And not having room for patients, patients out in the halls and beds everywhere. I was in there, beds any kind of anywhere, just push you out the way. You feel bad, but what could we do? Really and truly. With some people, I guess it was the best we could get. We couldn't even get *in* another hospital, so what you gonna do?

Sometimes I sit up and hear people group and grumble and mumble, even now. I say, "You're sitting here grouping and grumbling. Why are you here? Go someplace else if you're that dissatisfied. You come here cause you can't do any better so sit here and keep your mouth closed." I have said that to them, but I don't say it as much now, because why make a scene? Some of them would make me feel real bad, you know?

But the support staff, they need a change. I'm serious, they really need a change. They've been there so long they have what we call a burn-out. But, then too, there's some that are as sweet as they want to be. You just have to balance things. But on the whole, I think some of them need a change—not a rest, now, just a change. They need their jobs, but take another position for a while.

But I've even seen changes with the clerks. Once upon a time you was purely dirt to some of those clerks. [tight-lipped] "You take anything we give you." If you run up on one of them nasty clerks: "You ain't paying for it." I've seen a lot of that change.

Dr. Hoffman is just like what I would like in a son. He's a friend, he's my doctor, I can talk with him. Dr. Warshaw was the same way, she was my friend. She caused me to have my sanity today. [laughs] Really. I went through some problems. She really, really helped me through it, and Dr. Hoffman finished it up. [laughs] I tell people how long I've had Dr. Warshaw and Dr. Hoffman and they say, *"At the County?"* Because mostly you have the interns that leave on and go to study more, and it's another doctor. I said I have been through that too at the County, and I was shocked too to have a doctor this long—but them two has been more like my family doctor.

Even some of the nurses. That whole staff of nurses in that colon area, they all know me personal. I go back once a year to have a check-up, and they all say, "Mrs. Milam is here." It makes you feel good. It's a community there. I have a standing joke around this house: I say, "They know me so well at the County, instead of putting my whole name on my medicine, they just put Ida." [laughs]

The worst wait is at the pharmacy. You have to look at it...those people working it are under triple pressure, I think. Sometimes they have to send the patient back upstairs if the doctor forgot to put the signature on, or if the doctor forgot to put whether it's a cream or some kind of different thing. I'm saying what has happened to me. And you have to go back upstairs to try and catch your doctor to get this straightened out. But remember, they got your life in their hands. Sometimes we be tired from waiting upstairs, and you got to come down and be tired down there. But I've got to a place, by being a diabetic, I just stick me a lunch in my purse and take it with me, or I go around and get me a hot soup or something out of the canteen.

You have to look at it all different ways. People can aggravate you— the people there aggravates me standing up at the window. Standing up there, hollering at the people is not going to make them get your medicine no faster. I do agree we have to wait a long time, maybe too long— but I'd rather wait and get my medicine correct than give me something that's going to kill me. I'm gonna strike me up a conversation some where, somehow. And you get to talking and the time will pass. Up in the clinic I know people. I told Dr. Hoffman one day, "You like us old womens, don't you?" [laughs] We may not talk too much, but I see them, know them by face. They're all elderly, like I am.

Once upon a time, a doctor—you were just in his office and out of his office, just another number. Now, the doctors they give you more of their time. Not only my doctor, I've seen other people talking about their doctors. My Dr. So-and-so, I tell my doctor this, that's my doctor. Once upon a time, you didn't hear that.

I think there's more medicine in a doctor talking to you or telling you something sometimes than there is in their bottles and their pills. A lot of times, I go in and my blood pressure will be elevated, and he'll say, "What's wrong, Mrs. Milam?" He's gotten to know me well enough to know most of the time; I've either had a little stressful something here at the house or something. He'll say, "I'm going to go take care of this patient." I know how to meditate, so I'll just sit there awhile, and he'll take my blood pressure and it'll be altogether different, and then he'll know whether it's serious enough for a change of medications or not.

There's doctors here, once they get their training they could go somewhere else, but there are a whole lot of doctors I've seen for years—I know them by sight. Got their training, but they stayed. Now, I feel that's a dedicated doctor.

What you see in the newspapers about County doesn't really tell you...Oh, you know, I get *mad*. They don't show the good part: some of them know it and just don't want to give you credit, neither. There's a whole political thing. I don't know exactly how to explain it, but that's the way I feel.

Sherron Cleveland

Is ROBUST IN SPIRIT *and size. "As you can see, I like to eat,"* she *says, laughing. Her face is pretty and expressive, her stories are told with a theatrical flair. She raised seven children and is quick and proud to note that not one of her six boys has been in a gang or in prison.*

I WAS BORN AND RAISED IN CHICAGO. I WENT TO COUNTY HOS-pital as a kid. I was born at home, fifty-three years ago; but I guess, from infant on, most of my care as a child was there. I can remember going to County Hospital and sitting on these hard concrete slabs. I used to think they were really cool in the summer, because they felt comfortable.

I had a brother that was two years older than me—him and I were very close. He died at Cook County Hospital when he was five or six. This was around '43, I was three. He had rheumatic fever, and at that time they didn't know much about it. Until they did an autopsy after his death, they didn't know that he had it. I think that was my first thinking about not liking that hospital.

I had my first baby when I was seventeen, at Mt. Sinai, but my husband was still in school and we were on a limited income, so I ended up having to take my baby to County for medical care. I can remember the baby being full of a temperature and the treatment was to take your baby outside with no clothes on in the winter to lower his temperature. So you'd put a blanket around him, you'd go stand outside, you'd come back in, and they'd take his temperature. That was before the doctor ever saw you—that was standard procedure if your temperature was over a certain amount. They didn't do that at the other hospitals. I was always glad that the hospital was there, as I still am now that it's there, because so many people can't afford anything and something is better than nothing.

The doctors certainly seem to have a thirst for knowledge and a caring about the people they're working with. The patients don't get the same level of caring from the staff that works there as they do from the doctors. The nurses seem to want to run the doctors, because there's such an influx of doctors coming in, and as they're concerned for the patients and working and trying to do something—the nurses are busy back there, "He doesn't know what he's doing," and "That's not procedure." So there is a friction between the doctors and the nurses. It's not a blanket indictment. You have some very caring nurses and support staff, and you have some that aren't.

I would never talk to or treat people the way some of the people there treated patients. It was like, [haughty] "Obviously you can't do any better, 'cause you're here," and, "You will accept whatever I tell you and do what you're told." And it was like all of the adult people were children to a lot of the support staff. They did not treat you with respect, nor dignity.

When I had my second child, I was supposed to have him at home, but my husband panicked. We didn't have a phone, and I thought he went out to call the people from the center who were going to help. I was cleaning up—Oh God, between the pains—let me have everything ready before these people come. I was scrubbing, I was going wild. Anyway, my husband came back: "There's a cab out front. Let's go."

At that time, the fountain that sits in the vestibule was in the lobby area—it even had water in it once upon a time. Anyway, I got into the hospital and I got to the fountain and I grabbed it—and down on my knees I went! I was having the baby. Well, they crossed my legs on the baby, they messed his head up—I think they call it "coning." All of the back of his head was pushed up to the front. And I think that was one of the good experiences I had at County, I don't just want to say every experience I had has been bad. It was good because they *did* deliver my baby, they didn't let me deliver it out there on that nasty floor among all them germy people.

In '66, when my son James was born—I know, everybody opens ten centimeters before they deliver a baby, *most* everybody does. I don't: my body opens three, three and a half centimeters, my baby balls up out of the birth canal and shoots out. Every one of my boys did that. I went to County in labor with James. They told me I wasn't getting ready to have the baby. This was my sixth baby. I explained to the doctor, but he said, "You're only two and a half centimeters." I said, "Doctor, when I get another centimeter the baby is gonna be born." He told me, "You don't know what you're talking about—go home." I didn't go home—he saw me still there and said, "I'm gonna examine you one more time, and then you're gonna go home." He told me, "The baby is balled up in a knot, you're gonna be another three or four days, the baby is not in position. Go home."

I went to my father's house. He lived near the hospital. I went up the stairs, I went to get in the bed, I put my knee on the bed and I said, "This baby is coming out now!" My brother grabs me, helps me into the car, my brother can't get the car started. My brother is sixteen. I grabbed him, I said, "The baby's coming. Go in the house. You shouldn't be out here with me." He said, "Let me loose, I'll be glad to go." [laughs] I turned him loose, and he shot inside to tell my dad.

There was a lady standing on the sidewalk. I said, "Please come here, I'm getting ready to have my baby—help me get my bloomers off." [laughs] She said, "I beg your pardon?!" I said, "Miss, my baby's getting ready to come out. If he comes out and hits my panties, it could break his neck. You don't want to be responsible for my baby dying, do you?" She reached up, she grabbed my slip, my panties, and all, she *snatched* them. By the time they hit my ankle that baby's head came out. I had him in the front seat of the car, by myself.

My daddy called the fire department, the police. [laughs] They both came, a fire truck and a paddy wagon. The fireman came around on one side and the police on the other. One said, "I'm gonna hold the baby and he's gonna help you out." I said, "Can I see your hands? Neither one of you are touching my baby!" I said, "Take that paddy wagon and push this station wagon to the hospital, or get a doctor or a nurse out here."

We went to County. The same doctor came out and he said, "What did you go home and do? You went home and took something." I said, "I *told* you my baby was ready to come." So they clipped the navel cord, and they took the baby in.

They wheeled me in the hall and they left me there. Nobody came to see me, I'm bleeding like a hog. I called the nurse and said, "I just delivered and I'm bleeding." She said, "I'm busy." I said, "Could you give me a sheet or something, it's so uncomfortable, I got blood all back here." [motions behind her neck] She said, "Well, I'm busy." Another lady told me she was going to lunch, but as soon as she got back she would see about me. She came back from lunch and said, "I'll get around to you— you ain't hemorrhaging like you say you're hemorrhaging." I said, "I'm not? Miss, could you come here a minute. I just want to say one thing to you." I just did like this [runs hand up behind her neck and down through the air] and wiped it right down her. Then she raised up that sheet and she looked. She said, "Oh my God."

Then they started giving me some treatment, hooked me up to IVs. I'm allergic to penicillin, but nobody's asking me anything. The doctor puts some stuff into the IV and I started floating away. I said, "I'm getting very sleepy and I need to tell you something." He said, "What?" I said, "Please tag me because I'm allergic to penicillin." He said, *"What?!"* and he was turning the IV off. He said, "I just put penicillin in your IV." I said, "You're killing me." He went and got something and gave me a shot, and I came back. But that's how close I came to dying, because no one asked me a question—because nobody was really concerned.

In 1967, my father took ill and my stepmom dropped him off early in the morning when she went to work. I called over there looking for my father that evening. They told me, "He was here, but we don't know where he's at." I kept calling, and finally they said that he was supposed to be transferred over to the men's building, but he had never got there. I said, [voice rises with each word] "Well, I'll be out there and by the time I get there somebody *damn* sure better know where my father's at. And if you don't, just get ready for a press conference because I'm calling one.

You done *lost* a daggoned patient and he's *my* father." Oh, I went totally and completely *off*.

I want you to know, I had raised so much sand on that phone that when I got there, they were down there by the desk. "We found your father." My father had been going to be transferred like around three o'clock, when the shift was changing. Somebody had wheeled him in the underground to the elevator to transfer him, and he had laid there until six or seven o'clock! My father was too sick to get up—he had been laying there by the elevator, people going back and forth, and he was laying there. My father never recovered from this illness. I was very upset and for years I did not go back in that hospital.

When I didn't have a job and I didn't have insurance, that's when I went back, to get medication. That was in '90. They said something was wrong with my heart, and I told them yeah, I'd had a double bypass. At that time, I was working at County with the AIDS Legal Counsel—I was a paralegal and worked with people on getting their benefits—but my insurance was not in effect yet.

They put me in the cardiac clinic. They had this thing where they have a needle in your vein, in case something goes wrong and they need it quick. They change it every two or three days. The person who does that is polite and courteous and treats you like you're a human being. A lot of the nursing people on the cardiac unit were very nice, and the way the unit is set up, I think it's excellent. They have the desk there in the middle of the floor, they have people all around. You feel good there.

As long as I was on the cardiac unit I could cope, but when they put me on a ward I could no longer cope. The nastiness in the bathrooms, cigarette smoking in there, the nurses being way down, a block from me—the call button doesn't work. After I had come to the unit I got very, very ill and I could not get up out of the bed. They had started an IV that was supposed to be changed regularly and it had been in me for twenty-four hours. The floor wasn't open, like in the '50s—you had little cubicles with two people in there, and a social worker or something was talking to the other person. I said to her, "Could you please get someone to help me, I'm very ill."

She went out, a half hour or so passed. By this time I'm crazy. I get up, I'm holding on to the wall, I'm going down the hall. My doctor told me, "If you have any chest pains notify them immediately, I want you to have a cardiogram." I was having chest pains, I was dizzy, I was sick. I get down to the nurses' station and I tell her what's wrong with me. "You go back to your room, I will get someone there for you. Go back to your room." Anybody, my grandkid, five years old, would have said, "Sit down, let me get a wheelchair for you." I can hardly walk. I'm a cardiac patient, OK?

She didn't take my blood pressure, she didn't listen to my chest. I told her what the doctor said. I walked back and kind of slumped over the bed. The nurse came in, she took my blood pressure, she said, "Oh, my goodness, your blood pressure is very high! You haven't had your medicine today." I said, "Well, why haven't I?" "The pharmacy hasn't sent it up." "Well, would you get this IV out, it's supposed to be changed." "I'll be back."

She came back, she'd gotten my medicine, I thought she was going to change the IV. She didn't do it. When she gave me my medicine I said, "When will you be back to check my blood pressure?" "Oh, the medicine will take care of it, I don't have to check it." *Pardon me?!* Every place else I'd been they gave me medicine, they checked to make sure my blood pressure had gone down. I said, "Please get my doctor." He came, he talked to me. It wasn't like, "Hey, you got a problem here." [sighs]

About three hours later, they did take my blood pressure. I told the nurse, "Take this out of my arm, I'm leaving." I got up, I went to the phone, I called somebody, I said, "Come and get me out of this hellhole here." The nurse said, "You can't leave without signing the Against Medical Advice form." My doctor came back to talk to me. I said, "I'm not staying, I'm not signing—I'm not getting medical treatment here. If you want me to sign a statement saying I'm leaving here to go *get* some good medical advice, I'll do that." I didn't leave—I wrote this four-page letter. I gave the nursing staff a copy and sent a copy to the administrator. All of a sudden, my room was full of people. My doctor said, "If we transfer you back to the cardiac unit, will you stay?" So I stayed.

But mostly from the time my father died until then, if I went to the hospital it was because I had a cold—but for nothing that I considered serious. Or I went because I couldn't pay for my medicine, even though I was seeing a doctor somewhere else. I was using the hospital in a sense, and that was unfair. I guess that's the other reason I say that it's good that County is there, because a lot of people get released from what I call good hospitals but they don't have a way of getting their medicine.

I would fight anybody that would try to close that hospital, because it is a matter of life and death. But by the same token, if I were hurt to a point that I was gonna die, I'd rather lay on the street and die than go to *that* hospital. But I'm gonna go there on an outpatient basis, and I don't have a problem with other people being *admitted* to it, as long as it's not me. [laughs] I *have* seen concern from the doctors in the last couple of years that I have never seen in the lifetime of County, and I am willing to roll up my sleeves and work on helping that hospital—but I don't want to be its patient.

There are some doctors and nurses there that make you feel like everything is going to be OK, you're in good hands. There are some others there that make you feel like, [hard] "If you die, you're just another one gone—don't bother me, I'm waiting till three o'clock, when I can get my paycheck and go home."

I have very short tolerance for people treating me like an idiot. I don't have a lot of education, but I'm a self-taught person. I'm a paralegal, I ran for state legislator, I've gone to Springfield to address the welfare legislative committee, and I will *not* have anybody that I consider working for me—because, when you work for County Hospital, you're working for me—being insubordinate. Somebody pays dearly for every day you're in County Hospital, so I don't understand why they can't do a better job than they're doing.

Juanita Ousley

GENTLE AND REFLECTIVE, *her four children are grown. She is worried about health care reform: "I don't know how they're going to work it out so that everybody will have health care. What about the homeless people? I think I heard Mrs. Clinton say that everybody would contribute to their health care costs, but then if you don't have a job you can't contribute, so that means you're going to get left out of health care." She and Sherron Cleveland are close friends.*

I'M FIFTY-FIVE, AND I GREW UP IN CHICAGO. I USED TO COME TO County Hospital, to the Fantus Clinic, when I was in my early twenties, after I'd gotten married and began to have children. That was in the sixties. I wasn't very satisfied with the services because, during those years, each time you came to the clinic you saw a different doctor, whoever happened to, I guess, pick up your chart. So there was no consistency in the care that you got. The doctors were pretty good, but they couldn't follow up on you. This was in the GYN clinic and, you know, you kind of want to have your own doctor, but you didn't.

I remember coming to the clinic and I got a doctor—this was like 1964—and he wanted me to have an EKG. I didn't know why, because they didn't do a lot of explaining to you, like they do now. He wanted to do some more follow-up, because he thought there was something going on, and he was right. I didn't find out about it until twenty-five years later. If I had been able to follow up with him then, I would have known to change my diet and that kind of thing. No one else followed up on what he found out; there was no process to follow up with the patient.

The waiting in the clinic was much worse than it is now. I don't remember about the pharmacy. It seems like you had to wait, but not as long periods as you do now. Basically, I tried to get a babysitter because the kids would get pretty restless being out here that long—you could be here for ten hours for a clinic appointment.

After I got a job and we had health insurance, I didn't come to the County anymore. I went to my own private doctor. I worked for the State of Illinois. The position I had was eliminated, and after a year you don't have any more health insurance. One day, I began to feel very ill. This was two years ago. When my insurance ran out, I was in an HMO. Although you have your own physician in that HMO, you can't go there unless you have your HMO card, so I didn't bother to do that. I knew

156

better—I knew they'd turn me away. It wouldn't be the doctor, but the administration, and this is what they're all about.

Anyway, by then I did know that I had diabetes and a heart condition, but it was like I had a block because I didn't remember about the County. I just kept wondering, What am I going to do? I don't have any medication...Eventually my girlfriend said, "Well, why don't you go out to the County?" When I got so that I could not any longer bear being ill, I went to the clinic, the one where you walk in. The young lady that examined me, she told me that she would like to have someone in the Cardiac Clinic look at me. He called, and it was on a Sunday, I think. He had seen these tests I took, and he was very concerned. It surprised me—a doctor from the County calling you on Sunday?! He wanted me to come to the hospital. I did, and I went through all the procedures that were necessary.

I stayed in the hospital a week. It wasn't bad. Now, you don't have your own room, but you have a little small space. In the sixties I had been hospitalized, and *everybody* was on the ward, with the long line of beds that you see—looks like in one of those real old movies, OK? The curtain, they'd just pull it around, but you really had no privacy. This time I found it different, because you do have a little cubicle—it's usually for two people—and you feel different about it.

What I find now is that everyone has their own doctor. I had my own cardiologist, and he referred me to the General Medicine Clinic. I think it depends on your doctor, the kind of care that you get. I just think Dr. Goldberg is the best doctor, and I think my cardiologist is pretty good. So when you come you see your own doctor, you have an appointment—you're not sitting, waiting all this long time. And the care is consistent. There are a lot of things that go on mentally that will affect your health, like stress. So Dr. Goldberg talks to me about all things, the bigger picture—the total picture of the patient. My cardiologist doesn't; his only concern is making sure my heart is OK—but he's really good.

One of the things that I find much, much different is that even now you're able to call your doctor if anything goes wrong. It was not like that before: if something went wrong before, you'd just have to come out to the hospital, and there was no correlation between the hospital and the clinic. If you had to come to the hospital, they didn't get your records from Fantus Clinic to see what was really going on—it was like you were a new patient. Whereas now you can call your doctor, and your doctor can give some kind of instructions.

You know, when you're up in the clinic and you're talking to the different patients and they are referring to them, [pointing] "Well, that's *my* doctor there." I guess we have attached ownership to our doctors. I truly feel that when I see [laughs] *my* doctor, that I'm going to get good health care. But I understand that there are a lot of other things that he just cannot do with the other staff, in making the environment better and that sort of stuff. But he takes time and explains what everything is, and if he doesn't know he'll go and find out for you.

I recognize people in the waiting room and talk to people some. And especially in the pharmacy, that's where you really talk, OK? Because everybody is angry that they're waiting this long. They're talking about why it's taking so long and this, this, and this. And you're sitting there a long time, waiting for this medicine. You develop a camaraderie. The normal time you usually have to wait is three and a half, four hours. I usually bring a book, but I never get a chance to read it, because I'm busy talking to everybody! [laughs]

The doctors and the nurses seem to really care about the patients, but I think the ancillary staff needs some training. [laughs] Oh, they're the ones, they make you feel like you shouldn't be here. They're negative, there's that sort of thing, OK? "You're at the County, and I can treat you any kind of way"—that you basically have no rights. They just need some training. *Lots* of training.

What I've noticed in the pharmacy is there's maybe a language barrier. So many of the pharmacy workers are Asians, but I've never really thought of it in terms of culture because, see, the Blacks are like that too, OK? It's just there. With that pharmacy, I understand they have volume, they have to get it out. Maybe they should even have special people to deal with the patients, because the attitude that I see they have is that you have to wait because you're poor and you're at the County, and we do not have to be nice about it. That's what I got, not so much a cultural difference, because they all have that same attitude: "I'm better than you."

But basically the care that I'm getting now is good. I think now that if I went back to work and I did have health insurance, I would come to the County, because I'd want to keep my doctors. I trust them. It's just a different feeling here than it was thirty years ago. I would pay to come because of the two doctors that I have.

Betty Prude

SHE'S THE MOTHER *of five and, while friendly, has an air of not taking any guff from anybody. As we talk, little Betty, twelve, does a good job of distracting the next and youngest child, three-year-old Candice.*

I CAME UP FROM MISSISSIPPI WHEN I WAS FIVE YEARS OLD. My mother passed away at County in '59, soon after we came up. The County's got more to work with now then they used to. I don't remember it back then, but my grandma told me about it.

I love to go there, I always have. We get hungry, we walk down to a restaurant down the street, get something, come back. I know my way around. Now my sister, she don't like County—she won't go since my mother passed there.

[Patting Candice, who has climbed onto her lap] She's the miracle baby. I had a tubal ligation in '81, and I wasn't supposed to have no more. But we're happy, we love her. She's the joy of the house.

I had her at County. I was in a room with just two people, some of the time, and in a big room with a lot of people too. It didn't bother me. I had one person, a clean-up lady, she was kind of nasty. I had a C-section and, you know, the next day if you urinate it comes out, you ain't got no control, and I peed on the floor—it just came out—and she got mad. I said, "Look now, you don't be like that just 'cause we're at the Cook County Hospital." I told her off, and I didn't have to worry about it no more. I said, "Don't be treating me no any kind of way, because I can fight." [laughs] Next day she said, [simpering] "Hi, Mrs. Prude."

I been going to County for fourteen years. I didn't have no insurance— I had a medical card. My fourteen-year-old, he got sick—he was only seven, eight months old—and he was at Children's Memorial Hospital. At Children's, they started treating him for something he didn't even have—spinal meningitis. It was like a month before they found out what was really wrong.

He got an IV burn. They left a needle in too long, and it burnt his head. [points to a picture of her son with dark burn spots high on his forehead] He had IV everywhere. I said, "Take it off, I'm gonna take him to the Cook County." They said, "No, no," so I waited. They finally called some doctor. He had to fly here. When he saw my baby he just shook his head, said they should have called him sooner. He said, "God's really

159

with you." I know, 'cause my baby was looking like he was fixing to leave—it was that bad. I'll never forget it.

I took him out of Children's; a few days later he started vomiting again, and I took him to County. They kept him two or three days, no more problem. That's why I love County.

I'd heard about the County from other people—good things. I don't care that you got to sit and wait. If it's important, you don't sit there. I have been to emergency and got waited on right away, and the kids too. If I know I got to wait, I just go prepared. I walk around and talk to peoples, and it don't bother me—I'm used to it. I know a few people, other patients. I've been taking the kids to see Dr. Soter for fourteen years. That's *my* doctor there! She's real nice; you can talk to her about anything.

I tell them I ain't got no money, so I ain't never got no bill. I give them the medical card, and I tell them we're low income. Every time now, you have to talk to someone. We used to didn't have that, you'd just go right on in. But like Monday when I go, I got to go register. I got used to that now: "Go register first."

If I had insurance, I would still go to the County because I have been to other hospitals—I had a medical card or something—but it just wasn't right. They're talking about the County bad—*shoot,* the other clinics, other hospitals, emergency room, you sit there all day just like you do at the County.

And then what make it so bad, they don't even tell you really what's wrong with you. One time I went to Grant Hospital: I had an IUD and I couldn't even walk, it hurt so bad. They couldn't get it out, they couldn't find it. I went downstairs, called me a cab, and went to the County. I said, "Man, take me to the Cook County, *they're* gonna get it out." I wasn't there fifteen minutes, they called my name, they took it out. I felt like I was brand-new. I said, "Thank you doctor, 'cause I was hurting." [laughs] Sure was.

But they *do* tell you at the County—that's what I like about it. When I was in, in '90, they gave me a social worker to talk to, because I was pretty upset. I didn't want another baby—no, nuh-unh. So they sent her. And if they ain't nice, I tell them about it, say, "Look, you find me somebody else." One time since, I been there and I said, "I don't want to talk to her and I ain't telling her my business." But *this* social worker was nice—got me hooked up with the WIC program, and that's a big help. They tell you about different things you don't know about. The social worker talked to me the whole time, even after. It was a lot of help. When I got home they called me on the phone, see how I was. I felt good about it, I sure did.

They're talking about building a smaller hospital, but 525 beds, that's not enough. There's a lot of people go to the County—they *have to* go. And peoples come from all out of town, come to the County. I have sat there talking to them. I've met people, said, "You from *where?*" The hospital could be brand-new, but they need to make it big like it is now. With all them people?!

There's people that walks there, too, don't even have carfare. Especially at the clinic. I've bought a lot of people sandwiches and pops, because they didn't have no money. You'd be surprised the people you talk to in there. They is [big sigh] *hurting*. They *poor*. You be thinking you're poor, it makes you just want to shut up. [softly] A lady said, "I don't have no food, I'm so hungry"—and you can *look* at them and tell if they be jiving. You have to be careful about that too.

Emergency, checkup, whatever, I go to the County. My boy, the one that's fourteen, he got busted in the head, and that's the only place I thought about was the County. We *flew* there. And little Betty got burnt when she was four, on her arm there. Second-degree burn. They help you and show you how to do this and do that, 'cause I didn't know nothing about no burn, no way. They showed me what to do, and I had to do it for them, show them I could do it. They said, "You were supposed to take her to a hospital closer to you"—but I don't think about no other hospital but the County, whatever happens.

Curly Cohen

HE COULD BE A *tense, Chesterfield-smoking longshoreman. In fact, he's a tense, Chesterfield-smoking community activist, currently a resident of the mostly White Bridgeport neighborhood long associated with both mayors Daley (father and son) and with machine politics. He is on the patient-led advisory board of County's Fantus Clinic.*

I'VE BEEN GOING TO COUNTY FOURTEEN OR FIFTEEN YEARS. Dr. Bass is my family doctor: he's watched Michael grow up, and he's watching Zach grow up. I've never had health insurance—I've worked outside the mainstream always. I think, with no insurance, County's just where you went.

For me County is national health insurance, or let's call it "socialist medicine." It's what socialist medicine looks like: there's a ton of people, they give the best care they can give.

I just know from talk that you really get trained well there. How much you can do for two thousand patients a day is questionable. At Pres-[byterian] St. Luke's they have 250 people a month in their ER, and not a block and a half away they have twenty thousand people a month in *their* emergency room. Something isn't quite right about how medicine is distributed in the United States.

I know that if you have no real income and you have no real health insurance, where else do you go where you actually see the doctor and get the medicine you need and money doesn't change hands? That's paradise, isn't it? I think that's paradise. I mean, I've gone to speciality clinics there and you can *wait*. There are times we've waited six or seven hours. And then you go up and they say, "Oh no, we called your name two hours ago and nobody answered..." And you're getting ready to want to murder. [laughs] And so there's that. But just in terms of your basic having a doctor, that's paradise to me.

The Bridgeport Volunteers have an Emergency Assistance Program—low-income heating assistance—and we set up a table at HRD [the AIDS clinic] to help people fill out their forms, and then we set up a table at ASC, the Ambulatory Screening Clinic. There was just a constant buzz. My sense was that part of the problem at County is they have to stop thinking of it just as a health center, and realize that it's a community center where you can get health services. What's the real picture to me is: I'm bringing little Zach in, and there's older women and they're all looking out for him, the nurses are checking on him. You see this rapport between the people who work there and the people who go there. There's also a negative side, and there's tension—but as a whole, it's a community center.

Some clerks are extremely rude. The obvious image is that this is the last-stop hospital. You're here because you got nothing, so I can treat you like a piece of shit. My personal experience is that in a lot of cases you get what you bring to the hospital. I would say there's probably White folks that are already feeling edgy about going to County, and they go there and find themselves in a Black-majority situation and react rather than figure out how to be reasonable. And so I'm sure that tension exists. But 50 percent of the interaction is Black on Black and they don't do enough training so that someone feels welcome—and that's part of good health care, to make someone feel welcome. There's a shithead clerk in Family Practice, and I'll say loud, "I don't want to disturb you from going through your Tupperware book, but..."

I think that, as a whole, the weakness is in patient education. If patients are educated it's better. I like it when a doctor pulls out a book and reads the description of something. You want to give people information, not treat them as though they're mindless. If people had more information they'd figure out better for themselves. A doctor is like a fireman: you can only go after the problem, and so the idea is keeping yourself up. Even as busy as those clinics are, I think the nature of the training should include ways for the teaching physician to train them to be open to listening and talking to the patient.

I was in the Nurses' Residence, and what I really liked was there's this long corridor and graduation pictures of the nurses that they produced. Right around the time of the Second World War it was mostly White, there was maybe one or two Black women in the picture. And then it was half and half—and from then on, it's a majority Black women are graduating. You can see the real pride in the pictures. And I like going in there and seeing those old-time straight-back wheelchairs. It's like out of something else: and the peanut people are going through, and the candy people are going through, and the umbrella people are going through. The newspaper people come, you get your paper. It's just madness. I like it. Some people hate it, but I don't.

Epidemics

Dr. Demetra Soter

IS A PEDIATRICIAN. *Her office is a desk tucked into a corner of a large children's playroom full of, among other things, toys, stuffed animals, a toy kitchen range, and a slide. "I felt like a second-class citizen for a while: Oh, I don't even have my own office...But I looked at some of the offices, and they were dark and dreary, and this is wonderful. My plants are here, my posters, I have windows." By her desk is a bulletin board tacked full with pictures of children she's treated.*

I GREW UP IN CHICAGO. I'M AN ONLY CHILD. MY DAD WAS A doctor, but my mom and dad were divorced when I was young, and he basically had nothing to do with me, so I decided to do pediatrics or be a teacher—to take care of other kids. But teachers get children in gangs. They come in in a gang of thirty, and that's too overwhelming for an only child. If a parent comes into the emergency room with two kids, I don't mind; if they come in with three children, I start hyperventilating. I have to take them one at a time.

My own pediatrician was Robert Mendelsohn—*Confessions of a Medical Heretic* and *How to Raise a Healthy Child—in Spite of Your Doctor.* He was my pediatrician back when he was a traditional old doctor working on Michigan Avenue, and his brother was my pedodontist. My dad was supposed to pay all my medical bills—and he wasn't poor. He was a South Shore OB. When I was about sixteen I was looking through my dentist file and I found out that my dad had refused to pay all my bills. They knew my mom couldn't afford it. She was a single mom, from Greece, working full-time—but still, with child care and everything else...They knew she couldn't afford it, so they never told her that he didn't pay the bill; they just treated me for free. So it was like, where else was I gonna go? Plus, how can you tell somebody, "I'm not going to take care of your child," or "Don't you have the money for antibiotics?" I'd go broke in private practice.

There was no pediatric trauma ten years ago. And over 50 percent of the children in America die of trauma. More children die in America today of trauma—which includes burns, gunshots, falls, car accidents, poisonings, beatings—than everything else combined. These are national statistics. And penetrating trauma has gotten much worse recently, in the nineties. The seventies were a very violent period. The eighties—total, societal, America—were actually very nonviolent. The nineties have just blossomed with gun violence. I don't know about beatings and other things, but the gun violence had a dip in the eighties and it's now coming back up.

After I'd done all this trauma as a medical student, I went into pediatrics, and then I realized nobody knows anything about trauma in pediatrics. If you're lucky enough to go to a hospital where there's a pediatric surgeon, well, that's great, but there's only five hundred pediatric surgeons in America, and most pediatricians don't know anything about trauma. So I did a fellowship in several departments—Surgery, Peds Surgery, Trauma, Burn, and Peds. I also spent a month at Rehab. That's the other thing we don't see in hospitals—we don't see the aftereffects of our head injuries—I thought it was important to get some sort of sense of the whole picture. To us, what's a success story is not necessarily a success story: a child that should have died who survives as a vegetable.

Our families are good at taking care and following up. They do much better than I do. One of my little girls who recently died, she had a severe brain injury. At two years old, Mom beat her. Grandma took care of her. She was blind, deaf, couldn't swallow, but she always came in dressed to the hilt, with her fingernails painted. They just treated her like a normal kid, took her everywhere. Eventually she got too big for Grandma to carry and move—she was six—so they put her in a nursing home, and eight months later she died. The nursing homes can't provide the care of an intense family with lots of people to take care of her. It wasn't a bad nursing home, it's just the nature of…

I didn't plan to do child abuse. I wanted to do trauma and burn: kids that fall out windows and get hit by cars and injured in house fires, where you can work with the family. I finished my fellowship in June, and by the time the County Board approved all my papers it was September or October, and then the holiday season started. People don't handle the holidays well, and it turned out that half my patients were abused—and then I was ready to quit. Pediatric Trauma is a sad thing, and when you add in child abuse, then it becomes a very depressing field. I didn't want to go into a depressing field. I got ready to quit, and then the holidays went, the statistics got better—and I thought I could handle it.

Things have evolved. Like on the Burn Unit—instead of me being the only pediatrician, our children's ICU doctors see all the burn patients. I still do a lot of medical work, but I end up doing a lot of abuse and testifying in court. And we're doing a bunch of teaching. We teach at the Public Guardian's Office, trying to teach them the medical stuff; we teach at the state attorney's office; at other hospitals in the city and the state, teaching other doctors about child abuse. I do it, the people at Children's who do child abuse do it too. I don't want to be classified as somebody who "does" child abuse: I do trauma and burn, and because of it I *also* do child abuse. If I had to do child abuse full-time, I would be committed in an institution.

When you suspect abuse you report it to DCFS [Department of Children and Family Services]. It's up to DCFS to call the police; sometimes they do, and sometimes they don't. For example, we had a child with two skull fractures and a broken arm, and they didn't call the police because they thought it was only *one* skull fracture and a broken arm. When I called back and said, "No, it's two, please call the police," they said "Oh, OK." Most of the children we're talking about are toddlers, and toddlers are basically indestructible.

We had one little girl who fell sixteen stories out of a window, and she survived. She just broke one little vertebra. She was a nasty little two-year-old. [shrilly] "You stuck me!" No, I didn't, but I will if you *want*. [giggles] People think of children as little fragile creatures, and they're not—they wouldn't survive to adulthood if they were.

They did a study with two thousand children falling down a flight of stairs, and of the toddlers, none of them had life-threatening injuries—zero. It didn't matter whether they hit concrete, linoleum, cement, metal: it didn't matter what the stairs were made of. The older children broke arms, legs, but the young children were fine. So if you get a toddler with a couple of skull fractures, you get suspicious. Plus there's great documentation on what happens when an infant falls out of a bed, from studies done in hospitals where there are X-rays. They rarely get skull fractures. What's so nice about doing trauma is that, from the nonintentional trauma, you learn what sort of forces cause what sort of injury.

So we call in a report to DCFS, and they're supposed to investigate or touch base within twenty-four hours. Sometimes they don't do it for a week. One child we have now, the mom kept him at home with his leg contracted to a ninety-degree angle, post burn. For a whole year he couldn't walk, he wasn't at school. DCFS said, "Send him home, and we'll deal with it afterward"—but we said, "No, we'll hold on to him while you do your investigation." They're very overworked. Some kids where we feel they're very safe, we'll send them home, but we try to get them to do the investigation while the child is in the hospital. We'll tell the family we're waiting for DCFS to investigate. Most of the families are cooperative. They may protest, but they don't try and remove the child. And if the family chooses to ambulance-transfer the child to another hospital, that's OK, but most other hospitals don't want child abuse cases, because they just sit there and nobody gets paid anyway.

The ones that try and remove the child, those scare us. If they try to remove the child, if we feel the child's life is in danger, then we'll take custody. It's a legal thing. You call DCFS and say, "This child is in danger, I'm taking custody," and then DCFS has forty-eight hours to present their case in court. But we don't usually have to do that, and we try not to. We don't really want to get into a hostile situation with the parents—we'd much rather work with them. Most of our kids go home, eventually. It's an unusual situation where the children are pulled. Most parents are pretty understanding: they may be angry, but they understand, because they know they've done it.

We lost a baby the other day, four months old. He had a whole bunch of bruises and possibly bitemarks in the genital region. The baby was stiff when he came in; he'd been dead for about six hours. Mom and Dad were pretty together, it was Grandma and Grandpa who were the drug addicts—and they'd left the kid with *them*…It was real hard. It was the most upset I've seen any of our residents. One of our residents threw up, one of our attendings threw up, one just sat there crying. The nurse, she was so efficient, she was so good—and then afterward, I saw the head nurse walking around holding her. She was just zoned. It's very hard for people who have children to deal with it.

Ten years ago, the first time I testified in front of a judge in criminal court, it was about a dead child with bilateral subdural and retinal hemorrhages, and the story was she fell off a bunk bed. When you fall off a bunk bed you're not going to get hemorrhages on both sides, or retinal—there's no question about it. The judge gave the guy four years, but he'd only serve two. The reason the judge gave him that was because, *that* way, the other child would be old enough to protect himself when the guy came home. The kid would be *five* by that time…That same judge now has a good reputation on child cases, so in ten years I guess he's learned, and that's really neat.

And the juvenile courts are better. Before, if you were a judge who was crazy or a pain, they'd dump you in juvenile court because nobody watched over it, nobody cared. Now our judges are different, and they actually care. And now with the Public Guardian's Office, each child who ends up in court—so these are the most seriously injured—has a guardian, a lawyer for the child. There's a lawyer for the state, the state attorney; a lawyer for the parent, the public defender or the private lawyer; and a lawyer for the child. It seems like the first time ever that the women's movement and the children's movement—which used to be together—are coming to odds with each other, because people representing the best interests of the mom no longer always represent the best interests of the child. The National Organization of Women is not necessarily prochild, it's promom. That's why it's so important that the Public Guardian's Office is representing the child.

When Patrick Murphy took over, he started suing DCFS and opening up the courtrooms. Everything regarding DCFS is confidential. If I shoot you in the arm there's a police record, if you shoot your child it's confidential—it's DCFS. Some of our DCFS workers are really hard-working and dedicated, and then there's a few who are really bad. It's such a rotten job: the press hates you, the parents hate you, the children hate you. And you're overwhelmed and can't possibly do your job. You don't want to be in the position of sending someone home who later is killed. We had one where the kid was sent home and came back in burned, and then he wasn't returned to the family. *Then* we heard on the news that the mother and boyfriend killed a neighbor's kid they were babysitting for. It must be worse for the DCFS workers. At least *we've* got a lot of resources; *they're* forced to make medical decisions with not a lot of training and with a lot of pressure to close cases. I don't know why they do what they do, but I'm very happy that they do. I can't imagine a worse job.

I see nonabused kids, but even in our abused kids, most of our kids do pretty well. [pointing out a photo of a sweet-faced boy] His dad had horribly abused him and his brother. Now they're living with Dad's sister, and she's great, incredible. So, there's a lot of good outcomes. The little girl in that picture, she had been stabbed forty-eight times, and her whole family was murdered. She lived for eight hours with her dead mom, dead sister, dead dad...

I still remember that day—I was driving on Lake Shore Drive, stuck in traffic, and I got triple-paged to Trauma. She was conscious. They had to interview her before she went to the OR because she might never make it out. In fact, they lost her pulse and blood pressure in the operating room, so she did essentially die. So here's this little girl with her lungs and intestines hanging out, and I'm sitting there interviewing her. She was the only witness. But she's a success story. She's very bright and doing wonderfully. She's got a wonderful aunt and grandma.

Another kid that we had taken away, he was an asthmatic and whenever his alcoholic dad and his girlfriend would get into a fight the child would start to wheeze real bad. Bring the paramedics in, take him to the hospital, save the family. It happened about ten times, until finally they pulled him and put him in a pretty nice foster home. Now he's eighteen—he's been shot twice, just hanging around the street corners. He says he's not in a gang. [shrugs] So, some are good stories, some are bad.

They can live in foster care forever. This one family where the one child had been murdered, the other had both her legs broken, another had been starved to below birth weight, it's taken eight, nine, and ten years. Those children have been in the same foster home together for all that time, and it's taken this long to terminate parental rights and get them adopted.

I have regular patients too—families who work and have insurance and are loyal County patients, willing to sit in our clinic for all those hours. I think what happened with most of them was, I met them in the Emergency Room at some time or another and they just liked me, the place, and stuck with it. What's funny is that some of my normal patients—when they come into the Emergency Room and say Dr. Soter's our doctor, some of the nurses start looking at them funny, like, "What did you do to your kid?" But the parents all know what I do along with general pediatrics, so they all expect it, and some of them find it funny.

I like it here. I went cross-country skiing in the forest preserve with a friend of mine. Sher took over her daddy's private practice at Lutheran General. She got paged twice, and I got paged twice. Her pages were both the same mom trying to figure out the dose of Tylenol for her kid—healthy—that had, like, 101 fever. One of my pages was from the Medical Examiner's office, and the other was from the Trauma Unit. Even she was willing to say that my pages were much more interesting than hers. I'm glad people want to do normal child care, it's very important—and moms who live in the suburbs need pediatricians too—but I would probably climb the walls. And here, I'm doing some good.

Dr. John Hall

ASSOCIATE DIRECTOR OF *Pediatric Trauma. He's been up all night—on call and busy—and his eyes are pouchy, the whites laced faintly with red.*

I CAME TO COUNTY ABOUT FIVE AND A HALF YEARS AGO. CHICAGO was one of the first cities that mandated a pediatric trauma system as well as an adult trauma system. Dr. Reyes, who is chairman of the department here, is really the person behind that happening, with the Board of Health, at that point. And he asked me to come in to run the Pediatric Trauma Center.

There's a spirit, camaraderie around here, that you don't see a lot of other places. Sure, things are very frustrating, slow to move, it's very ponderous. Things work at County pace, versus the private practice pace. Everybody has a bad day, obviously: the elevator operator has gotten yelled at, and fifteen other people are snotty with everybody else because of it. But the next day they're, you know, fresh and refreshed, and wonderful to everybody. Every day, you'll hear somebody say, "I'm going to quit, I can't take it anymore"—but they're here. I think there's something here that's not seen most places. Most people realize that what they're doing here is needed, and they do a good job of doing it. They're tired, they'd like to do better.

I have two areas of focus. One is, I run the Pediatrics Trauma Center. Dr. Reyes is in charge of it, and I do the day-to-day running of it. I also do general surgery. When I burn out I go back and do hernias and stuff with adults, and relax. For kids I see we have, along with New York City, the highest number of gunshot wounds in the United States. We do kids up to age sixteen. I had one child last week that got shot in the chest, who came in three months before—shot in the chest too. It's frustrating when you see these kids that know they're not going to hit their sixteenth birthday—and they probably won't because of the violence in their area. That's frustrating.

Also, you see, for example, kids that fall out of windows, and we try to present changes as to how to prevent that, ideas to the city and so forth, which have slowly been taken up on recommendations. New York City took the lead with that program, "Children Can't Fly." They made those childproof bars—that the fire department can remove from the outside, but kids can't fall through—and had them put on all the high-rise buildings. We here—also doctors from Children's Memorial and the University of Chicago—have given data to the city to do this, and slowly it's being done. Several of the high-rises have the windows now, and they're planned for all of them—at least for the Housing Authority high-rises. I mean, these people have to have their windows open, because there's no ventilation other than the windows where they live. The rooms are small and their beds are against the window—just because that's where it fits: the kids roll out the bed and out the window. That's frustrating.

And then we see kids that are hit by cars, in car wrecks, and et cetera, et cetera. So, that's what we do here. You get discouraged sometimes. Having thirteen-year-olds or ten-year-olds...I had a ten-year-old with an Uzi. He'd gotten in a machine gun fight with another ten-year-old: they were guarding the turf for a drug dealer. I mean, that's *frustrating*. I think there has to be something done in certain segments of our society where kids get love from home and don't have to go to the gang to get love and attention. Until that time happens, the kids are going to join gangs, because they *do* get the attention and the affection they need from joining. I think that's without a doubt. There's Black gangs, Mexican gangs, White gangs, and we see all of them.

There's a part of society, though, that don't care about their kids. Or, maybe "don't care" isn't right, but are too busy...I had a young boy the other day, fourteen, who was shot. The nurse psychiatrist was talking to him: he's fathered three different kids whom he's not seen, he doesn't care about seeing. To him it's a macho, I'm-a-man image. I have thirteen-year-old girls that have babies whose mothers are twenty-six, twenty-seven, whose grandmothers are thirty-nine. I have seven-year-olds, five-year-olds, taking care of two-year-olds. Some of their moms are stoned-out drunk, but a good majority of their moms work. There's no place else besides *their* mothers, their sisters, their brothers, their older sons or daughters who are wise to the world, for watching their kids. I think that they have to be able to work, but also have to have some type of system where their kids can be watched while they work.

One of the advantages of working at County is that malpractice is far from our head. We give medical care as we think medical care should be given. Tests that are ordered in the private world to cover yourself aren't done here unless they need to be done for the patient's care. I think our health care costs at County are a lot cheaper than elsewhere. One of the things that everybody is praising, the Canadian system, two of their provinces have set up contingency fees for lawyers, which should probably be there: people can go to a lawyer and say, "Hey, if you win you get paid, if you lose you don't get paid." So those two provinces' health care costs are estimated to equal ours in five or six years, while the provinces that don't have that have stayed very low. I think that part the Clinton plan has not focused on.

People who say that malpractice is not a lot of health care costs are just looking at *that* part of it. If you look at the tests that don't need to be done, from an odds basis, if you look at a one-in-a-million case—should *every one* of those million have an expensive, thousand-dollar CAT scan? Can you do something else to help make those odds? In the real world, you have to do that CAT scan on those million people. But here at County we watch and observe them, we can take care of them other ways. We don't have that cost basis, I think. When I worked in Rochester, New York, I saw patients come down from Canada for dialysis because, there, it wouldn't be done because of their age or their health. So yeah, there is rationing of health care. In Canada the CAT scans aren't done on those million people, because, odds are, if you are that millionth person...too bad.

I think that there are some advantages in America. Everybody has access to the best medical care that they can get, on the whole. I personally think that the county hospitals that I've seen give very good medical care, as good as any private hospital I've seen. The problem is that there's a long, long line to get in that door. I think Mrs. Rothstein's plans of opening up smaller secondary centers—clinics—around Cook County is a very good idea—to get those things in faster, and to use the present County as a tertiary referral center for more serious illnesses. Obviously in some places, smaller towns, you can't have a county hospital system, so a second system has to work for the smaller areas, where people can be funded and can get good medical care. But in major population areas, I think county hospitals give better care, because here everybody is equal. It doesn't matter who they are, they get triaged by the severity of illness. And every private hospital I've ever been to, they triage by the wallet as well as the severity of illness—a wallet biopsy.

I think Americans aren't ready for some of the changes. [sighs] Americans feel, "I'm seventy years old, eighty years old and I have a disease, or if I'm thirty years, if I have a disease that's 90 percent fatal, or 95 percent fatal, but there's one chance out of a hundred that I may be cured of it, or have another year of living, then it's my right to have a million dollars spent for that one year." Most managed care countries don't give you that choice. The best for the common good, not for the individual good.

I've had patients that have a *zero* percent chance of living—patients who are in different disease states, or terminally ill—more than a couple of weeks or a month after the disease, yet we pour a lot of money in trying to make them that one exception. Burns, one of the major advances in treating burns is that, in the past several years, it's become recognized: if somebody has 100 percent or 98 percent third degree burn, they're not going to survive. They're usually awake or alert initially after the burn, just because of the state of the injury. Now people are starting to say, "Hey look, Mr. Jones, we can either spend lots of money and try to keep you alive and it's going to hurt like heck, or we can make you comfortable and let you die in peace and dignity without doing that."

And I think a lot of other diseases haven't reached that state yet. And I think that has to be done.

Dr. Roxanne
("Rocky") Roberts

ASSOCIATE DIRECTOR OF *Trauma and director of the Intensive Care Unit. "Every time I'm on call and I'm up all night I think, I'm too old for this. I was on call last night, that's why I look so bad. That thing [points to couch, piled high with sheets, blanket, and pillow] rolls out. So depending on how busy we are, that either rolls out or it stays like that. I got to sleep last night. [laughs] I was very lucky."*

THE FIRST TIME I WALKED INTO THIS BUILDING I WAS SCARED, absolutely scared to death. I was twenty-five then, it was 1980. It's also a cultural difference: coming from Seattle—people are really different on the West Coast than they are in the Midwest. So I was coming from that more mellow, nonaggressive environment into this type of setting, inner-city, multicultural.

My ultimate goal was to be the ideal internist who can operate. The surgeon always seemed to me to be the renaissance doctor. Actually, at County Hospital, that's what the surgeons are pretty much forced to do, because they are primary care doctors, they're not just consultants—so they see the people right as they come in, and they manage all their medical problems as well as their surgical problems.

When I got here, I did general surgery and then rotated through the speciality surgeries; I did that for five years. I did my Trauma rotation in my second year, and that's when I really fell in love with it. Coming up at that time, surgery was very conservative and very closed. Not that people weren't friendly, but as I looked at it, only the exceptional woman really made it to the top in surgery...White male doctors, older and conservative—which made it pretty inaccessible for me, I thought. So when I looked around, a lot of the younger staff people were Trauma people; they were friendly, and it was a very open group. You were given a lot of independence, which I liked, and I felt like what I was doing was important—like *I* was the one who was going to make a difference for this patient. I also thought that there was a real need to take care of these patients, and that violence was just increasing, you know? And that some of the private hospitals were closing their eyes to this problem. I bonded to the patients and to the staff here.

I think we need to take a leading role in prevention—certainly as far as intentional violence, because that's what we see mostly. We used to see people who were shot once who would come in, and that was pretty easy to take care of; *now* you see people with the automatic and semiauto-matic weapons, they're shot ten or twelve times. They're really sick, they're in the Intensive Care Unit for so long. And the really scary thing, too, is that people come back: you operated on them a year ago and they're back, shot again. It's a frequent event, it's not unusual. And that's what really made me think, Jesus, what are we doing? We're patching this guy up, sending him back out, and he's coming back in, shot. The third time he comes in he's going to be dead. That's it: nobody survives more than three of these. It's really terrible. You feel you're not doing anything. In fact, in a very cynical way you're adding to the problem, because you're just sending him back into the same environment to get shot or to shoot somebody else or whatever.

The medical solution wasn't the only thing—it was very frustrating—but also the age of these kids. It really breaks your heart. They're chil-dren—they're *babies*. What's happened is that, in the old days, the gang members used to use, as runners, older kids; now that they've found out that a lot of the sixteen-year-olds are being prosecuted as adults, they use even younger kids. So now you see young kids come in all shot up—even ten-year-olds. It's so sad. The families are so devastated, the parents are so shocked. You know, there's a lot of love in the families.

It seems like, from my culture, which is White middle-class, the fami-lies are small. They don't have the big extended families. Here, you have somebody who is injured, like little Johnny—and, *boy,* aunts and uncles come in, the cousins come in, everybody comes in. It's this big, extended family with a lot of love for this kid. It's very difficult to go out and to talk to some of these families. When they saw this sixteen-year-old kid, he was going out to school and going to meet his friends after school to play basketball or whatever, and then suddenly the hospital calls and says, "You better get in here. Little Johnny's been seriously injured." Last time they saw him he was running around right as rain, and suddenly he's deathly ill.

These kids, everybody sort of thinks that because of the kid's back-ground, they're really assholes or something, nasty people. They're sweet—most of the people that we see here that aren't drunk and stuff, they seem like really nice kids. You just wonder what happened. Did you provoke somebody to do this or something happened that got out of con-trol? What were you *doing,* packing a weapon out on the street? You think, This is a nice kid. It's shocking. It seems like it's almost a culture raised on violence, and that people are a lot less sensitive. I think the more you see guns and people have guns and they're out there...and TV. And young kids don't have the idea that they're ever gonna die; I don't think they connect pulling a trigger with the fact that somebody is going to be seriously injured or dead.

There's a lot of times when patients are very drunk or they're violent when they come in. The hospital staff are not that experienced with tying people down and, in order to take care of the patient—if they're incompetent or violent toward the staff—you really need to take control of that patient. Oftentimes, a lot of these people are calmer once you've put them down, so to speak. A lot of people in shock are actually not very cooperative because their blood pressure is really low, they're not thinking clearly: they're fighting for their lives, and sometimes they're fighting *against* you. So the security officers come up, and they help us. Sometimes just their presence is enough and the people calm down and let us take care of them; other times we actually need to put on physical restraints. They have to be still for us to help them, and they might hurt themselves if they're not. They might have a spinal cord injury and, just by moving around that much and being that agitated, it could be dangerous for them. It's our last resort. We try to spend a lot of time reasoning with the person—it's just wrong to tie somebody up, you know? You'd like to be able to have a nice relationship with them so that they're consenting to their medical care, but sometimes we can't wait for that.

Once the family arrives, then we try to get the family involved: "Can you calm down little Johnny, please? Come in and talk to him, tell him he's going to be OK. Just get him to let us take care of him." The family can really help to calm them down. Grandmothers, mothers—they're the best. We have these great ladies who are actually Patient Care Attendants. They're not really nurses, but they're these Black ladies who are older, who have kids of their own, and they come in and work up here on the unit. I tell you, if you need a surrogate mother figure for some of these kids you just call these ladies over and they come over and whisper in this kid's ear, and they just cool out. Or when you have to tell the family bad news, they're always really good with the family members. They're from the same background culturally, and they can sit there and hug the family and be with them.

When we lose somebody, the doctor is the one that has to tell the family. It's very difficult—it's not like the patient was a grandpa who had bad heart and bad lungs and, yeah, he was going to go any day now. This is a kid who was absolutely, perfectly healthy, just starting their lives, and suddenly they're just...gone. [shudders] Even after all these years, it still gives me chills. I think that's one of the most difficult parts of our job. I try not to cry...Sometimes it really breaks my heart.

A lot of times when the patients come in they're in extremis already, so they're probably unconscious. You don't have time to relate to them like a patient or a person, because you're on automatic pilot, and you're just *boom, boom, boom.* You do your stuff, and you try to save them—and then it's over and you look and you think, Jesus, this kid was probably just finishing high school or whatever. You look at the clothes laying there...And then somebody tells you the family has arrived and you have to go out and talk to them.

When you see the family, it really brings it in. And they tell you, "He just left"—he was going to church or doing whatever he was doing, and suddenly he's gone. And they're angry a lot of times with you, although I'm surprised that we're less a focus of their anger and hostility than I would expect we would be. Really, the families are pretty cool and pretty accepting. That fills me with a sort of gladness...that they can accept us, come into a totally foreign environment—surrounded by most often, a group of White doctors, and most of us young-looking—and have the confidence that we really did the best for their relative. That makes me feel very good. You know, you'd like to be able to save everybody, but that's not the way it works. There are some people who all they can expect is to be on a ventilator the rest of their life. Not that any of us should judge the quality of life that somebody can have, but that depresses me, and I think, Jesus, maybe it would have been better for this person if they just hadn't made it in the hospital or we hadn't been so aggressive. But it's not our call.

In surgery, there's a lot of blood around and because of AIDS...[sighs] I think that certainly it makes me thoughtful and a lot more conscious about the good old days when you used to walk around and you'd be covered with blood and you wouldn't really think about it. The bigger risk is actually hepatitis. Our patient population has a lot of that too. I think we've all become more conscious in taking necessary precautions that we should have been taking all along, but everybody has a heightened awareness about it. And with the new OSHA regulations, we've got plastic booties, impermeable gowns, we double-glove now, we wear goggles. And we wear that stuff even down here in our Resuscitation Area, so we try to protect both ourselves and our junior staff, especially. We're very conscious about needle sticks and picking up sharps and making sure that all of that stuff is taken care of appropriately. During a resuscitation, people are just grabbing, putting IVs in, there are scalpels everywhere—there's a million ways to get injured, so I think we're extra-cautious about that. The group of us know that we're higher risk than most people, and we all sort of deal with it in our own way. All of us have taken precautions and tried to be safe surgeons, if you will. But it doesn't totally eliminate the risk.

I think part of me has become used to the intensity, to all of it, a little bit, which is scary. I always want to remain as sensitive as I can, but part of me gets sort of toughened to it and sort of used to it. I try to think of the stuff that we're doing to prevent this person from coming back in, and the interventions that we're making in a positive way. It still gets to me. But I think every person has their own way mentally to distance themselves, and not to get drawn into the grief of having to take care of these kids who are shot up. You'd be incapacitated if you got swallowed up by that.

I think that, sometimes, when you get beaten down because the volume is just so great, and you're on call a lot, and you're just moving constantly, and it's like, "Jesus, another guy's been shot!" and you're exhausted and you've got to go down and take care of him and spend a lot of hours on your feet…Then you need to have some time off, take a deep breath, take care of yourself. Because if you don't take care of yourself you're not going to be able to come in and give it your all. You gotta guard against cynicism and "this is never gonna end…" "These people"—which is the worst phrase—continue to kill themselves and shoot themselves and here I am, all alone, abandoned [laughs] to hold back the tide. You can get really carried away, and you just gotta stop yourself from doing that and go, "OK, time for a little break."

Places like this, where people would be inclined to be altruistic—they aren't going to come here or stay here for the salaries and that's why we have such a large turnover of our own attending staff. People come here for a couple years when they're young: they get the training that's needed— and that's fine with us, we're happy with that, we realize what's going on— and they move on. We feel like we're spreading the good news. We're spreading the County word and the Trauma doctrine. We're training people and then sending them out to be good surgeons, and hopefully they'll go out of here with a little bit of our attitude about people. Hopefully.

Dr. John May

IMAGINE HIM AS A child and The Andy Griffith Show *comes to mind: he could've been Opie's cousin, or a nice neighbor boy. He is an attending at Cermak Health Services, and he volunteers at the Human Retroviral Disease Clinic at the hospital.*

IN MEDICAL SCHOOL I STARTED VOLUNTEERING AT A SOUP kitchen on the West Side, at Henry Horner Homes. While I was there I met a man who works with street gangs, Brother Tomes—he's employed by Catholic Charities here. He goes out to demonstrate that someone loves and cares for them; he doesn't try to change the gang members or interfere in anything, but he lets them know that someone is concerned about them, interested in their lives and opinions. Once a week I'd work at the soup kitchen, and once a week I'd work with him. We went through Cabrini Green, Henry Horner, Robert Taylor, and so on. I was just outraged to see some of the conditions—probably from relating to my background in Racine, Wisconsin, where things are clean and nice, and coming to Chicago and seeing such inequality and suffering. I remember coming to the soup kitchen and mothers saying, "Oh, there was this stabbing last night, but the paramedics wouldn't come, and we kept calling." Sometimes they come, and the kids throw bottles at them and rocks. Sometimes I'd take the train down there and walk six blocks to the church area and I would be stopped by police officers who'd say, "You shouldn't be out here."

All these things just struck me so…How can this be? And as I then got to know the people who lived there I found some wonderful, beautiful people. People with a tremendous capacity for love and care, who had a lot of hopes—and mostly just a lack of experiences or opportunities that seemed to be responsible in large part for their plight. I developed some good friendships—I guess you have to use the word a little loosely—but relationships, at least, with some of the street gang members and so on. It taught me a lot about the streets and what the realities were.

When I finished medical school I was ready to quit, but what I ended up doing was going to Ghana, West Africa. It was sponsored by AMSA [American Medical Student Association], a program to inspire us to careers in international health. It was a wonderful experience, too, to see poverty in a different way: there everyone is poor—there's some disparity certainly—but overall people are poor *together.* There's a lot of pride. Here in the United States, poverty is really seen as an indignity.

When I returned, I found out about a job at the Cook County Jail as an AIDS educator, a health care educator, teaching the inmates about HIV. I thought, Hey, that sounds nice. I really enjoyed that atmosphere. This was in '89. I started seeing that there were a lot of things I could do if I really completed my M.D. training. All along, I'd been thinking that if I was ever going to do residency, County would be the place. After my residency, I wanted to go back to the jail, but I wanted to keep a tie in with County—which we are at the jail, we're voluntary attendings at County. We rotate through here on ward rotations once a year. And I decided I wanted to keep a tie here even more by coming to this clinic. It's called the HRD Clinic, but it's the HIV/AIDS clinic. I think certainly at the jail that's a big problem, so I wanted to be up-to-date on everything that was happening—we treat at least a quarter of all the HIV-infected persons in Chicago. A lot of the times, we'll initially diagnose someone at the jail, and then it's a shame to just empty them out onto the streets without a follow-up. I'll say, "I will see you at my clinic on Monday at County." We share a real important role there, as far as providing good public health policy. We treat at least a quarter of the syphilis in the city, a quarter of the TB and all that. Those wouldn't be caught otherwise, if we didn't have these screening systems.

Part of what I saw at Cook County all the time was diseases or processes that could have been prevented, such as drug abuse: complications from injectable drug use—abscesses and endocarditis, an infection of the heart which comes from injecting through dirty skin or needles. It will cause the heart to fail, or cause strokes in the brain, lung clots, damaged kidneys. And the treatment of that disease is six weeks in the hospital with antibiotics. When you're a resident, you hate to get the call from the Emergency Room that you're going to have an injectable drug user with a heart murmur and a fever, because you *know* it's going to be endocarditis and they're going to be on your service for six weeks. They're usually not the most pleasant patients in the beginning, because they're withdrawing from their drugs or whatever; and usually they have very poor access to put in intravenous lines. You might have to put in a central line, which requires a lot of extra maintenance. It's really a burden. And it's a large proportion of the patients here. People would just be amazed, if we did a bed count, how many are in here because they're using drugs.

And then alcohol...We have so many complications, whether it's cirrhosis or DTs or aspiration pneumonia from seizures from alcohol. And then a large part are related to smoking cigarettes. And, then, diseases not only related just to lifestyles but to poor access to care: people whose diabetes has never been controlled because they could never get to a clinic properly, people who had high blood pressure untreated for a long time and who then develop a heart attack or a stroke. So it's very sad.

You look at the majority of all the patients that we have treated and you think, There probably could have been a way this could have been prevented. Then you look at the enormous effort that you personally have to invest, that the hospital invests, that the taxpayer invests, and realize there has to be a better way. In our primary care, we did a lot of domestic violence. We started talking to our female patients about abuse and seeing how that may play into symptoms of their illnesses. And one day I heard a lecture about trauma as a health problem, and suddenly it all sort of clicked: we need to address the gunshot problem and violence as a disease, and not discount these young men coming in with bullet wounds.

I was impressed how, if we got an alcoholic patient admitted to the hospital with an aspiration pneumonia, the standard of care was that I would sit down and talk to them about their alcoholism before discharge; or have a social worker talk to them about A.A. or so on. But then I noticed in the Trauma ward, you get a young man admitted to the hospital with a gunshot wound, basically they'd patch him up and send him out the door, quite often to get shot again. And these weren't nameless faces that I would see in the Trauma ward: they would be some of my friends that I knew from the West Side. Through these years now, I've known five people from there who've been killed. So that's been my new push, that we can do this from a public health perspective. Actually, for an African American male, aged ten to thirty-four, homicide is the number-one cause of death. And so why am I going to sit and talk to a young man from the West Side about cholesterol when he has a very high chance of being shot. And, certainly, all my training in medical school was about that—cholesterol and exercise and heart disease, and *not at all* appropriate and relevant necessarily for the day-to-day lives of everybody I see.

I did a study where we counseled young men coming into the ASC [Ambulatory Screening Clinic] with whatever problems. Usually it was a skin rash or an STD or an upper respiratory infection. And while they were there we counseled them about six preventive medicine issues: smoking, drinking, drugs, safe sex, seat belts, and firearms. And at the end of the visit someone interviewed them and asked, "What do you remember that the doctor talked to you about?" And the thing that they remembered most was the guns, the firearms. And the thing they remembered second most was safe sex. And those are the number-one and -two causes of death. The age group was sixteen to thirty-four! At that time, that was the number-one cause of death for *that* group—now it's ten to thirty-four. It wasn't even that you had to say that much—just to bring up the issue of guns, or, "Have you ever been shot before? Do you carry a gun?" Suddenly the patient became more engaged, more interested, they sensed that you were caring.

And we were saying, "Not that *I* can change anything or make a difference here." We know the problems are so large, and a lot of it has to do with poverty and racism and the whole field, but *you* yourself have some individual control over the situation. I always used the analogy: "You might not think we have any control over whether we're in a car accident or not, but certainly we do. We cannot drive drunk, we can obey the traffic laws, and so forth." We still might get hit out of the blue, but we do have *some* control, and the same is true with gunshot wounds. If you have a gun or carry a gun you're much more likely to be shot; the same is true if you use drugs or sell drugs, if you use a lot of alcohol. Most people are shot by someone they know—usually you're in a fight or in an argument. All those things are preventable. I think just to start raising the awareness, eventually it's going to start having an effect. Words from a physician evoking care and concern may ring in their minds for some time and may effect, eventually, behavior. Smoking, too, or drunk driving: We've been able to make inroads in those things, and it's due to the sort of full-court press of a public health approach to these issues.

I attended conferences and talked to people, and one thing I found with all the interest in this issue is that I didn't see any messages out there about it. In fact, the only messages that society does provide *promote* violence—movies, television, and so forth. I did some work at Austin High School during my residency program, and I saw signs on the wall like BRUSH YOUR TEETH, and on exercise and nutrition, but they weren't right for the kids. So I decided we need to develop some messages about violence and violence prevention. I got some of my friends together, and we decided to start our own little company, develop some posters, and try to promote them to clinics and schools throughout the country. We finally developed eight posters.

The signs went up a month ago on buses and trains. How it affects people individually, we haven't been able to measure exactly. But any time I see a young person and they see the posters and we talk about them, they know what the message means. And I think they're somewhat comforted that society is finally announcing that gun use and violence are not acceptable anymore, and in fact are preventable. It shows that society cares about this problem: we're not going to just throw our hands up and let you get shot every night. One time I was riding on a bus on California Avenue, I sat behind a young boy and his mother, and one of the signs was up on the bus: it showed two hands shaking, with the caption PEACE IN, and right below it is written PIECE OUT, with a gun and a line through it. He was about five years old, and he pointed to the sign. Now, he could have pointed to any sign on the bus, but he pointed to *that* sign, and he said, "Mama, what does that say?" She was somewhat preoccupied and just said, "Oh, it means don't play with guns." But he kept looking at it, and it hit me that this young boy knew that message was for *him*, you know?

Dr. Ron Sable

COFOUNDER OF THE *Sable/Shearer Clinic at County and a tire-less activist: against war and for social justice, human and civil rights, and public health care. When we speak in June of '93 he is forty-seven, HIV-positive, and feeling the effects of the disease. He coughs often, but his eyes are clear and bright—the kind of blue you'd want to find lapping at the sand on a South Sea island.*

I WAS BORN AND RAISED IN KANSAS CITY. IN 1968, I HAD APPLIED for and got a kind of conscientious objector status that is peculiar, where you serve in the military—I was a medic. I came back from Vietnam pretty discouraged about the value of doing anything. It seemed like there was a kernel of genuine worth in medicine, and so I sought to do that. I didn't like medical school very much. I felt kind of out of it, and I was beginning to deal with being gay—I came out in medical school.

When I first came to work at County in '76, Quentin Young was the chief of Medicine. In my internship I was still interested in family prac-tice, but my friend, Naomi Kisten, had this notion that we should do a shared-time internship. In 1976, this was fairly pioneering. We were selected for one job slot, and for two years we worked alternate months; we split the salary and both got a package of benefits. I think most people feel that you can't learn without suffering, but for me, after the army, I felt like this was my real life right now: I wanted to have time for living.

In '81, I finished my training and became an attending. I worked half-time at the jail, and the other half of the time I worked at Fantus Clinic, doing outpatient care. I met my current lover, and the first report about what ultimately came to be known as AIDS came in June or July of '81. Within a couple of years, we started the clinic here—there was that much work to do. I got drawn into the electoral stuff—ran for alderman in 1987 and 1991—and I started cutting back on my time at the jail. From '87 on I've just been at the hospital, where I work part-time.

A big part of why I chose to work at a public hospital was derived from my belief that health care is a right. *Nobody* should be turned away because they can't pay. Certainly, I felt very strongly about the AIDS pro-gram in that regard—that people were here with difficult, complex prob-lems. Some come by choice, but many come because they have no place else to go. I think we all feel strongly that they deserve as good care as anybody else. In many ways—in terms of the medical expertise and all—

that does happen. I mean, it's still not a pleasant experience to be hospitalized here. And, speaking as someone who's taken care of people in the hospital here and has himself been hospitalized at other places, it ain't the same. We have room to go there. But the Clinton administration we're dealing with now is light years improvement in that regard.

The first case of AIDS showed up in the General Medicine wards. It was a pretty complicated and puzzling case: the guy was in and out of the hospital over a period of time. Renslow Sherer had a lot of the early cases assigned to him. I guess, by '83, there were enough people who needed someplace to be followed that we said, "Let's do this clinic." In 1983, Renslow and I pretty much did everything: we saw the patients at the clinic in one clinic session. We called it the Sable/Sherer Clinic, to identify it without stigmatizing it.

From early on, some of the patients' needs were clear: they had not just complicated medical problems but also legal problems, housing problems, employment problems, all that stuff. And so, making sure that your service either had access to or could directly provide all those things was something that was always on our minds.

County's administration at that time didn't do anything to support us: the program was basically built with grants from outside, and County didn't have to contribute. I think they were as reluctant as any other hospital to get labeled as an "AIDS hospital," or to accept the public responsibility for that. New York has been overwhelmed, and it's sort of crushed under the weight of this and many other problems. San Francisco was always looked to as the model, because you had a much more open and sympathetic government structure, and a lot of people who came together in the community to raise money and provide services—education as well as care services. But I think we sort of beat our heads against the wall, dealing with a lot of public officials, in the state, the city. The county...I'm not sure how distinct the effort was at the county level. I don't think we ever expected very much, and therefore we didn't push.

In 1987 they basically tried to fire a doctor who had AIDS. It had been known for some time by many people here that he was sick. There's such a progressive and enlightened viewpoint in virtually all of the Department of Medicine—and in most of the other departments—that I don't think there were any serious questions, even in 1987, about the safety of his continuing to practice. It was typical of that administration, coming down on somebody or behaving in an inappropriate manner. He fought it with the ACLU's support, and he won—but by the time the case was actually settled, he was pretty sick, and I'm not sure he ever worked beyond that.

By contrast, the way I've been treated by the administration here has been like night and day: people are bending over backward to accommodate me. There was never any question about continuing employment or seeing patients if I wanted to. And this administration has held our program up as a center of excellence, instead of pushing it aside and not paying attention to AIDS programs.

I had a General Medicine clinic—diabetics and hypertensives I've been taking care of for fifteen years—and the rest of it was HIV. I'm out of the clinic work now, and sort of being a consultant, trying to make our clinic work better—that's my first task. The patient care at the time was very draining and, at a certain level, risky: I got tuberculosis last year. Thankfully, it was the regular, garden-variety kind that was sensitive to drugs; there's some very bad, very nasty TB out there. It's a concern for health care workers generally whether their patients are infected with TB or not, but in particular HIV-positive workers have a major vulnerability. And working in an HIV clinic, with its population, there's a much higher incidence of TB. So, for those reasons—but primarily because of the way I was feeling—I knew it was time to change the focus of my work.

A lot of the people who are drawn to AIDS work are infected with HIV and know they're infected—I think that's always been the case. [softly] It probably provides some additional strain, but I don't know...I guess there's just ways that you figure out to protect yourself, to build up some defenses against—you kind of distance yourself from a certain part of it. It's like anybody who takes care of terminally ill people: you can't feel every loss in the same way. It's too much.

In many ways, one of the biggest tragedies of AIDS is that it arose just as Ronald Reagan was being elected for the first time, and it suffered from the neglect—the grotesque neglect—of that administration and the one that succeeded it. And there's *still* this notion that sex is bad and dirty, and abstinence...you know, "Just say no." It's so obviously inadequate and wrong that it's incredibly sad this view has prevailed.

The rhetoric you hear about how the government has blood on its hands because of AIDS deaths that could have been prevented is not rhetoric—that is *absolutely* true. Jesse Helms is directly responsible for deaths of hundreds if not thousands of people, because he blocked the funding for prevention messages. And the messages that *were* funded were framed in a way that people couldn't even understand what they were saying. [sighs] But hopefully it's something of a new day. Certainly, the people in Washington who are very involved with this feel that having a president who knows people with AIDS and who is publicly employing people with AIDS...that's a big step.

Frankly, I don't feel very optimistic at the moment. We're years away from a vaccine; there may never really be a cure. More and more people, I think, realize this as a chronic disease to be managed—hopefully for many years—but never eradicated as a virus. If you look at it from a world perspective, this virus is decimating Africa, and this incredible epidemic is poised to decimate India and other parts of Southeast Asia—

where people have a tiny fraction of the resources that we have to deal with it. It's a major problem that's going to be with us throughout all of our lives. And it's probably only the beginning.

I think we're probably entering an era where it won't be bacterial infections that are the problem, it'll be viral. There's a lot of other weird viruses out there, and some of them remain hidden—especially in jungle and rainforest areas, where there's a complex ecology, there have been devastatingly deadly outbreaks. Most of them have been very confined to one village or one group of people, but there are some other nasty critters out there, and they just aren't...we don't have people in contact with them.

This virus is spread by sexual contact and through blood, and it probably broke out of what was some confined area and spread. But we're not at the end of the millennium: we have to deal with the fact that man lives in a still hostile environment, in some ways, and that there are no magic bullets. You know, you can't intervene *here* without there being a consequence *there:* we're part of an ecology that includes viruses, that includes plants and animals and whatever. And AIDS is not God's punishment. I don't know, and I hate to say it, but I'm not terribly optimistic. At least, in the immediate future, there'll be more and more cases, it'll be more and more stress to provide for their needs—and it'll be probably a few years before we have more effective treatments for this.

We have memorial services every three to six months for anybody who wants to be a part of it. There are times when we've read lists of names. There's usually a place where they have a kind of banner and people will come up and write names of friends that are important to them. And those banners have been kept. It's just a pause to reflect on people you've cared for and people who are no longer here. I think they do what they're supposed to do—give people a moment to pause and reflect on all this.

I think these kind of events, like the AIDS Quilt, are a very powerful message. Working on the quilt at different times, it was very powerful: I felt like I was individually memorializing all of these people. It personalizes it in a way. It's not just a disease, it's people—real people.

Ron Sable died of AIDS on December 30, 1993.

Dr. Mardge Cohen

DIRECTOR OF THE WOMEN and Children's Project. She is petite and powerful, and seems, even seated, to be moving forward at breakneck speed. She and her County Hospital–employed husband, Dr. Gordon Schiff, have two children. "It's a little too rushed than you'd want anybody's life to be—especially when I see the kids rushing. [laughs] I said to my daughter, 'You're a little too tense, you take things a little too seriously.' And she said in all seriousness, no irony, 'Where did I learn that from? How did I get like this? How did I learn to be so intense?' [laughs] I didn't discuss nurture and nature with her at all. I said, [totally hyper] 'Let's just figure out how to be less intense.'"

I CAME TO COUNTY TO DO AN INTERNAL MEDICINE RESIDENCY in 1976. I've been here seventeen years all total this June 30th. For the last five years, I've been doing a lot of work with women and children with HIV infection. We created a program here which certainly was unique when it was started, and now it's been replicated in many other places—to take care of families with HIV infection in one site, with a multidisciplinary, multicultural grouping of people, and to care for the medical and pyschosocial problems that families with HIV have.

When the HIV epidemic started growing during the 1980s, it became clear that the majority of people affected by HIV—which were men—lost their insurance, and they needed to come to a public sector–type place. The public sector all over the country was bearing the burden of HIV disease. There were fewer women and children at that time—there still are—but those women and children often were going to hit the public sector first. They weren't going to lose their insurance, because they never had any to start with.

Ninety percent of the pediatric patients are kids of color, 80 percent of the women are women of color—so you were talking, from the beginning, about a group that never had access to other institutions. And some of the community-based HIV groupings that are more accessible to people were started, for the most part, by gay men on the North Side of the city. That wasn't where women from the South and West sides—who spoke Spanish, or who used drugs—went. And even if they found the way there, when they got there they found the issues a little different from theirs: it wasn't issues of "How do I take care of my kids?" or "How

189

do I get the Department of Children and Family Services [DCFS] off my back?" It was about how to use alternative nutrition.

So it was very clear that women and their kids would be coming to a place like County. The disease in women was framed as a transmission issue: "Women pass it on to men, let's worry about the men." They could pass it on to their children, too, so we should prevent *that*. But what about the women themselves and the disease? It absolutely reflects what was and *continues* to be medicine's approach to women's health.

We found that the women were just like any other mothers: they cared about their kids, and they'd bring them back and forth. So they didn't have the time and energy to *then* figure out how to get their own care in another setting—more appointments, plus all the psychosocial appointments, all of the entitlement appointments...People had figured out that there were twelve to fifteen needs that had to be filled by different agencies. They'd have to go from one part of the city to another—it couldn't even be done in one area. And that's daunting to people, especially if they're sick.

In July of 1988, we started seeing the first patients in the clinic with the idea of building a program in mind. We were able to access private money: we got a grant that began in March of '89 and lasted for three to four years, and that allowed enormous growth, with more staff. So we've now served over 850 people—families with HIV infection. Thirty-one people do the work, and, of those, four are employed by Cook County Hospital, twenty-seven are grant funded. Public hospitals have had the large burden of HIV care, and because there was private funds available from the artistic community, the gay community, there have been partnerships. You know, cardiovascular surgery isn't run on soft money; people don't have to sit and write grants. It takes a lot of time, and I think that's a ridiculous approach to providing health care to people.

The disciplines of obstetrics and gynecology, pediatrics, family practice, infectious diseases, internal medicine, all come together to deliver comprehensive care providers to the women and children, families that we see. Probably always—but I think, with HIV, it's particularly important to have a real strong team approach, because, emotionally, it's a wipeout to deal with...To have other people helping is a way to have people stay with it. And the clients have so many needs it's better to have more than one person trying to fill them.

For people who are infected, we offer a full range of services. It means the kids see the doctor, their partners see the doctors, there are psychologists, case managers who do all the entitlements—like getting on public aid, getting on disability, getting your phone, your utilities, getting a house, getting food, transportation back and forth—basic needs. Ten to 15 percent are homeless, 20 percent don't have a telephone. We have a lot of Spanish-speaking workers at every level. Our approach is to have all those services available at a single site—a *very crowded* single site.

An enormous amount of health education happens for people at Cook County Hospital. We've staffed the Obstetric and Gynecology wards—so, for everybody at risk either in terms of drugs or sexually transmitted diseases, or with an interest in HIV education and counseling, it's available all the time on those wards. Testing and counseling is available. We staff those wards, the Prenatal Clinic, the Outpatient Clinic for Sexually Transmitted Diseases—we're on call for anybody else who needs to be seen. We have a special person who does adolescent work in the schools: she trains kids specifically to be peer educators themselves, as well as doing general education for the local school council and the faculty and kids in large settings. That's a very exciting part of it. Plus we get speaking engagements all the time for everywhere. We also train peer educators—we've trained more than seventy-five women, most of whom are infected. The women are just dynamite at what they do, and are the most effective at getting the message out in almost every setting you can think of.*

We also have a support group. We've seen an enormous amount of strength that individuals have gotten from the group, to the point where we think it's an essential item in delivering care to women with HIV. People are still very isolated about it, and many women have told nobody else that they're infected. And we've seen them then be able to go to the agencies and the Department of Children and Family Services and disability and so on, and demand what they're supposed to get. We have a caretaker support group for people who are taking care of those who are infected; we have a Spanish-speaking women's support group. We have a parenting class—because a lot of them had their kids taken away because they were in abusive situations or they were abusive or used drugs, or whatever it was. They get told they're infected, many get their lives together, stop using, and want to reunite with their families. They said, "If you start a parenting class for us so that we could show that we were serious then maybe they'll let us..." And we did. DCFS funds some of that.

At County, I'm also in the Division of General Medicine: I supervise patients on the wards, I have my own clinic of General Medicine patients I've been following all the years I've been here, and I do all the regular

---

* Sonia R., a peer educator for the program, talks about the experience: "The first time we didn't get anybody—nobody was interested. At first I was, [tentatively] 'Hello, my name is So-and-so, would you like to...and it's really for your own good...'" After a while I'm thinking, No, these women are going to be going home, laying in bed, back here in nine months—and they ain't going to know *diddly-squat* about what they're letting come in and out of them. So I was, [firmly] 'And I need you to come back to the end of the ward here, and I'm going to do HIV/AIDS 101 with you, which means I'm going to educate you a little on basics. I'll be waiting for you back there. I'm getting everybody.' And you know, you get a lot of these women, street smart, they give you that look. Some of them would end up going to the bathroom and staying there, hiding. I don't know if it's denial, 'if I don't know about it it's not going to hurt me.' But a lot of them were very open to it."

teaching stuff. I like all of it. It's a real privilege, and I think that might not be possible at other places. I'm part of that crew that came because Quentin Young was here, and I think, coming as a group, you didn't feel isolated—like you were the only one who cared about this stuff, or you were special, so therefore everybody else wasn't.

There's a lot of ways that this stuff measures out. It's important if you're doing it in a more collective fashion—which was just a given, at that point—that allows people to maintain a lot of energy and spirit and commitment. The place has that mentality of "we're the underdog, and we're all in it together," so that always brings its own kind of spiritual energy.

Dr. Mark Sherman

HAS A SKITTISH MANNER. *While speaking, he frequently waves his hands and arms around and jiggles in his seat.* "Sometimes I wonder why I'm working here, the amount I make. Why am I working for so little? But then when I look at how many poor people there are in the world, it's like, "Well, I'm rich!" Someone told me I have to stop comparing myself to the Third World." *[laughs] He is a psychologist.*

I'M ORIGINALLY FROM CHICAGO, AND I GREW UP IN THE CITY ON the North Side in the "Gilded Ghetto," the Jewish neighborhood in the city. I went away to school, and traveled around as a hippy for a while. Once I finished my Ph.D., my research, I thought, OK, what am I going to do now? I started looking around for jobs and there was a job here. This was in 1979.

It's not like I wanted to work here. I thought, Oh, I don't want to work there, it's just going to be…[scrunches up face] I came here because I thought it was good to go on job interviews and polish up your interviewing skills and I got real energized by this place. I said to my friends, "I'll work here for a year or two, it'll be a good experience, exciting and stimulating, and then I'll figure out what I'm going to do next."

At the end of '83, Ron Sable was talking about the AIDS clinic he and Renslow Sherer had just set up. He asked if I was interested in working in the clinics with them, setting up groups for people dealing with AIDS, their families, lovers, professionals, people in the community—and I did it.

This place is at a certain level of chaos. Part of the frustration of County is space, at the Sable/Sherer Clinic and everywhere: there's not enough space, and what space we do have is inadequate. Essentially, with the ethics of my profession, I probably shouldn't be doing a lot of what I do here, because there's no confidentiality in a lot of the settings: in the clinic I'm in with Ron,* there is no room for me—I, like, hang out in the hallways. Depending on my mood, I am into it, I find it frustrating, insulting. [laughs] Whatever. And some of what I'm supposed to do, I won't do. Because to me I won't ask certain people certain things in the hallway. I just don't think that's right, I just don't think that's respectful. A lot of people I know who've left here, some have left because of that: "I don't want to treat patients that way, and I don't want to treat my profession

---

* At the time of this interview, Ron Sable was alive.

193

that way." Even *this* office is considered a prime office, just because it's an office—because it has a door [laughs] and on a hallway that's quiet!

With what my work is, I think it's harder for the M.D.s and the primary care people: my goal isn't to cure that person, so I think I have a less difficult time in some ways. I'm trying to help people—whether it's HIV, AIDS, or any other situation—deal with what their life situation is and deal with their feelings about it, come up with some solutions, help them move on. So it's a little easier for me, because I'm not trying to make them well physically. But it's still frustrating and difficult at times.

It's this cycle—my cycle: sometimes it's much harder, sometimes not as hard. I'm in a difficult cycle now, because some of my co-workers have died or are sick, and that's not easy. [long silence] It's not easy. I care about my patients and get involved with them, sometimes too involved with them. I thought, Well, this should be easier. But obviously, there's a big difference between people in your life and people in your work life: there's some kind of protective thing people do, whether they're aware of it or not, with their patients. I know that now. The bottom line is that they're not in my life in the same way that colleagues and friends and family are. It's hard when people you care about die—and I've felt that with patients too—but it's real different when you lose someone that's more in your life.

There's a certain kind of thing we all probably do, which we're not aware of, because we know these people are sick and are probably going to die at some point. And, depending on where you get involved with them, it may be closer than not; I know with other people in my life who've gotten sick, it's been harder for me, because this isn't supposed to happen—they're not my patients. [laughs] And there's been some interns that have told me they're HIV-positive, and I've had a more difficult time dealing with them than with other people. The same with some co-workers. It's not supposed to happen.

I've gone through extremes at times of, "Nothing is important, so whatever I determine is important is important." It does help you to be much clearer on priorities and what you do and don't want to do. But sometimes just the opposite—sometimes it's like, "I just don't care. Do you want to go to a movie, do you want to stay home? I don't care—none of it matters. I don't care what restaurant we go to, I don't care what movie we go to. I don't care." I sit here. [slumps back in chair] I don't like when I'm in that stage, but I have been in it.

One of the frustrations of working in this, for me, is that AIDS just keeps spreading and spreading and spreading. People don't like thinking about drugs and people using drugs and shooting with needles. And they don't like thinking about sex and different kinds of sex and talking about safe sex and...This society is *so* hung up—and it is *this* society, it isn't "the world." I don't even think it matters at this point whether you think it's OK to give out needles or whatever: just decide and do something.

But this country, everyone likes to pretend that this really doesn't exist—or if it does, it exists down over there, around the corner, in a neighborhood you don't have to deal with. And in other countries—countries that acknowledge they have a problem with drugs and either give out needles or have treatment programs—they have ads on buses and on TV and everywhere, in schools and...But here, when the patients want to go to a treatment program, there isn't one. It's crazy!

County attracts lots of people for different reasons. Some of them are very committed to the concept of this place and treating people that can't get treatment other places, and some people are just collecting a check. It's part of what makes this place a difficult environment, because it's such extremes. I'm sure that's true in most places, but it's *certainly* true here, and sometimes it feels like the extremes are, well, more extreme. There are some people here who, I think, are near sainthood in how they are and how they treat people, how they are professionally—and that makes the other extreme seem worse. But part of what I love about this place is—and when I was talking about all the great people that work here, I didn't mean just the medical people: some of the soul of what this place *is* are the elevator operators and the Transportation people and the people in housekeeping...

There's this woman on the AIDS unit in Housekeeping, and one of the patients just went on and on about how the most important person to him was this woman in housekeeping, who every morning had a smile and would open the blinds and say, "Let God's light in." She was just full of energy and joy and caring about patients. And that goes up and down, all the strata of people here. And that is part of what's great working here—the people you run into who are like that.

Dr. Bob Cohen

ATTENDING, PULMONARY DEPARTMENT. *When called about the interview he says, referring to hospital administration, "They don't usually send anybody to talk to me"; when told they* haven't *sent me, he's incredulous. "You mean they haven't asked for a list of who you're interviewing?!"*

I CAME TO CHICAGO TO GO TO MEDICAL SCHOOL AT NORTHwestern and saw what very wealthy, elite medicine was like. I met a professor there and he was very active in INCAR, the International Committee Against Racism, and the Progressive Labor Party. He started explaining some things politically that opened my eyes, and then suggested that I come over to County and take a look at it here. So I got on the El [elevated subway] and came over here to do a clerkship, and I've been here since 1981.

My feeling is that, as a communist, my main purpose isn't in being a doctor—my main purpose is to organize people and try and fight for a communist revolution and fight for a better world. I'm not going to be able to do that as a private practitioner in business, because I'm not a businessman. So if I am going to do it, I've got to be at the best place for a doctor—and there aren't many places. It's very difficult, I think, for a doctor to be an organizer—certainly if you're in private practice or at a little hospital. I thought that a hospital like Cook County—which is multiracial, its house staff from all over the world, a very integrated work force—that this was the place to come. Also, it's a place where health care is really not very good, and there are lots and lots of weaknesses that need to be fought.

The membership of INCAR has grown quite a bit. We have hundreds of members here, and we have a publication, the *INCAR Arrow;* it comes out every payday. It's come out now for ten years. People just call it "the paper." It's got articles and letters written by hospital workers about their jobs, about what's happening to them—their complaints, their hopes, their struggles. And then it has editorials: the editorial committee writes about what they think is going on in health care, world issues. It's very, very popular among the hospital workers, from what I can tell. Even the guys from Buildings and Grounds, who tend to be mainly White workers—political patronage employees, some of them— all pretty good guys: they used to not touch it with a ten-foot pole, now they read it avidly. And administration sends their secretaries and folks down to get one, to make sure they have one. It's really become the voice of the workers at the hospital.

We've been able to organize patients to come to demonstrations, to fight for more staff. We have patients that are members of INCAR, and we have patients that contribute to the newsletter often. A lot of times, the nursing staff or hospital staff will solicit articles from a patient if something bad happens.

INCAR tries to build up an organization that is multiracial, international, that has all professions except for administration—we don't want bosses in our organization. One of the things we do, one of our main issues—aside from fighting and organizing people to protest for better job conditions—is fighting for more staff. Jobs is the number-one thing here at the hospital. I think that INCAR would take the position that the hospital is mainly run by the people that actually *do* the work: the dietary workers, Transportation, Housekeeping, Nursing. Less so the doctors, they don't tend to do as much useful work, they just *organize* work. And the hospital administration, their big thing now is a new hospital—well, we don't need a new hospital as much as we need to have the old hospital *staffed*. They're going to build new buildings and tear this down. They love contracts and patronage, but they don't like to hire workers that actually do the work. That's one of the main things that we've fought for over the years, and we've been able to build a base of support for it among all these workers.

We do social activities, to try to get people to know each other and trust each other, because the main way the hospital administration prevents us from doing things is by splitting Filipino nurses from Black nurses, or splitting RN from LPN, or LPN from nursing assistant, which we call PCAs here. They've been able to get Indian therapists to fight Black respiratory therapists; they've been able to engineer all these racial and job differences between work forces and emphasize them. Sure, they existed already, but the administration tends to favor one group a little bit to get anger and discontent, and we try to break that down. One of the ways that we do this is by social activities like the bowling league, or we have a talent show we put on every year, which is attended by hundreds of people. We have doctors getting up there and trying to sing, or Housekeeping workers and Dietary putting on a show.

The hospital has a horrible history of encouraging racial tension. What they do is pick, say, a nursing coordinator of whatever race and then they tend to try and hire only that group of people from that unit. It used to be seen a lot in the intensive care areas. For example, Trauma has a history of being mostly White nurses. The Burn Unit used to be run by a Black guy, and it used to be mostly Black nurses; the MICU [Medical Intensive Care Unit] was run by a Filipino woman, and it used to be all

Filipino nurses. Wherever you had a boss of one particular race or other, they tended to give favors to that particular group, and that created tension among the other people.

There's one good example where we were able to break that down—the MICU, in '85, when we were able to organize the nurses to refuse overtime to protest the horrible staffing. They had one nurse with three or four ventilator patients at a time. We put out a newsletter that was in Korean, Tagalog, English, and organized all those nurses; a committee that included Black, Korean, and Filipino nurses refused overtime, demanding one nurse for one patient.

We have very corrupt and some horrible supervisors in some areas who do this playing of worker against worker—using race and all kinds of things—and the administrations do nothing about it. INCAR says that the only race is the human race, and we really firmly believe that racism is the biggest thing holding us back. I think you can see that here at the hospital, how race is used to divide people. We do everything that we possibly can to overcome that.

The only other organizations are union. I think there are seven different unions, maybe more, and they're all organized by job—and the jobs, generally, are all segregated by race. The majority of the RN staff is Asian; there are some Black RNs. The majority of LPNs are Black. Hospital workers in Local 46, one of the main unions representing the hospital workers here, are mostly Black workers. So the unions are fairly stratified by jobs, and there isn't that much crossover. And certainly across the professions, the unions have *no* interest in organizing any kind of industrial union—in other words, *all* the hospital workers together in the same union.

We've actually tried to organize an INCAR union here, with some level of success. We're calling it the Anti-Racist Union, the ARU. And we actually got enough signatures to certify an election against Local 46—which is mainly Housekeeping, Dietary, Transportation. They took us to court, saying that we were a company union, because I am an attending physician, and as an attending I represent administration. We brought in hospital workers who testified that, far from me being able to coerce on the part of the company, they thought it was a liability to be seen talking to me. [smiles]

The unions here are very political and, often, what I would call "company unions." It depends on which one, but unions like Local 46 are historically Democratic Party–controlled unions, and they were the main vehicle for giving out patronage jobs at Cook County; they still are. So those unions, we would fight them openly. Some of the other unions are trying to fight a little bit more—but there aren't very many of the unions here that are particularly radical. *Strike* is a dirty word, and in general they just fight for a few pennies, wages; they don't fight against layoffs or things like that.

They recently had a huge cut in jobs, in May, with an early retirement incentive—and they eliminated, I don't know, somewhere between five hundred and a thousand jobs. In order to pay for more administrators and for studies of new hospitals and things like that, they're eliminating jobs! If they build this new 525-bed hospital, they'll pay for it through job cuts. Then they'll have a beautiful hospital that somebody got contracts to build, and there won't be anybody left to work there. They have all the big doctors around here getting on TV and talking about how wonderful that is and how terrible it is that the plaster here is peeling, but the fact is they've rehabbed this hospital enormously. They've put a huge amount of money into the Trauma Unit, the ER, they've got brand-new Burn, Neonatology. They've got some beautiful areas. They put millions of dollars into new fire-control devices, they've got pipes and sprinklers. You can do things in an old building. The bottom line is the workers. But they do like to build things, because they raise bond issues which gives interest to investors and bankers, and contracts to political contributors.

I think the public hospitals are pretty political in general. I know some people who work at L.A. County Hospital—people in INCAR, actually—and some people in the New York hospitals, but Cook County is right up there: it's very intimately tied in with the county politics and city politics. So you learn a lot about politics working here. There's enormous stress put on the hospital right now in terms of infection control, because Governor [Jim] Edgar controls the Illinois Department of Public Health—which is the inspecting agency—and he's running, in the primary, against [Richard] Phelan, who is the County Board President. So they're inspecting the hell out of County for infection control, which maybe isn't bad; maybe we'll get some infection control done.

But anyway, a new hospital is good business, but lousy for...I mean, it *would* be nice to have a new building—if they gave us a new building *and* the workers to staff it, with all the beds that we needed, that would be wonderful. But I'm not going to hold my breath for the new hospital. As a lung doctor, I know *that,* physiologically, is not a good idea—I might die first.

I've been taking care of tuberculosis as a specialist since '85. The lowest rate of TB incidence, nationally, was 1985. After that came the resurgence of tuberculosis—due to poverty, homelessness, unemployment—as well as coinfection with AIDS—which has all come together to make this epidemic spread like wildfire. We've always seen a lot of TB here at County anyway, so for us there was never a point where there was no TB—it never left the cities. Then with the resurgence of TB we were hit with many, many more cases, and the hospital was unprepared to handle it in terms of the number of isolation rooms, which is how you have to handle these patients in the hospital. And then I noticed that in my clinic lots and lots of house officers and employees were coming to me with positive skin tests, and a few were coming with active tuberculosis. It was one thing when they caught it in the community, but another when they caught it here because of bad or insufficient isolation practices. We knew that it was happening because we were putting people with open-cavitary tuberculosis in open wards, coughing into the middle of the room with lots of people and patients.

I guess in about '90 or '91, we decided to study house staff. I worked with some colleagues on a study, looking at how many of our house staff converted their skin tests while they trained here. The study was published in the *American Review of Respiratory Disease,* the main journal of the American Lung Association, and it made the front page of the *Chicago Sun-Times.* I was quoted as saying that the hospital had lousy isolation practices, and that it wasn't doing enough—so people in the administration were unhappy with me, again. But that resulted in some attention being paid to it: they kind of remodeled a few isolation rooms. I would say that the TB issue here is an example of the hospital's usual practice of not doing the right thing or paying attention to what needs to be done to protect the workers and the patients. TB is an occupational infectious disease.

I think the thing that people don't appreciate is that TB was not eliminated because of the development of antibiotics. The myth is that they came up with these fancy wonder drugs and modern medicine took care of TB. Well, the fact is that TB was declining before the invention of those drugs in the thirties, because of better housing conditions and better nutrition. TB is caused by poor people being all crammed up in tiny little living quarters and breathing the same air, having poorly ventilated living spaces, and then not being that strong; and by their bodies being weak because of malnutrition or other diseases or other problems. That's how you spread TB.

Well, that sure is coming back—homelessness, people crowded into shelters. We have one shelter in Chicago that's had thirty cases of TB: it's an incubation chamber for TB. And then we have massive unemployment, we have substance abuse and alcoholism and drug use, which weaken people's resistance to TB. We have AIDS, which also weakens people's resistance to TB. And then they're all crammed up, and *that* spreads TB. We're seeing more TB among kids, which means that it's recent transmission—nobody can say that it's "reactivation." One thing that people say is new about TB but isn't new is drug resistance, and then something called "multidrug resistance." The bug doesn't respond to the standard medications: it gets resistant to one or more of them, and that happens because people take their medicine intermittently. Bugs get used to it, and then you have TB that's untreatable. Eventually, we'll get back to Charles Dickens's times, when TB was a disease you could watch people be slowly consumed by—they used to call it "consumption"—but you have no medicines to treat it with, so it becomes an untreatable disease and an unpreventable disease. We're swiftly heading back into the nineteenth century in terms of tuberculosis.

The CDC [U.S. Centers for Disease Control] came out with new regulations over the summer which state that hospitals at high risk, which we certainly are, should have their whole work force tested semiannually. It's not rocket science to do that: you gotta hire some nurses and people to do the skin test. It's just a question of staffing. It still isn't happening, although they're trying to get around to do that now, or so they claim. I haven't seen the data yet. I'm not sure I *will* see the data, though I'd like to. I might hear about it, through the grapevine. [sighs]

The biggest failure in TB treatment is finding and providing housing and nutrition and support for people to finish the course of their medicine. It takes six months of medicine to cure TB. You got a homeless guy—if you send him back out on the street with his pills, you ain't gonna treat him and cure him. You need to find homes for people who have TB, so that they can heal and get better. I don't care how many fancy medicines you have, or how many fancy blood tests or other kinds of tests—you're not going to get rid of it until you provide people with those things, which, ultimately, means jobs. They gotta have a way to support themselves.

That's why I think that my being a communist is more important than my being a pulmonary doctor. A lot of people are approaching it from the point of view of being pulmonary doctors and trying to make things better by developing new medicines—say, figuring out how to give an injection that will last for six months, so that a homeless guy can be injected for six months and get better. People are working on that, very hard, and have big money from the NIH [National Institutes of Health] to do it. There's one solution they're working on: it's called "depot medicine"—you inject it, and it deposits a dose under the skin that will be long-acting. That way you don't have to worry about finding the guy. He can sleep on a grate, and that stuff will percolate in his body and the TB will go away. I don't think anything is going to get rid of TB until we can improve people's living conditions.

I think a lot of the liberal docs here—very, very nice people—work very hard to fix the system. I work hard in my eight hours to really try and take care of people the best I can, but I still spend a lot of time trying to convince people that they have to get rid of the system. I don't think it can be fixed.

Quality Struggles

Dr. Gordon Schiff

DIRECTOR OF GENERAL MEDICINE, *Clinic Section. He is a tall, spider-thin version of the absent-minded professor. "There's this quote from Rudolph Virchow that politics is medicine on a larger scale...If I can put my hands on it." His office is jammed with a bookcase, file cabinets, books, folders, piles of papers stuffed everywhere. "Actually, what you're looking at is a very neat, obsessive-compulsive person who's gone over the edge."*

I GREW UP ON THE SOUTH SIDE. MY FATHER WAS A DOCTOR who worked at Michael Reese. I began volunteering in the Emergency Room at County when I was a premedical student.

When the hospital was built, in the early 1900s, it was modeled after the Columbian Exposition architecture—the big columns and all that stuff. It was budgeted for $3 million dollars, but it cost $4 million, and they ran out of money. Most of it was spent on the façade of the hospital: there were supposed to be four wings on the back, but they only put two on. There was no money left over for medical equipment. So even at the opening in 1914, the hospital—which is the one we still have—was a complete scandal and an embarrassment. By 1932, the American College of Surgeons, the forerunner of the Joint Commission on Accreditation of Health Care Organizations, found this place to be a disaster: they said the long wards were "completely antiquated for modern hospital care." It was designed by an architect who had no experience in designing hospital architecture—so the hospital was flawed from the start, and this is the same building that we're taking care of patients in today.

The nurses' station is almost a city block away from patients at the end of the wards; there's no telephones for the patients. These are the kinds of things that we've been demanding for years. There's a few payphones outside the wards, but even *they* are a block walk. It's that kind of lack of respect for patients as people—really a measure of their political powerlessness in this society—that shows they're not the really valued customers, to use this modern-day "quality improvement" language. In the old days, the customers were the patronage job seekers and the contractors—and even the medical schools, for training and research. In the eighties, a new customer of the hospital became the accreditation body: we basically had to please them and the taxpayers, in the sense that we don't want to drive taxes up too high. Obviously, we have an obligation not to misuse taxpayers' money, so I'm not saying that they're not one of our legitimate customers. But when you think about who really should be conceived of as the people around whom we design the services and our decisions are guided, it ought to be the patients. Unfortunately, they were a low priority.

One of the things I always need to stress—and I do this with the medical students—is how really wonderful the patients are at this hospital. There's the stereotype of the typical County patient as somebody who's a homeless, alcoholic drug abuser—and now with AIDS or TB. Most of the people I take care of are working or have worked most of their lives: they built this city with their hands. These people are very grateful for our services—they're very appreciative, they're very decent, articulate, interesting people. They're very kind. And even the ones who *are* shooting drugs or victims of alcohol, mostly when you piece things together, are people who at some point in their life had it more together and, some circumstance—they lost their job or...There but for fortune go I.

A patient may come in here who is dirty or in DTs—they're delirious from alcohol withdrawal. Within two or three days, that person is the nicest, most decent, finest person. And here they come in and we treat them like...they're in leather restraints, violent and irrational. We put them on a ward where there is no privacy, just stretchers strewn around. It's *still* like that on our admitting wards. So there's the dehumanization of the patients, from the conditions from which they come to what *we* put them through. But despite this, the patients' humanity shines through.

A medical student who'd also worked at Rush and Mount Sinai said, "All the time I was at County, I never heard a patient referred to by these pejorative words—gomer or scuzzball." Words that aren't even fit for print, part of that gallows humor of how undesirable patients are referred to. But here, where so many of our patients are less than fully cleaned and all those things, the staff never refers to the patients in those ways. There isn't that kind of antipathy—and it's amazing, because there's so much of what *is* bad about County that does get internalized by the staff. Unfortunately, we get used to patients waiting fifteen hours for their X-ray or their prescription. We say, "That's the County..."

I have something right here on my desk. [digs into pile of papers] A worker at County brought a friend of hers to have her prescription filled, and she ended up being abused at the pharmacy window. She was told, "If you don't like it you can leave. Don't raise your voice. Don't interrupt." Sometimes you feel like you have just got to go up there and scream, "This has got to stop!" in order for people to be treated differently. Many of the people who try get burned out and leave.

There's another group of caring people who just somehow try to make their peace with that. You just cannot flip out every time poor care happens—though, probably, you've lost some of your humanity by making such accommodations. There's another group—and I don't think it's actually all one group versus another, as these attitudes are widely distributed—where people just get completely resigned. They're just here punching a clock, getting a paycheck, they really don't care. The lower people are on the employment ladder, the pay scale, the more alienated their response. Because they have so little control, so little ability to feel like they're even making little tiny changes.

The point is, there's this constant Catch-22: someday we're going to have to get a new hospital, but the someday never comes, because we have to deal with the crisis of this month so we won't get disaccredited. It creates a sense of hopelessness and resignation and frustration. The question is, "Are we captains of our own destiny?" I mentioned the customers, who, for our hospital, are often the private hospitals. This hospital exists in many people's minds—and, of course, in terms of the political clout they have—only to the extent that we serve the private hospitals: we're here to absorb their deficit, their bad-debt patients. It's like a ship being battered around from one place to the other, rather than setting a course and sailing in that direction. Even if we don't have a lot of power, a lot of wind, we could chart a course if we were captains of our own ship—and be more than just the mirror image of the rest of the health system, there to fill in gaps. We should be here with a very forward-looking mission of our own.

The current leadership has that more positive vision rather than just the negative. Nobody is talking about what's going to happen to the public sector when this whole competition thing is unleashed: basically, you're going to destroy some very fragile support services. I'll give you one example. We take care of a lot of HMO patients at County, but not by the HMOs' choice...well, maybe by the HMOs' choosing to deny access, but not by explicit design. At one point we figured out that we provide $150,000 to $200,000 worth of free HMO care annually: the HMOs go around signing people up, Medicaid pays them X number of dollars a month for this, and then the patients come to County—either because they always did, or they didn't know they could go to the HMO, or they even tried going to the HMO and were told, "There's nothing wrong with you, we're not going to take care of you," or just didn't treat them well. So they come here. So here the HMO is being paid the money and they're providing no care! *We're* providing the care and not getting any money at all. Then they turn around and say the reason the County shouldn't be funded is because we're inefficient!

The issues that concern me are access and quality. In the early eighties we did some research on dumping. I did a study on ambulatory dumping where we interviewed five hundred people sitting on the bench here in the Emergency Room—not the ones being dumped by ambulance, but the unofficial, never-counted, walking ones: somebody broke their leg, went to another hospital, and was told to go to Cook County Hospital tomorrow for follow-up care. The person will come here thinking they have an appointment, and they find themselves waiting with the other thousand patients that come to the Emergency Room each day.

Another interest of mine is quality of care, in terms of technical medical quality—that we're giving care with a good outcome. When we put somebody under general anesthesia, whether they wake up or not, for example; or when somebody has a heart attack, that we give them state-of-the-art medical care. And that doesn't come automatically. It's a real struggle to provide these quality services: it means you have to be introspective about the kind of things you're doing. You also need data, which we tend not to have. County is a place where you don't have to search very hard to look for problems to work on. It's not like we have to do detailed studies to know that we've got a problem down in the pharmacy with waiting times, which also turns out to be related to dispensing errors. Pharmacists are giving out more than one prescription per pharmacist per minute, OK? We don't have enough *space* for all the drugs. And these are all things that have medical consequences.

Many of these problems are not unique to County. They often feel like they are, and it's very hard to distinguish which ones are. It feels like the X-ray radiology clerks are unresponsive, or fail to find the X-rays you need—well maybe that happens 10 percent of the time here, but it might happen 6 percent of the time over at Rush. Some of these are things I call "state-of-the-art problems." This week, the Illinois Department of Public Health is in here doing a surprise inspection, and they found there were missing drugs on the wards—2 or 3 percent of the drugs on the floors were missing. I would be surprised if it was that little, since we have a much higher percentage of patients whose medicines don't even *get* to the floor. All hospitals have these kind of problems.

I currently chair the hospital's Quality Assurance Committee. Before, the whole idea of quality assurance was to find out, for example, where the problems are in cardiac arrest, who these doctors are who don't know how to do it right, or on which wards is the equipment broken—rather than looking at generic issues, the system issues, and then bringing people together to work together on these things. The former approach makes people defensive; but saying that the problem really isn't bad apples but system design...There may be ward clerks who have "bad attitudes," who don't want to do their job because they are very alienated; but the way to really improve the care from the ward clerks or on the wards is not to go after the bad apples, but to try to identify these systemic causes that underlie some of the problems.

The real research lab of the 1990s is the health care delivery system—taking care of people and learning from *that*: How do we really know what we're doing is right? How do we collect and learn from that, and how do we understand outcomes? My idea of research, what academic medicine should be, is merging clinical practice with these questions. The U.S. government has just set up the Agency for Health Care Policy and Research, which is beginning to make an investment in the field of health outcomes research and practice guidelines.

Almost everything we do here—the scientific basis of why we do it, how we do it, how we could do it better—is totally underdeveloped. On one hand, that's frustrating for patients. There's all the stories—you know, a woman who goes to six different doctors about whether she should take estrogen and gets six different answers. It's easy to say that part of a problem like that is just the sexist health care system—it doesn't care about women's health, et cetera. But the next step, really, is to understand the controversies and the limitations of our knowledge. Once you *recognize* the problem, well, that's only the beginning. We need to create an information infrastructure to harness what we're doing all the time for learning. And, it turns out, we're doing a huge amount at this hospital.

You could say, "Well, Cook County Hospital isn't like a *real* teaching hospital—it has inferior quality, it can't attract American medical graduates." But it's *here* where the action really is: the huge clinical volume of things we do, and the enormous public health significance of the things we do in terms of HIV, TB, sexually transmitted diseases, substance abuse...Someone might say, "Well, these are just poor people's diseases, and we're going to turn our back on them." But the whole fabric of society is being torn apart by all these big problems.

Martin Luther King marched for civil rights, but if you really look at the quality of life—which is, after all, what health care is about for Black people—it's definitely worse than it used to be in Chicago, whether because of gangs, violence, or poverty. We can't turn our backs on the problems; we may want to close our eyes to them, but the realities won't let us. So it's not just that we're being forcibly reminded of it against our will; this really is our commitment and our raison d'être.

We've got many religious people working here. Hospitals used to be run by Sister This and the Order of That; but now you look around, and hospitals have turned themselves into for-profit entities. Everything you do for a patient here at County is a public service, whether you're emptying their bedpan or giving them directions. It's not like you're helping some board of trustees or owners of a proprietary hospital to get rich or gain a better profit margin. Everything you're doing is literally, by definition, a public service. That feels *right*.

Carrie Bennen

ASSISTANT DIRECTOR OF *Quality Assurance. She is reflective and forthright, and it is her nature to fret over things and seek to fix them. "My aunt, who is a nurse, had gone to Cook County. She said that if you're a nurse, you're going to have a good job: you'll never be dependent on a man to keep you going, you'll have a certain amount of security in your life. And that was a real big influence."*

I WENT TO COUNTY FOR NURSING SCHOOL. THAT WAS THREE years—'74 to '77. I went back to a regular university to finish a degree later, at night. There's this big movement to say that nurses without a bachelor's degree aren't well-rounded enough to be considered a professional, like that you don't have as many liberal arts classes, that you didn't take statistics and things like that. It's a sore point for those of us who did our basic education without that. We put in more hours in our basic training in three years than they did in four.

I learned to do nursing in another era, where the standard was different, where part of your day you planned to spend just talking to the patient and making them feel comfortable. What do they call it? Spiritual wholeness and well-being, things like that. Making sure that they're not frightened of what's happening, that they understand. The personal touch is being removed from the system: because it's not measurable, it's not part of the equation. And that's one reason that people are leaving nursing. If they're going to expect you to be a technical person, then you may as well go into a technical job; but if you went into this profession because of the personal side, then you're not going to get any fulfillment out of it, and then you'll leave.

That's not just public health, that's more everybody across the board, and nurses are leaving like you wouldn't believe. To me, we were taught a totally different frame of mind in nursing than what they teach now. Now they teach nursing as systems, and it's a very structured way of decision-making—it's very bottom line. You have very strict structures that are preestablished in textbooks, and things they expect you to do. What you end up doing is having to become an overachiever and overgiving through the system, or figuring out what we call "bypass systems." [laughs]

Within our place, if the system won't let you function, then you build a bypass. You just figure out a way to do it. You can come in a little early, work a little longer through your lunch—you find a way to make this thing work faster, so that you have more time to do what you feel that you need to do. A lot of people say, "Well, I'm just a robot here. I'm just doing a job, and there's never enough time." What did I read? Eight out of ten nurses right now feel that they don't have enough time in an eight-hour day to finish their work. But that's not County, that's the whole system.

Whenever people want to cut money—and this is one thing in the public health system, and any public system, that I really have a problem with—when people talk about socialized medicine and the health care system, putting that under the government, you think back to what happens with education, with the criminal system, the highway system. You start out, put it under the government, because that's the best way to do it, right? It's just too big for anybody private to handle, and you guarantee that we will do these things. But as soon as the decisions get difficult, we lower our standard. We lowered the standard in education: when you run out of money, instead of finding more money or fixing the system or finding what is the cause of the problems in the system, we lower the standard. Now, is that how people want their health care to be administered?

Health care used to be something that was top of the line, everybody was very dedicated. It's becoming a real business: you have productivity levels, you have schedules of how fast you should get people in and out of hospitals, there are set numbers. If you have someone come in with appendicitis, they should be gone in seventy-two hours or they—insurance, the federal government—aren't going to pay you. It has caps on every diagnosis. It's called DRG, "Diagnosis Related Groupings": you don't bill for what you did, you bill for what was wrong with the patient, and the government presets how much money it's going to cost you to provide that diagnosis with care.

You have to put in an appeal as an "outlier" if there is some reason that you can't follow that standard. An outlier is someone who lies outside the normal. Say you have a little old lady that comes in and she had pneumonia: they diagnosed her with pneumonia, they say she should be out in four days. Well, suppose she has a bad heart, or she's got diabetes too—things like that. You're going to have to put in writing that she has these other diagnoses to get it extended. If you don't get all of that in four days, no matter what you're doing with her, they cut her off. Now, at County that means nothing, because she doesn't go anywhere. At other hospitals, it would mean that they would discharge her or transfer her to County. Or they would send her home, even if she wasn't ready to go home. And there's no backup systems—there's no backup system for a little old lady whose kids don't live nearby anymore. Thirty years ago, the daughter would take a few weeks off work and stay home with Mom. That doesn't happen now.

People want to talk about socialized medicine models, they want to talk about Sweden. They don't realize that all of those systems have an

element of rationing, that they won't provide certain cares that we provide—they just *won't* give them. For instance, in this country—and this
is one of my pet peeves—we have all these neonatal centers for premature babies. By law in the State of Illinois, for a baby born over five hundred grams—which is about a pound—we have to go all out. While it's
possible that some of them will survive, they have a 90 percent morbidity
rate—or they'll have eye damage, ear damage, they'll have mental deficiencies, things like that. They'll have long-term, very severe health problems. But it's not impossible that they'll survive.

In Britain, they don't resuscitate under nine hundred grams—it used to
be nine hundred, I can't say what it is now—which is about two pounds.
Because those are the babies, you're assuming, that come out with fairly
healthy lungs, fairly healthy eyes, the brain is more fully developed. Investing the money to help *that* baby is going to provide a whole lot more in the
long term. Whereas investing a half a million dollars to keep those five-
hundred-grammers alive for a year, well...But you can't tell them, "We're
not going to do it." People just don't have the heart to do it as long as
there's the technology that *allows* us to do it. But does that mean that we
have to do it? That's something nobody is willing to deal with.

I've worked at a lot of different intensive care units. At County, I
worked three years in the Burn Unit when I first got out of school, and
then I worked in the private sector for eight years. I went back to County,
and eventually I went into pediatrics, because if you do your job really
well, chances are the kids will bounce back and be normal, healthy people. If you do your job real well on an eighty-year-old person who is on a
respirator and who has brain cancer or a massive stroke, no matter *what*
you do, that person is not going to improve—which is not what I trained
in intensive care to do. Some people say, "Just because she's eighty doesn't
mean that you can't go all out." Well, that's something that I didn't want
to be caught up in. And then the advent of bringing AIDS patients into
there. I have a real problem with people with terminal illnesses soaking
up so much of the resources that are so scarce now.

People think that health care money is a limitless thing, that people in
America will just continue to write the check. Well, we're getting to a
crisis point where the checkbook has only this many dollars in it, and no
matter how much you shift it from column A to column B, the money is
still not any different. And why is it so hard for us to say, "There's nothing we can do. We *can't* do this—we *shouldn't* do this."? At County Hospital, the worst part of it is, there's no one you can say no to without
being politically incorrect. There is no one that the County Board could
say no to. If they say no to cancer patients, if they say no to AIDS
patients, if they say no to the elderly, if they say no to the premature
babies, they'll have somebody angry. And nobody wants to hear that—
nobody wants to hear the hard truth.

I am sure that if we took all of the money that we spent in intensive care on the people, say, with terminal cancer, we could keep another public health clinic for children open just in our County Hospital. But instead of saying no to people that we know we can never return to a normal life, the Chicago Department of Health has closed public health clinics. I mean, where is the leadership? You are prolonging death and not prolonging life. Because it's easier to close the clinics, saying, "They can go to County Hospital," than it is to say, "No, we can't provide high-cost care for the terminally ill."

I left Pediatrics because I got stuck with a needle on a patient we had just drawn blood from. The kid was wild. He was tied down, restrained—he was a drug user. I had handed off the sample of blood to this doctor, in a syringe, because he hadn't been able to get the sample. I drew the sample for him, because I'm pretty good at drawing blood— normally, that's his job to do, but he was a junior doctor and I figured, Well, this kid's wild, let me do it. I did and handed off the thing and, well, he left the needle in the bed in a piece of gauze, and I didn't know it. I'm cleaning up afterward, and I pick up this piece of gauze. I normally go around and pick up all the papers that we've left on the bed doing the procedure—I crumple them up and put them in the garbage. And I get this needle stuck in my hand—it had fresh blood in it. We didn't know that he had AIDS, that he was HIV-positive. I wasn't too concerned at first, I mean, people get stuck; in ICU, Trauma, whatever, you get stuck, you get splashed, you get blood.

When I found out the kid had AIDS, I was hysterical. The thing is, I knew more about it than the hospital health service that was supposed to be handling me—and this is something that is *very* sensitive if you put this in a book, because that's something that's a problem in hospital administration. It's like, how involved do they get in this? Do they go all out and try to help you and kind of admit fault and then put themselves in a liability thing? Or do they let you handle this on your own? So the hospital and the County are in a bad position.

So I can see that the administration would have to be on the defensive, but it doesn't help those of us that have absolutely no risk factors in our life to be met with this defensive attitude. You're saying, "Tell me, what's my chances?" and all this stuff, and they're saying, "Well, you need to go to your own private physician." Well, don't you understand?! I don't *want* to go to my private physician and have this in my permanent health care record! And I know for a fact that if this gets in my record and my insurance company finds out about it, I could be dropped or I could be turned down for life insurance. You have to think about all these long-term things. In every hospital, and at County, I know that a lot of people get stuck. This was two years ago, so I'm clear now.

Since then, I've been in Quality Assurance. I monitor primarily the medical staff and the support services, but mostly the medical staff; there are mandatory monitoring functions within the hospital that are required by law, federally and statewide. You have to look at infection rates, death rates; you have to look at procedure rates, things like that. Statistics—I look for system failures, I am not so much concerned about how one person made a mistake. People will make judgment errors. As long as when they look at the death they say, "This was a judgment error, I've talked to the person." We *are* a training institution—and there are acceptable failure rates in certain things. If you're going to put a catheter in somebody's heart, ninety-nine times out of a hundred everything will go fine, but one time in a hundred the person is going to die. You could have your tonsils out, and one time out of a thousand the person will die under anesthetic—it doesn't mean that we did something wrong. We may have, I have to look, and I have to see if it's something that can be prevented.

My whole focus is a systems-oriented approach in that I group things. If I find a certain area is having repeated problems in a certain thing, or if I find that we're having a certain kind of problem—but that the basis for those problems all seems to be in the laboratory where the doctors are making decisions...They may be bad decisions, because maybe the lab tests are always coming back late, or the X-rays aren't ready, or they tried to get this person to surgery, but they couldn't get him through CAT scan...In Quality Assurance, we don't work with patients, we don't work as doctors and nurses, so we can stand back and say, "We work with all of the systems, and this is what we see." For example, we see that we have a real problem getting equipment that we need, but because we have to go through the County purchasing system...If it's over so many dollars, you have to put it out for bid, and if you do this then you have to do contracts, and every contract has to have so many affirmative action positions and blah-blah-blah. But this is a piece of essential medical equipment, and we can't wait two years for you guys to vote on it—so how do we work with the system to make sure it works?

Somehow the hospital always keeps going, because, even though the system is not set up to work, bypass systems always make it work. And you have a certain number of people that will overcompensate to make the system work: they're the real power within the place. But they're starting to complain that their bypasses aren't working anymore, because it's getting more tense. It used to be that you couldn't get things because the delivery system was bad or the ordering system was bad; now you can't get things because it's just not there. Used to be, if you knew somebody in purchasing, you could get it—now you can't. The money is really drying up. They have more people going to County Hospital, they have fewer public health clinics. They have a higher acuity of patients, but they cut the budget last year. The bypass systems just can't even kick in anymore.

I used to get such a kick out of watching *M*A*S*H*. It was like working at County: none of the rules made sense, none of what you did made sense. It was like, "Hurry up and wait! But you better do a damn good job and everything else." But at the same time, you always persevered and you always came out, and damn, our statistics actually came out better than the rest of the country. And we'd be like, "Well, how did we do that?" [laughs] And the thing is, though, it's like working in a war: you have limited resources, but a few very strongly dedicated and functional people to keep the system moving, where you're always getting more and more dumped on you, with less to work with, but somehow you make it work. That's how a lot of the people that ended up at County are— they're overachievers—but that can only go on for so long.

If you look at the public health system as in a crisis or like in a war situation or a disaster—disaster is a good analogy for it—you know that somebody has a massive injury, and he may still be alive—but you're not going to put all your energy into him. Now, at what point do we determine that this is a disaster? And when do we start saying we don't have unlimited resources? Once you do, then you have to get into the resource-allocation thing. Someone has to start setting priorities. If the eighty-year-olds are going to be your priority, fine—but don't go on TV and complain because the kids aren't immunized. And you can't say we're going to immunize all the kids while you close the public health clinics. At what point are we going to go tell everybody, "We've got to double the health care budget for a couple of years so that we can get these people healthy with family doctors, and at the same time increase their food stamps and at the same time increase their education?" You can't fix one without fixing the other, and everything is so interrelated that people don't want to hear it.

Another systems problem is we have this humongous hospital, with thousands and thousands of patients and hundreds of doctors and thousands of nurses, and we don't have a centralized computer system! The smallest hospital in a small town will have that hospital computerized from the pharmacy to the laboratory. We have a computer in the pharmacy that talks to pharmacy only. That's where we have the biggest problem—there are things they just cannot find.

Here's one we get into trouble with: we have a lot of kids come in with *bad* bronchial colds. And it's very hard, because the kids haven't been getting vitamins, they haven't been fed real well, they have a high chance of having pneumonia, they're real susceptible to viral infections. Well, you have to do a chest X-ray and a culture. If you go to your normal hospital, they'd send you over to X-ray, take an X-ray, wait in the ER for twenty minutes. The doctor would say, "Here you go, take antibiotics, go home." It takes us three days to get the X-ray because—well, you gotta wait in line to get into X-ray, then you got to wait in line for them to take it, then you gotta wait in line for them to get the results into the computer. They don't have full-time chief radiologists on duty around the clock, because it costs a lot of money—those guys make $150,000 a year. Can you staff them seven days a week, twenty-four hours a day? No. So the X-ray will just sit there waiting to get read. If it's done on the weekend, they don't have any typists to put what he says into the computer—so the ER doesn't know that it's OK for you to go home. A diagnosis could take days, and so we end up with all those kids in the hospital because we don't know if they're well enough to go home.

Or suppose he's *just* sick enough to be watched, and he needs a little oxygen—so we put him in the hospital. Well, after twenty-four to forty-eight hours with antibiotics and oxygen, then we'll reshoot the X-ray. It *still* takes us three days. Well, you know what happens? We have those beds filled. The government says, pneumonia in a child is only good for two days. The hospital eats the last three. Appendicitis, same problem—and we do this on so many of them.

They say County Hospital is a hospital that has to live by the standards of every other hospital. Well, we're not in with the same people or the same system that everybody else is dealing with. It says that if you fall down and break your leg and they put a pin in, you should go home in five days, right? And you can go home in a wheelchair with so much equipment, and a nurse will check you after a week—that's paid for. Our people, we're going to send them to Chicago Housing Authority with a wheelchair that will get stolen and an elevator that doesn't work. We're going to have to keep them for *three weeks*. We got a kid that has pneumonia, it's getting better. If he was in a normal environment where the mother was going to be with him around the clock to give him his antibiotics, check his fever every four hours, as soon as he got worse bring him right back, you'd send him home in three days. But if you're sending the kid home, and Mom is living in a shelter and doesn't have busfare back and forth to the hospital…Or you can't be sure the kid is going to be fed correctly, or that he's going to get his medication, or be kept warm enough…What do we do? We put him on social hold, meaning because of social reasons you can't discharge him. And then we have to have a social worker verify for Medicare that it's not safe for him to be discharged—but that's a judgment call, and half the time Medicare doesn't pay for it.

I see more nurses now that are overworked and overextended, and they've gotten to the point where they don't complain anymore, because they see that that's a part of the system. They really have to be nudged constantly—they're just *so* used to making do and being told, "We don't have any help for you." And if you speak out and say something, they can't do anything to you. They can try to make your life a little miserable, but it's not the same as someone saying, "I'm your boss, and you'll do as you're told or take a hike." I've had people at other jobs say, "You're *only* an employee. There are other jobs—if you're not happy, then leave." Whereas at County they're not going to do that: they'll listen to you complain.

In fact, we have—it's the *strangest* thing—members of the communist party stationed at the doors every other Wednesday. They hand out their literature, their socialist stuff. They're members of the hospital, they're physicians, talking about the administration is a bunch of capitalist dogs, and County workers should have four-day work weeks and this and that. It's tolerated—it's...like when the big abortion thing hit. We knew that there were prolifers with Operation Rescue on staff in the hospital. They actually hired additional security guards just to protect the employees working on those floors from the hospital personnel who were turning their names in to Operation Rescue. And they know this.

It's a world that people don't understand. It really is like a microcosm of society: you have elite groups and the lower groups, it's like a little study in microeconomics. It's really a reflection of what's going on in this society: education, economy, family breakdown, the whole thing is just built right into it. And that's where we have a hard time reconciling whether or not you can set the same standard. And if we're going to be a socialized medicine system, does that mean that, to be fair, the standards would all be lowered to meet a minimum standard?

Working the Building

Wally Gannon

HE'S FROM CHICAGO *and worked as a mechanical engineering assistant at County in the early eighties. "Even though I would never go there myself because, with medical coverage, I'm in the position that allows me to go to a good hospital, a clean hospital, a kept-up-to-date hospital. Even though I have that freedom, I still say thank God for County Hospital. If I ever get shot, stabbed, or burned, take me to County Hospital."*

WHEN I STARTED IT WAS THIS BEEHIVE OF ACTIVITY—THAT'S the best way to describe it. The thing that I noticed instantly was this incredible separation: the doctors didn't speak to the help in the hospital, they only spoke on occasion to the administration, the head nurses, the head of Housekeeping. Or to our department, which basically handled all repairs in the hospital—it maintained the mechanical operation of the complex. And there were these class separations, definitely. These union people who were in my department looked down on everybody else in the hospital, because we were union, we were getting scale—all of us were making more than the bulk of the doctors who worked there. Doctors don't get paid a whole heck of a lot until they've been there awhile. Then you have the nurses, who made less. Then you had the Housekeeping people and so forth. And then there's this uniform distinction too: in our department you had to wear work blues, Housekeeping wore green, doctors wore white, administration wore ties. [laughs]

My department was predominantly White, predominantly Irish—and out of that, a good percentage were from the Old Sod, so they still carried their brogues and all that with them. The rest of the trades that were there, like electricians and plumbers, you had Italians and Poles, and so forth. When I left, I'd say, there were probably a dozen Blacks out of 120 trades people. Everybody got along, you had to work together. Our common denominator was that we were all trades people, and we were all union.

We were smack dab in the middle of the world's largest hospital complex. There's something like 170 something medical buildings there, between all the colleges, the state, and the city, all the stuff combined. And here we were: the eyesore in the middle of all this. [laughs] But it's a marvelous building. When you look at it, the way this thing is built, it would probably withstand a World War II atomic bomb. The walls are four feet thick in some places. It's really an attractive building when you stand there and look at it from architectural and construction stand-points. But you go into that building and you're really looking at a med-ical museum: there are still some places in County Hospital where there are open wards. You look at that and you think of consumption and Jack the Ripper, turn-of-the-century London health care. That's the old days. [laughs] And it can't really accommodate the leaps and bounds that med-icine has taken. It can't accommodate it, and you can't bring it up to code fast enough. The maximum that they can possibly do is just enough to meet the minimum requirement, because it's an antiquated structure. Here's the other thing too: the strictest codes in this country are in nuclear power plants, the second strictest codes are in hospitals. We were lucky over there...Certain code violations are grandfathered in, just by the grace of political pressure.

Basically, our job would be doing things like going through the build-ing, checking all the mechanical operations. Anything that involved motors, they were greased and oiled, filters were changed in fan units. But we wouldn't always have what you needed—sometimes you're out of stuff for a long time. As a matter of fact, when you put a window unit in, or when glass broke in certain places, for example, it was replaced with Plexiglas. Well, there was one point where we didn't have Plexiglas for nine months. Then you'd get the sheet metal guys, and you'd put a piece of sheet metal in there, which isn't transparent. But that's what you did—you had to make do with things.

There were times when it was almost impossible to move through that building to get to a work location, because it would be so crowded. And you were maybe trying to move a large piece of equipment through there. Elevators are tied up all day long with the people that are lucky enough to be ambulatory. I've been on an elevator with somebody who's carry-ing a filthy piece of equipment from something that's just been disman-tled, with a person laid out on a gurney, being fed intravenously—with two other people talking about how they're going to get laid after they get off work, and some other person with a food cart! And all this is on one elevator. There's this conglomeration of everything happening in one little space at one time. It's just ridiculous.

Sometimes we had to fix things around patients. If you could, you got a patient out of the way, but sometimes you were right there near a patient, and you never knew what patients had. I remember one time, turning a corner and seeing a guy sitting on a bench right by a pay-phone—they had these payphones at the end of each ward—and this guy was sitting there, on the phone talking, and I looked over and he was *yel-low!* I said, "Oh shit," and pulled back around the corner real fast.

And you know, when we go into an open ward where thirty people are laid up...I think that really slows down the recovery process. There's no dignity in recovery in a place like County Hospital—it's an assembly line of patients up there. The dignity of recovering, the dignity of being sick...You don't think of that as being a term, being sick and having dignity, but when you're sick, you don't want twenty million people looking at you. And when you're laying on an open ward and you're looking around—and you're not looking at other healthy people, you're looking at other sick people—it's demoralizing. Almost every patient has a radio or a TV from home next to his bed. And, here, these people come from congested neighborhoods, they're poor—they come to the hospital, they're put into a congested ward. It's impossible for them to rest! I used to walk onto some of these wards, and I'd see someone out to the world with three or four TVs blasting all around. The need to rest was so great they could overcome that.

And then you have patients dealing drugs in the hospital. I remember a patient, he was in a wheelchair, the guy had three beepers. He was in what they call the "day room," which is a little alcove at the end of each ward, and there's usually a TV with lousy reception mounted up there on the ceiling. They're back there watching TV, and this guy is saying, "I'm waiting for that motherfucker to call me." And then, beep-beep-beep-beep. Hey, speak of the devil! The guy is wheeling off down the corridor to the payphone, got the thing on his lap, he's looking at the number, and his other pager starts going off. [laughs] He says, "Bring it on down—I got four people here that would be interested in that." I can hear this stuff, you know?

One day I'm walking down the hallway, and I go to make a phone call, and this guy goes, [sharply] "No, no." He's on crutches, leaning against the wall like twenty feet away from the phone. I look at him and go, "What?" He says, "Nuh-uh—I'm waiting for a call." I said, "Well, you're not going to get to the phone from over there." So I come over and grabbed the phone—he says, "I'm telling you, motherfucker!" and he comes at me with the crutches and stuff. "I'm waiting for a call and it's important." So I put the phone back down, and sure enough the thing rang two seconds later. He goes to the phone, and he glares at me: "Now I be talking—walk away." Making demands, chasing the employees away. [laughs] Oh yeah, you have that stuff there.

There was one doctor there, an attending; we called him "Jekyll and Hyde." This guy was the king of bedside manners: I saw him work one day, and the way he comforted this patient was just amazing. He talked to this patient in really a caring way, almost like a family member. Then this guy was in the hallway and I saw him talking to some nurse: "When I tell you to bring that plasma down there, you get it down there, you piece of shit." Then, a couple of weeks later, I'm in an area where he is, and he's dealing with a patient—and I've got to get something. I'm actually a good twenty-five feet away from the patient, doing a little thing, nothing complicated, nothing noisy, nothing dirty—something that would only take me ten minutes to do. I could hear this guy comforting this patient: "I know you can't get around. Can I get you something from the library?" Couldn't be sweeter. When he was done, he came over by me and he stood with his back to the patient and leaned over to me and said, "I don't ever want to see you up here working when I'm near a patient! You got a lot of fucking gall." He says, "All you assholes got a lot of fucking gall working around patients. Get the hell out of here right now!" I just kept working.

The morale in that hospital, it's nonexistent. It's just bad. I remember that from day one: the people that were showing me around said, "If you can't do this, then don't do it. If you can't get to it, fine—who gives a fuck? It'll be there tomorrow." That was their attitude. By the time I left there, I hated everybody I worked with, I hated the entire hospital, I hated the patients. I felt the same way everybody else did: you looked, you saw a patient, you said, "Oh my God, another one"—you just *hated* seeing them. It just...I don't know. See, it can border on racist, I guess, when you start to talk about it; I guess I never really measured it in that way. I know that for a lot of the White people that worked there, they looked at it and just said, "More niggers, more niggers, more niggers." That was their attitude. You go up on the maternity ward and you see a million Black babies up there, and you'd see what seemed like a million mothers that were teenagers—and it was just like...You looked at it and said, "It's out of control."

I don't think I'm a racist, but I can see how that can happen. When you're around people all day long and your co-workers are saying, "Look at this nigger, look at that nigger"...Rather than freak out and say, "You know, you're a racist asshole"—and then suddenly have everybody you work with shun you—you find yourself in that weird position of going, "Yeah, I know what you mean." And just agreeing with them in such a way where you don't make a commitment verbally like, "Yeah, you're right, that nigger."

I heard it from patients all the time that Filipino nurses showed no compassion with the Black patients. They had a tendency, if they were drawing blood or administering something intravenously, of just stabbing a Black person. Their excuse was—and I heard this from the Filipino nurses—"Black people's skin is so thick, you have to do that." And there, you look at a case where stereotypes breed themselves—like my just saying right now that Filipino nurses have no compassion for patients. Maybe at County Hospital, the bulk of those people that work there over a period of time just lose any compassion, and that particular group per se—yeah, it just seems to be that the Filipino nurses lose their compassion. But to even say *that*, even if it *is* true, it's a stereotype. And you'll find that happening at County Hospital: every group hates one another. The White trades dislike all the Blacks that are there. The Blacks there dislike—even within the blacks you'll find lighter skin blacks dislike darker skin blacks. And "I grew up on the South Side, so therefore I hate the West Side brothers," and vice versa. All that crap. It's classist...It's speciesist...whatever.

I just felt that it was a place where nobody gave a shit. The customers were people that nobody gave a shit about in their daily life, and now here they are sick in this hospital and not many people really give a shit about them in there. You can't generalize. Some doctors certainly cared about their patients; some doctors and nurses looked at it as a nuisance, but it was their job. That's a shame when that happens. When you're in a place like County, the majority of people would rather not be there, but they're there because that's their livelihood.

A lot of stuff just becomes rote for people. They take their break at the same time every day, they eat the same thing every day, they sit with the same clique when they have their break or their lunch. As far as the class distinction goes, you really had two classes of people there: you had the doctors, and you had the workers. And then you had that nebulous class which we call "the administration." And then, within all those groups, you find people trying to think that they're better than somebody else: the nurses always felt they were better than the service staff—the janitors and all that. You know, "You're just a janitor, and I'm a health care worker." You found that. And then the janitors were like, "I'm an environmental services worker, you're just an elevator operator." There was always that separation, a pecking order. And the trades, "We're the trades people, you're nothing." It's just the way people do that in their everyday lives; we always look for some little tidbit to make ourselves feel better. And when you get a bunch of people together, then it becomes a class distinction.

There's a lot of people that do good work there, and there's some of them that can joke, "I got a jellyroll [easy] job." They laugh because they know the perception of the place, so they make jokes about it. But, yeah, throughout the hospital there are people in every department, within every little regime, who are just coasting through, just eating up the clock, as they say. There's department heads there that just shit on their employees. There's an old saying at County Hospital that if you like the job you're doing, and you let them know you like the job you're doing, you're not going to be doing it the next day—boom! They move you to a shitty job. That's the whole thing: they don't want you to be happy, they want you to be on the edge.

And the health care is racist. It really is. Because the County Board doesn't appropriate the proper amount of money for health care there, it's looked at as racist. They keep hemming and hawing about building a hospital. And as every year goes by, you're talking about more money tacked on to the cost of building a hospital. Where's that money going to come from when it's time to build it? Now, that's racist, because the clients of the hospital are predominantly poor, Black, Hispanic. The bulk of Cook County voters don't live in the Chicago area that is serviced by County Hospital.

I got fed up with it and had a better job offer elsewhere, and said, "The hell with this," and got out. Everybody that I talk to that I'm still friends with there are just killing time. They do their job, they're there, but it's just a place where they work. There's one guy who every time I talk to him, he'll say something like, "Five and six"; the next time I talk to him it's, "Five and one"—five years and one month to go until he retires and draws his pension. It's just time, as they say over there, till they pull the pin.

Working the Staff

Jewel Fowler

SHE SEEMS SELF-ASSURED *but a little shy. Once she starts talking, her delight in the wonders of human behavior shines through. She has been a secretary at the hospital for fourteen years, and is both a union steward for, and the secretary-treasurer of, her local. "When I started here, I had no medicine terminology, and it was rough in the beginning. What was rough was all the different accents in the department. My boss is from Australia, we have a doctor here from India, from Iraq. Really, there was no one here from the United States when I started. Now I understand every last one of them, but it was hard at first."*

I'M IN AFSCME, LOCAL IIII — IT'S CLERICAL AND ADMINISTRA-
tive. Nurses have their own unions here, and we have Local 46 which is Housekeeping. The ward clerks, they have a separate union, and then there's 73 that has the technicians. And there are trade unions here too—the painters, electricians. Everyone is unionized besides the attending doctors. The residents and fellows, they're unionized. The administrators that are on a certain level, they're not unionized. We encourage people to join, but it's still a choice thing. What happens here now, is we have Fair Share—so if you do not choose to join a union, you're still paying something that's going to automatically be taken out of your check, because when we negotiate we negotiate for every person that's covered under our bargaining unit. So really everyone is unionized, whether they want to or not. We don't say, "Because this person don't want to be unionized..." because County is across the board: what we do for one, we're gonna do for all.

If a Fair Share member gets in trouble, we have to represent them, but what happens usually—I think it's their conscience or whatever—the first thing they do is they sign up. They come to us, because they need our help—and they will sign up and become a full member. That's how old-time members get signed up. And eventually you do get in some type of trouble and you might need union representation. You could apply for a promotion and your director might choose someone else, but yet you fit the minimum qualifications. I can type ninety words and you can only type seventy, but if the job calls for sixty-five words a minute and you've been here longer than me, you deserve the job.

We represent the members any way we can. It's our job to see to it that they are being treated fairly in their department. We have a contract made up with County, and we have to make sure that management is sticking to our contract. Like when I told you about the promotion: you know, because they like this person better, they will get the job. Same with sick and vacation time—some people is turned down for vacation so this one can have it. Christmas is a big vacation. Everything around here really has to be done seniority-wise. That's one big thing that we do have in our contract.

And then we have employees that get in trouble. [chuckles] They get in trouble, people don't come to work, they call in sick a lot, and there's rules about that. If you keep abusing your time, you're taken to a hearing, and we represent them in hearings. And if the employee warrants discipline, we have to make sure that the discipline is not too severe. The hearing officer listens to the supervisor and then listens to union. If your supervisor don't like you then anything you do you'll get in trouble for! Sometimes we allow the person to speak, sometimes we don't—it depends on what happened. [laughs] Most of the time, when an employee is totally guilty, like we have employees falsifying time cards...You know, they'll come to work, and some of them are on drugs where they go to lunch and don't come back till the next day. Some employees we advise, "Don't say anything, we'll do all the talking for you"—because they're guilty. We can't even argue attendance, it's in black and white: either you were there or you weren't there. So we really throw them on the mercy of the hearing officer, letting them know they're aware of this problem, and they'll try to clean it up. We talk to them and let them know: suspension leads to discharge.

Because of the contract, it's hard to get someone fired. So when an employee gets fired it's because...Like we have employees that fight— that's automatic discharge, that don't go through the procedure. We had many employees that fought this year. Fighting over boyfriends, you know? [laughs] What's hard is when we get two people in the same union: one always talks hard against us, because they're saying this one got treated better. All we want to know is who started it.

But before you get fired, you must have a hearing. What happens is, if we don't like the hearing officer's decision, we appeal the case, and they send someone in from downtown to hear the case over again. That's when it takes forever. We've put in lawsuits against County, because we have a procedure clause in our contract: thirty days is the longest it's supposed to take for you to give a decision. They don't do it. We've had employees off from over a year to almost two years. In order to get fired around here, the hospital director must sign that letter. The director is busy. When they get around to it, then they'll look at the letter. We can't do anything without a letter—the decision has to be sent before we can appeal.

It's better for an employee to try to stay out of trouble. The majority of the time, employees don't realize—they look at us like we can work a miracle. We can't do that; the only thing we do is make sure that you're being treated fairly in whatever goes on. But if you have an attendance problem that's your problem: the only person that can clean that up is you. We try to explain that to them, but we have had employees get upset with us after getting fired, went downtown and filed unfair labor practice against the union. We go to court and have to bring our records and show how we represent these employees. So we have to be careful too. We have to do all we can for them, because when they get fired then they're going to blame someone. And there are cases where we make a decision whether to arbitrate or not. We go to arbitration, we get a lawyer that has nothing to do with County, nothing to do with the union, and they hear the case. That's the last resort. If we feel we have a good case, then we'll get an arbitrator. We have a committee that discusses the case, looks it over to see, you know, do we have a winner?

In our part of the union alone there are eleven hundred employees. It's like a city here. This hospital is not like other hospitals: first of all, well, you can *see* that. Did you have a pass or something when you came up here? *Anybody* can walk up here, you know? Whereas at other hospitals, you don't have a pass, you can't get through security. This hospital is so open, and some of everything goes on here. You know, in the morning when you walk into the main building there's the homeless people sleeping out there, or they're around the corner. We have all kinds of strangers walking these buildings. Sometimes, I'll be up here and no one is...the building sometimes is isolated. I'll see somebody strange in the building, and I call security and they all come over, and it'll be someone that has no business here. People have got hurt. People will come in and take your purse. Everything goes on out here.

Other hospitals aren't so visible. And employees know, they take advantage of the system. We have these contracts set up between County and the union that help make sure everyone is treated fairly, but then you got people that take advantage of it. That's why you got people who say it's hard to get someone fired around here, because a lot of people...We have a department where they have employees that maybe don't come to work like they should—but they don't jump in and try to discipline them. We have a lot of departments where they're not used to trouble, so they give you another chance; they try to talk to you, and this goes on for a year or two, and then you're taking advantage of them. They should have fired you, but they don't know, they try. It's hard—you don't know who to give a break to, who not to give one to.

When you have an area where there's a large group of people working together, there's going to be problems. Problems with overtime—it's not done fairly—this one is coming in, they're picking this one particular employee, she do all the overtime, the other one's not even asked to do it.

We have to come in and tell them: set up a roster, go down the list. It's simple, but it's not done. [laughs] People have their picks and chooses. You're doing someone a favor when you're giving them overtime. A job comes up, everyone feels like they deserve this promotion. Then there's tensions by the person that did get it. No one wants to respect *this* one, because [with attitude] "I worked with you all these years and all of a sudden you gonna tell me what to do?!" That's the kind of stuff going on in a large department. It's always something.

The hospital meets with the unions one at a time. Everyone has their own little agenda, but there are some things that we have to be together on. This is a rough negotiation, because County employees have never paid health insurance before, plus County is talking about building a new hospital. That means a cut down in your bed size. We have Provident Hospital over there, which they're hoping will cut down on patients here, so that's gonna mean a shortage of employees. What we try to use when we negotiate—when we think they might want to lay people off—is we had a lot of employees that retired, so you need to count them positions as part of your layoff. We look at stuff like that, because when these members start getting laid off, they're going to come running to us—and what can we do?

County is just like Peyton Place. Anything goes on, everyone's going to know about it. [laughs] You know everything about everybody. This one broke up, and these two are fighting over that one—it goes on all the time. You see two people talking together, have lunch together two days, the next thing you know they're going together, you know? That's the rumor. People keep up with everyone's business around here. They really do.

One thing they try to stress on us, as a union steward we have to set an example. My record is clean. [giggles] I can't be written up all the time, getting in trouble and expected to represent people, because they'll look at me like…'Cause anything you do around here, it gets around.

Coping with People

Michael Martinez

There is something truly buoyant about him, as though nothing could keep him down for long. He works at the hospital as a clerk while going to school, to get a degree in psychology. "I'm from Chicago, born and raised. Born at Cook County Hospital. When I was younger, I had swallowed bleach, and I think I went to County then—but otherwise I didn't go there."

I'M A CLERK 3. THE GENERAL DUTIES ARE JUST GREETING THE patients, making sure that the doctor is aware the patient is in. In your smaller clinics it's easier to do that. In General Medicine, we have almost thirty doctors each morning and each afternoon. I greet the patient and give them a card that tells them what room number. Then they generally step on the scale and press a button—which is patient participation, I call it—and the weight is spewed out on a sticky pad, and I stick it on the chart so that the doctor sees it.

The system is get 'em in, get 'em out. You know patients just don't understand—and maybe *we* don't understand—we see thousands and thousands of patients a week and so, you know, it's blurred. You see patient after patient after patient after patient, and you tend to forget that this is maybe the first time the patient is here, and the patient is sick or maybe they've had a rough day. You want to be as sympathetic as you can, but it's not always gonna happen. Let's say the patient waits from seven until nine-thirty—you're one of those rare cases where you're first in and first out. Then you go to the appointment system, and they will make an appointment for you to return—you'll get everything stamped and then you will go downstairs to the pharmacy. Therein lies the big wait.

If you get down to the pharmacy between nine and ten o'clock, [snaps fingers] you will be out like that. If you get down to the pharmacy any time after ten o'clock, you will wait four hours. They will not tell you that they are out of anything, you will be told *that* when they call you to give you a prescription. That would make you *angry.* So John Raba formed this thing called the "outtage list": the pharmacy would write the list up, and it would be dispersed to the floors. But if your doctor doesn't look down to see what's on the paper before he writes something…And it happens. Pharmacy is supposed to call up and try to get a hold of the doctor to prescribe something different. It *doesn't* happen. The patient is given the thing, they're sent back upstairs to find the doctor to get it rewritten to take it back downstairs, and wait...If you want the system to work, you do everything you can. I've filled out phony appointment slips because they forget them at home, or you know...

I basically feel that patients should be given their dignity and their respect. It doesn't matter whether they can afford or they can't afford to pay for the services. They are there for a purpose, you are there to do a job, and you should both do it with dignity and respect. It doesn't always seem to fall out that way. [laughs] Ninety-five percent of the time, yes, it does, but when you go through County as a patient you're hardened also—you're hardened by these people that treat you badly, you're hardened by having to wait, you're hardened by everything in County. You're a victim of County. There are some times when patients have come to my desk and they're the first ones to attack. And I have to be the one to say to them, "Look, *I* haven't done anything to you." Most people at County are there because it's a job, it pays the bills. And they've been hurt and screamed at by patients, and it's just formed a hard shell.

I can see that happening with me, and I have seen my fellow workers...[sighs] I've seen them be nasty to patients, tell them to go away, that they didn't have the time, and all of this they're doing with their head down. [hangs head, pretends to concentrate] Not even looking at the person. So that's where the dignity comes in, because a patient *feels* like they're no one, and is being told by this person that's sitting there that they *are* no one. No one needs that. Eye contact is very important. The other two clerks I work with, one of them's been there for thirteen years and the other one, on and off for twenty. Basically, their thing is, they've been there a long time, they know how people act, they're hardened— they know just to be quiet. There's a huge wall between them and the patients. They're very nice, very sweet, but they just don't say much.

I did start losing it out front. I was snapping at the patients, and I had to rein myself in and say, "OK, calm down." It was like a patient would say, "Do I press this button?" I'd say, [wearily annoyed] "How many times have you been here? Well, if you've been here before, then you *know* you have to press the button, right? Please step down." I think it was a combination: the fact of also being in school and...I woke up one day, and somebody had said to me, "You know, So-and-so died." One of the AIDS patients had died. You get this bond with them. When I first started somebody said to me, "You know, we have an AIDS clinic today." I would do my job, and I would see the devastation on peoples' faces—and I had to be nice, I had to smile, I had to make it seem like they were...living.

What got to me was one of the men was dying, and the dignity...[chokes up] He got up on the scale from the wheelchair, did the nine yards. I had a little woman that came up to me and said, [nastily] "I want to see my doctor *now!*" I thought to myself, this woman who is living and breathing and capable of doing so many things is sitting here, bitching and moaning about seeing a doctor—and this poor man is dying, and knows he's dying, and he's doing it with such dignity. I couldn't say it, and I think that's part of the reason why I had to get away from the front desk, because I knew that this was breaking me up on the inside. And when they told me that this person died it really hurt. [eyes tearing] It just devastated me and I thought, Well, it's time to move on. You've done your time in the trenches, you've done your time at the front line, it's time to move on. I think it's the basic need not to be hurt, not to see the devastation. Now, if I was a doctor, that would be different; but as a clerk and as a human being, I don't think I want to be exposed to that anymore. It's not that I'm giving up, it's just maybe I can do it in another capacity, to help them. I think that's what broke my back. I thought I could handle it, but I can't.

One thing I don't like, County is run on the bullshit of seniority. I'm one of those people that believes it should be done on merit. Whether you're there a year or twenty, if you do your job and you know how to do your job, that's merit. If you think you deserve this because you've been there twenty years, that's not how it goes. But County gives you that message, that *is* how it goes. You don't have to think about your job, you just have to go through the motions. You read this board, you're allowed to go and apply for these positions, but 90 percent of the time the positions are already in mind for somebody else, and you know that. You don't know it the first year you're there, but you learn. [laughs] It's a patronage type of thing, and that's the way that the system has been for years and years and years.

Right now I'm in the middle of a squabble. I'm in Local 1111, and I resigned as of December 13th in a heated moment over misdirected quotes and miscommunication between the top administrator and my administrator and myself. So I resigned, and I was informed that I had five days to rescind my letter of resignation, and I did that. The administrator called me at my home the day before I was supposed to return to work and said to me that she would strongly suggest that I not come back to work, that she wanted to leave it the way that it was. I've been out of work for seventeen days, and we're *still* fighting over this. She has yet to call and make a meeting with the union, any representatives, myself, my administrator. She's dug in her heels. Because of the holidays, the union is sort of dragging their feet. I just called them today and said, "Pardon me, either shit or get off the pot. Are you going to fight for me?" So I'm in limbo. I would like to return to County and continue to do a good job for County, but it just doesn't seem like County wants that.

I may come back to it at some point after I get my degree. If you feel like I do, that I'm a people person, that's the first place to go, back to County, to help the people.

Michael Martinez was later reassigned to the Dermatology Department. He then applied for, and was accepted as, a senior clerk-secretary to Dr. Gordon Schiff in the General Medicine Clinic.

Dr. Vinay Kumar

HE IS A SERVICE *doctor in the Ambulatory Screening Clinic and seems both solemn and somewhat fragile. "I was born in India, in the place known as Kanpur. That's the place where I did my high school and my bachelor's degree in science and medical school. That's the place where I came from."*

I STARTED HERE AS A RESIDENT IN '88, JULY, DID MY THREE years training in Internal Medicine, and since that time I've been working in this area. I used to be a surgeon before. When I moved to this country I had trouble getting a surgical residency program, so I just moved to Medicine. They call me a Service Attending Physician—my job is to provide direct care to patients. I'm a fully trained and board-certified physician. The attending position, their job is to supervise residents, they move on the wards and do administrative stuff.

Mostly people who have no insurance, they come here. And not only does this hospital serve the people from the County of Cook, it serves people far, far away. We see people coming from Indiana, DuPage County, Kane County. I've seen people coming from Wisconsin, the Milwaukee area, coming all the way here because they couldn't afford the medical care in that area. People have told them the only place you can go, Cook County.

We take care, from seeing a patient with a common cold, coming for over-the-counter medication, to patients who are really sick with pneumonia who need to be admitted into the hospital. A lot of people who come here have been stricken with the HIV, and have a problem. A lot of people, they're Medicare patients, they see the doctor outside, their Medicare cover their doctor's fees, but it won't cover their medical bill—especially medication. They like their doctor, but they will bring the prescription all the way here to get the medication refilled, and then they don't want to go back to their doctor again. A lot of time we see people who've been referred by an outside doctor who need a CT scan, an MRI [Magnetic Resonance Imaging]. They can afford the doctor bill, but they cannot afford all these tests, so they bring the slips, they want to get it done here. A lot of time, I think, they *rely* on—you don't have a job, no money coming—so whatever money you're saving in some way, it's like earning money. When they come here, they waste a whole day, but at least they get medical care and do not pay anything a lot of the time, because they can't afford it. A lot of time they may go to emergency room, private hospital, and they do basic thing, and then they tell you go to County for the rest of the treatment.

Security is a big problem here. Sometimes patients get very mad, angry, when you don't do what they want. They will come for Tylenol 3, some medication which is restricted. They blame the doctor here, "Why they not giving?" Sometimes they want to abuse the medication. Sometimes they may need it, but there are some policies from the County Hospital—they cannot provide all medication to everybody. They get mad sometimes, they become volatile, and we have to call security. It's happened to me, and it happened to one doctor here. The patient came, he was very angry, he really became wild. There was a patient who came, he showed the doctor his knife, he want to cut his wrist off because he's feeling depressed and suicidal. You can see, people can walk in with any kind of guns and knives and there's nobody to check.

There's always anxiety to see what kind of patient it is. More anxiety can happen, the younger the patient: they're more volatile than a patient who is middle-aged and older, who are more mellow, they talk nicely—and what you say, they listen to you. But the younger patients, eighteen, nineteen, twenty, they sometimes get volatile. We serve the poor neighborhoods here, and people are very unhappy with their lives, and the frustration has to come out somewhere. The first thing is not to argue too much. I usually tell them, "Listen, let me talk to an attending, the senior doctor. Tell your story to him and if he agree, then OK we'll do it." Sometime they say, "I want this thing, I want that thing, I want Tylenol 3, I want Valium." And if you say, "No, you can't," or, "No, I don't see any reason to give all that"—they get violent.

People come here thinking that County should fill them up with what they want, but the County has a policy that we have to justify whether they need it. If you don't think you're justified or if you're just demanding, or you want to abuse the system...Some people sell—I've seen a patient who come in the last one year, eleven months, 230 times, the last time we counted! For what? Every time he comes, he has a different symptom. Every time he comes, takes a lot of medication. A lot of people we see come eighty, ninety times. And because there are so many providers in this area, you can always see a different doctor. Sometime it is because he has so many different medical problems that he has to go different clinic, and that's why; sometime we see a young healthy man who has no problems, but he has so many number of visits—and you look in the computer, he comes here every two, three days. One day he'll come here, one day he'll go to Emergency Room, then he'll come here again.

I think 98 percent of people come for genuine reasons, 2 percent abuse it. I don't know if they sell it or—I don't know what they do—but they take away all medications. I've heard that some pharmacies outside maybe buy the medications from these people. This is just heard, I have no way to substantiate. County have to end up spending all this money for nothing, which they could spend somewhere else. I feel responsible to County. I don't feel like giving medication to somebody who is trying to abuse the system. The County is here to help people, and County money is taxpayer money. Somebody is paying it—there's nothing coming here free.

There are packed in so many things within that fifteen-, twenty-minute time to see each patient. As a doctor, I have to first pick up the chart, go outside, call his name three, four, five times, so he can come. I bring him, seat him and talk to him, and then arrange other things. A lot of time we want to give—especially the females—we want to talk to them, to see they're not being abused or beaten by their husbands or boyfriends. There's a Hospital Crisis Intervention Project, which is mainly trying to find out if there are females being abused. [pointing to a list of crisis centers available] We see a lot of females having a lot of symptoms we don't know why they're having, but we don't think they have any disease or physical problem. But it may be something going on in the family. Sometime you get a reply, "Nobody hits me, I hit them back"—people sometime if you ask feel offended. But sometime you can pick it up, people who are really being abused...Sometime they come and they start crying and keep telling what's happening.

It's much harder to pick up things in the non-English-speaking population, because I cannot pick up the subtleties. When you're talking through the interpreter, you don't know what emphasis she's giving to particular words—so you can miss those things in the Hispanic populations and other populations which don't speak English. It's hard to get a translator here. Maybe sometime you can get a Spanish-speaking translator, but we see a lot of people who speak Polish, and it's very hard to find interpreter. A lot of times we have to go through the phone, have two phones, and talk to interpreter at home—that's how we do a lot of time. It's very hard. Most of the time, people don't want to volunteer to talk about it when their husband is beating them up, they don't want to tell that there's abuse going on. We can ask a couple of questions, but if the patient doesn't want to tell, there's no way you can push it.

You come across a lot of curious things. In one country where you think "thank you" is a good thing to say, in another country people may not be like that way. I was in England, and there, if you do something for anybody, a little thing, you always get a very polite "thank you." Here, people don't give that word. I see in a day, ten, twenty-five patients—rarely I get one or two "thank you." But I know that's the way it is here. Whatever you do for them—you do chest X-ray and find out things—hardly ever you can get a "thank you" here, any patient. Initially it hurt me: I'm doing all these things for him, running around, and he have no way of, to reply back. That's the only thing you need, is to say "thank you." A lot of times a patient comes and they want a medication, and I say, "We cannot give you." They immediately burst into using all kind of...they start cursing you here. [laughs] They don't even consider you a human being sometimes. If you don't do what they want, they are very angry. They have all four-, five-letter words they can use for you—start shouting-and-thumping kind of thing, very demanding. If you are working here, you have to take all of it. You cannot change their behavior in a fifteen-minute time.

They may be grateful, but there is a lack of language. Like a patient come to me, and he have bad pain, OK? An educated person will say, "Doctor, I have a very severe pain, it's causing me difficulty in sleeping." But here he'll say, "Doctor, four-letter-word pain, four-letter-word hurting me, four-letter-word." He want to say same thing an educated person will say, but he have a lack of language, a lack of vocabulary. You may get frustrated, you want to tell them—I sometimes tell them, "Listen, you want me to help you, stop using these four-letter words!" He'll say, "Oh, I'm sorry, doctor." He probably didn't mean to...it's just a natural way he's talking, his lack of vocabulary, he'll use a four-letter word. A lot of time people appreciate you, but they don't know how to express it.

I've seen, which strikes me, a lot of people have good insurance, Medicare. They are Black people, and they will come to County: I say, "Why don't you go to private hospital?" They say, "I like County." For them, this is the best hospital they have; they want to come here, they don't want to go anywhere else. Probably, they have a kind of affection for County. When they come here, they feel they getting respect and nobody shunning them out. Sometime people don't tell you that you're not welcome: a lot of hospitals, they go—the nurses will in a way tell them...you don't have to tell them but in the way that the people behave, show them that they're not welcome. This they don't feel here.

If they build a new hospital or not, as long as the people are the same, it won't make much difference. See, I'm here because peoples are here, people who need medical care. I won't be here if they're not. If they make a way-fancy hospital, that's very good, but it won't change things. Nothing is worse than what is here now. No older building they could find than what we have now [laughs] They can make any building, it will be better than this.

Moving People

Dorothy Wilson

ELEVATOR OPERATOR. *She seems patient, not easily flustered.* "I came to Chicago from Mississippi when I was seventeen. I wasn't familiar with the hospital until I started working here in '83. I was working at Sears and Roebuck, and I was laid off. I'd been out of work for a year, so I came here and did volunteer work for four months, hoping to get a job out of it, and I did. I've worked in all the buildings here, but I like the main building the best. It keeps you stimulated. [laughs]

IF A PERSON STEPS ON THE ELEVATOR AND THEY DON'T HAVE a pass, well, then, you have the authority to ask them to step off to go get a pass. But if a problem occur, then you have to call the officer to come. A lot of your problems, you can handle yourself—it all depends on how you handle yourself, and what person you're dealing with. You might come to me angry—maybe your mother is very sick, or your husband just didn't do something you wanted him to do—and at this moment you're angry, so you come to me nasty and rude and all that hostility in you: I'm gonna get it. And then if I can't maintain, then we're just two people standing there being nasty. If she calls me a bitch, and I turn around and I call her a bitch, then we got a problem. So I just have to be the bitch for the day, that's all. [laughs]

If a person comes to me and I see that they're angry, then I break down, you know? I be their little punch bag, whatever. You be nice, you just let them say whatever, get it out, and don't come back to them with something nasty, and it'll work itself out. Sometimes, people will say they don't have a pass—they'll say, "Well, my mother is in Trauma, she just got shot and I'm not going to get no pass. Take me to see my mother!" You say, "Well, ma'am, hospital policy states that everyone must have a pass. Go to the information desk, and they'll give you a pass right away." Most of the time that works, sometimes that don't. Most of the times, *then* you need help.

There's a phone on the elevator and you call. Most of the time, you get most of your help from the other people on the elevators. If a person comes up with what everyone can see is an off-the-wall story for why they don't have a pass, then they help you out. "I got an emergency up on the fifth floor, I got to go." And usually the person will step back off the elevator. If there are two or three, especially with the younger crowd, you have a problem: they'll try to pass the pass to each other. The excuse that most of the people use for not having a pass is, "I left mine upstairs." [laughs] But after you operate that elevator for so long and you deal with so many people, you pick up so many different kind of personalities—and you can almost tell if they're lying or not.

When I started, it took me a long time to adapt. I had never seen anything like it. At most private hospitals the elevators are quiet: you may see one or two visitors every now and then. [laughs] When I came in, it was *wild*. Now, Trauma has their own elevator, but during the time when I came they were using elevators 6 and 7 to take patients up to Trauma. They would call and let the operator know to clear the elevator. Working those elevators was frightening, because you saw so much. When you first see this, it do a little something to you—but after a while it was just like nothing, you don't think about it. Only thing that will bother me is sometimes I'd think to myself, If I open this door and they bring a stretcher on, will it be a relative of mine? That would bother me sometimes. Here you get to learn, and you get to understand a lot of things real quick—basically death or killing, because you see it all the time. Here. If you were somewhere else, you wouldn't see it that often.

You have to use your own judgment—especially if you're in tight with all these people, and they're going to crowd in on you at one time. It's a distraction, having ten or fifteen people standing there waiting, because out of that ten or fifteen, five may not have a pass. While you're asking these ones for passes that *do* have them, the others are all around there in back, trying to sneak in behind the others however way they can do it. Then once they get in the back and it's crowded and you ask, "Sir, do you have a pass?"…That's when this behind-the-arm thing starts, and you got to be looking very closely to catch it, if it's crowded. You got to be on your toes.

The two elevators on the end, they're just for freight and to take employees only to the seventh and eighth floors. But employees will still come to you and want you to take them here and there. When you refuse, they're angry because they may be in a hurry—and then when they come to the center elevators, those're full, they're tight, people waiting…So I guess they say, "If I run down here right quick, I can get where I'm going." Sometimes they get real angry—the doctors, everybody. And, then, some of them can be so sweet too. That's why you have to be flexible, because all people that approaches you are not the same.

People ask me, "How do you stand it?" or "Don't you get bored?" or "Why don't you read something?" "Where's your radio?" That gets on your nerves, because you might have to hear that from fifty people. By the time you get to the thirty-fifth person, you're angry—so that person probably gets a nasty response. Then they'll say, "Ew, she got a nasty attitude." But I don't, it's just because I done heard this so many times until now, I got to release it. Dealing with the public is hard. You got to keep the mind going, because a lot of time if you don't, you'll do or say something before you think: sometimes you can just say the smallest thing, and someone will report you. Every person feel that you should just be all smiles—they don't stop to think or understand what you're going through for the eight hours. No one thinks about it. *No one.* [laughs] If I'm slow, don't have to look for too many passes, then frankly my mind's back at home. We're not supposed to have books, but if a book do happen to just walk past your way, you know, and you catch it...[laughs] and you read a paragraph or so. During the time you're reading, you blank everything out. You may lose your attention for a minute, but you can't lose it for that long.

There's two bells. One regular, just for waiting for the elevator, and then you have your emergency bell for all floors, and that can be a problem—three long rings. So you get a transporter or a doctor or whatever there with a patient, and they ring it: *ring, ring, ring.* Now you put all the peoples off because you have to go to an emergency for the third floor. The third-floor emergency is three short rings. No one's there—so you go back and pick up the people you left. You know, people play with the bells all the time. You load all the peoples up again, three short rings come right back. So, you go back to the third floor—but nothing is there. Now you got to use your own mind. Where is it? When you get to seven they're angry, but they didn't ring the bell right. "Well, I'm going to write you up because I rang three long rings." What can you do? Sometimes you get away, sometimes you don't—sometimes you be believed, sometimes you don't. Sometimes you hear the emergency bell, put people off, rush to the floor and see an employee standing there. "Oh, I need to get down to warm my sandwich." You know, something like that. Now you're ready to...Oh...[shakes head]

Sometimes you just have to stop, walk around the corner, and get you a soda. And they don't understand that: "Oh, the operator stepped off." Or you got to go to the washroom—I do have a bladder, you know? I have one, just like you. But people don't understand that; they feel like you're just supposed to be there. You're not supposed to be angry, don't get upset, just treat peoples nice. You can do it for a while, but somewhere down the line, before the eight hours is out, you've got to explode. Some days you can get through it, it's OK all the way. You might tell another operator, "No one made me angry today." [laughs]

When I train people, I try to eliminate telling them about the bad parts, because then that's what they'll be looking for. You don't really want to be looking for that, because it's coming anyway. [laughs] I tell them, if you talk to the people nice, they'll come back with something nice; and if a person comes to you hostile and talking crazy, then just don't say nothing till they finish. Sooner or later, if they don't go get the pass, they'll walk away and go somewhere else, because they can't get what they're looking for from you. Basically, it works out, because we don't have that many problems. Sometimes we have to get the officer, but it's not that often.

I learned that it all boils down to how you treat people. Most people respond to you the way that you respond to them—most of them. And a lot of people can come to you hostile, and, sometimes, talking to them nicely—it's all they need to hear. This is what they want to hear, is a nice word. I can do it, because I don't have a hostile heart. But if your heart is cold you can't do this job, you can't do it as well. You got to have compassion, and you got to be able to apply it when needed.

Richard Love

He's a husky young man, serious, but quick to laugh. He and a friend are working on starting an accounting business. Working at the hospital is what he's doing in the meantime. "I'm an In-patient Transporter. You get to wear the ugliest thing they have. [referring to his burgundy uniform] Nobody likes it. They give it to us so they can spot us."

Besides being born here, i'd never been to county before I started the job. I would see it on the news.

When you start here they don't even let you move patients for about a month. You just get to pull the equipment, walk around, learn your way around the hospital. I was here three weeks when a police officer was killed—over here on the West Side somewhere. A guy shot her. I was working down by the Emergency Room, and they came through with her. I could see the blood jumping out her chest—she was already dead, but her body was still functioning. I went and threw up, then I had to help take her to the morgue.

My first assignment was the ER, and it gets busy. You never know what's going to happen next. Last week I was working, I had to take a patient from Trauma. A guy was in a car accident, a motorcycle versus a car, and his arm was in the sink in ice. When they took the helmet off of him, I looked at him, and it was a guy that I went to grade school with. You know, working here is one thing, because you can go talk about everything when it's done—but when it's somebody you know it really hits you differently. His cousin came running down the hall, asking where was he. He was dead. I couldn't tell him he was dead...He lost too much blood. [pause] There was nothing that could be done. I couldn't tell him—that's something that's best left for doctors to do.

That Emergency Room is quick, everything happens so quick. You have to stay on your toes. I was going over to check the NSU [Nursery Service Unit], and at the back door of the Emergency Room the lady got out of the chair and got on the ground. I picked her up and put her on the stretcher, and I was saying, "Don't push, don't push." She pushed, and the baby shot out—and I blocked it with my legs from hitting the ground, like in hockey. I just stood in front and closed my legs and trapped him up against the stretcher.

I have a pretty strong stomach now. I don't know if that's good or bad, because, you know, you can watch somebody die and then go get lunch. It doesn't even bother you like it should, like it should to see a dead body. You shouldn't be able to just go out and get you a sandwich.

I talk to people while I'm transporting them. Everybody has a different conversation. Some people make you laugh. Nobody wants to be in the hospital, so you try to treat the patients like you would want your parents to be treated, with respect and everything. And 95 percent of the people in here, they do a pretty good job—not only transport co-workers, but other hospital personnel. This place can be really trying sometimes. There's never enough time; elevator service is not that great, and it's not really the fault of the operators. There's no priority. There should be a patient elevator and an elevator for everybody else, but there's not, so you just have to deal with it. You're laid out on a stretcher and everybody is leaning over you, trying to see what's wrong with you—unless you have a mask on, and then everybody is trying to turn away. This is a place like no other. It reminds me of *M*A*S*H*, that TV program.

We need a lot of help right now, and I don't know if they're hiring as many people as they should. I don't know if it's some money problem or whatever; all I know is, we need some more help. One weekend we showed up to work, we had six people to work transportation for the *whole* complex—every building! And there should be fifteen, at *least* fifteen people. Out of that six you had to send two to the ER, someone to the Clothes Room, someone has to go up to the fifth floor for the OBs, and it was like three people to move the rest of the patients. That included the transfers and X-rays and *everything*. That's just a typical Saturday, Sunday.

We get a tough rap. The dispatcher sits there and answers the phone, with five phone banks going off every two minutes. Everybody needs a transporter, and they don't have enough to send. You would have a foul personality too—yeah. "Soon as I can," *click*. You just don't have enough people to send to do the work. Most of the transporters, we like to get the work done, we *want* to get the work done. Every once in a while, you might have a bad day, you might not be up to par. You need to take you a break or two, and that's understandable because everybody goes through that. You get into it with some of the residents sometimes because they're busy, you're busy: they'll see you walking down the hall and, because you don't have a patient on your stretcher right then, they think they can just, "Come here, do this." Just, "Hey you!" Everybody will run out in the hall when I'm coming down from lunch, and they'll all swamp me at one time: "Love, we got a patient to go." Then you go off on the nurses a little bit, because they don't seem to understand that there's just one transporter against seven people. It's crazy! They can see it and won't understand it, so how can you explain it? [laughs]

It's not the sick people that depress you, it's the hospital. It's the lack of help you have, it's the frustration you feel when you know that these patients need to be moved, and there's just nobody to do it—and *every-body* is jumping on the first person in this burgundy that they see. And that gets to you. We just do the best we can. But you know what? The hospital shuts down if there's no transporters or no ward clerks, because the doctors, they can transport, but there's not enough doctors to do the transport. And they wouldn't have the slightest idea what to do with a chart. If they had to do the job of a ward clerk for an hour, they would quit! Sometimes the clerk, she might be working Ward 41, and she might also have to work Ward 43. Back and forth, admitting patients and discharging patients and scheduling exams—it's hard. You take the transporters and the clerks away from the hospital, and they're in *big* trouble.

The nurses and the doctors, they deserve a lot of credit, and I understand that they went to school and that they dedicated whatever number of years to be that—but I'm no less a person just because I'm a transporter. They do give *individuals* respect. A lot of the doctors, we play basketball and football and everything, so I feel like they've exerted themselves to trust me and befriend me in whatever way.

After I worked in the ER maybe a year, I worked in the OR. We have a lot of same-day surgery patients. You get those special patients where the doctors are like in moon suits—there's a lot of things that happen up there...I've watched them do hip replacements: they were knocking the ball joint out in the hip, and he actually had a hammer and chisel. He was whacking it, and you could hear it, *whack, whack, whack*. It's not like watching it on TV, when you can look in the room and watch them do a surgery. Sometime you stand there, and you might have some work to do, but you get caught up. It's the same way in Trauma. Sometimes you come in, for a car accident or something, and it's amazing to see a doctor actually stick his hands in somebody's chest and massage the heart. Until you see it...Some of us, it fascinates us, and some of us, we just do our jobs. I don't know which one is the better. When you just do your job, then you don't get so intense about everything you see.

Sometimes I wish I didn't get so intense...a lot of times, actually. Christmas Day, two years ago, a lady had twins, stillborn. I had to take them to the morgue. They wrapped them up in...like when you go to the store and get a dollar's worth of cheese, and they wrap it in that paper. I walked down with twins in my hand, taking them to the morgue. Then you open the door, and you see all these...There's a lot of them, you wouldn't *believe* how many it is. Stillborns, maybe fifteen inches long, just wrapped up in paper. And they look like you just went to the store and got some bacon or something.

I can do just about anything, but I really hate going over to Peds. When you see the babies with the needles and everything sticking in them—it tears you up. Here's this baby, three days old, tubes in their noses, needles in their arms and on monitors and everything. We had one baby, he wouldn't quit crying. One of his parents had tossed him into a wall and his brain was swelling—it was pressing up against his skull and it caused pain, and he just cried. I don't think he was two months old. I had to take him over to the CT scan room, and he cried all the time. I took him out of the basket and carried him in my arms. I left crying, it tore me up…so I don't like to go over to Peds.

A lot of patients, you get attached to them. One guy, Percy, he was in the hospital for maybe eight months. He couldn't swallow—his esophagus was big as a dime. I don't know what they did, but his reflex was in the side of his neck, and they rearranged everything inside so he could swallow. Percy knew he couldn't win, but he tried to do everything they asked him to do. You get attached to them, because every day you come in, you go up, and when you're up on Ward 60 you stop and say, "What's up, Perce?" Then one day you come, and he's not there: "What happened to Percy?" "He passed away." It gets kinda tough, because you get used to seeing them. The only thing you have to make you feel good is that the people appreciate your taking care of them. You don't get a kind word from anybody but the patients. Everyone else is, "Just the transporter." You're *just* the transporter!

I went from the OR down here to Endoscopy. They say I'm not permanent. They won't give me the weekends off, but I've been up there for three years—that sounds pretty permanent to me! [laughs] You never know what you're going to see. We came in one day, and we had a lot of police up there. One guy had swallowed about sixty balloons of dope—heroin—he got sick at the airport, and they had to bring him out here. You walk in, and you see the FBI and the Chicago police. I walked in the door, turned around, and walked out. [laughs] I didn't know if they were there for me or not. I mean, when you see police, you just turn around. We've pulled shampoo bottles out of people, bowling pins…potatoes, light bulbs. One guy comes in maybe once every other year, with a potato—a whole white potato! And then one day he had the potato sliced! I kid you not. They put me out because I laughed: the doctors said, "Rich, you gotta go." [laughing] "Foreign body," that's all the report says. [laughs] It's so crazy when you see it and hear it—you just sit there amazed.

I can't stand soap operas, but I watched *General Hospital* when I was a little boy. I think County's just like it—love affairs and everything, you name it. Matter of fact, I was married and I *did* meet my wife here—she was a transporter! We didn't get along, so we decided to part. She still works here. It goes on. You flirt. What else you got to do? You got three thousand women to look at. You see people dying all day, and you need some relief, so you flirt.

There's nothing wrong with this, but it's just, pushing patients is a dead-end job. We're not paid as much as at most hospitals, even though we see probably three or four times the volume that any other transporter sees. One clerk, she told me, "You changed a little bit." It wears you out, every day, day in, day out. She's been here about twenty-five years, so she said she done already went through it and recovered. You don't have the smile on your face, that's basically what it is. Because when you're new here it's like *wow*, you're smiling, because everything is so new and so exciting. And then you see everything repeat itself every day, and it wears you out. The aggravation, waiting on the elevators, arguing with doctors and nurses if you do this or that, and the four or five long trips...you name it. And maybe that's what changes your personality some too, because your body is so beat up. It just wears you out.

Guarding People

Caroline Morgan

SHE LOOKS STERN *in her police uniform and pressed white shirt, but in fact she is kindly and reflective.* "*I became a police officer in 1983. It was just about the time that Reagan was president, and many jobs that had been available were closing down, and the job market was pretty tight. I started venturing out to see what there was. I'd always wanted to work in a hospital—at one point in time I had planned to study nursing.*"

YOU HAVE TO GO TO POLICE ACADEMY FOR ABOUT THREE months. We work only on the complex of the hospital. When we get off, we're still police, but we have to lock up our guns here when we go home.

We're paid very low, and as a result we get a big turnover—I guess because it's a hospital, but that's not necessarily a good reason. We're providing the same kinds of services as a police officer on the street: we do have to lock up individuals, and many of them are very hostile. Officers have been hurt or nearly hurt. There have been occasions when these individuals attempted to take the gun. A person could die—when you have the same kinds of hazards involved, then you should be paid comparable, I think: equal pay for equal work.

I hadn't had much experience with County before I started working here. I got sick once and came. It was a trying experience. I liked the doctors and I liked the service and all that, but I remember the same thing I hear now, often: "I've been waiting eight hours." That particular night I had waited something like eight to ten hours in the ER: I came in about four, and I didn't get out until about twelve at night. At that time, I had lost a job and didn't have any money. I had gone to this private doctor I was seeing when I had the other job and I had money, and he had told me what he thought was needed. I said, "OK, Doctor, that's fine, but at this point in time I don't have any insurance. I'll be happy to pay as soon as I get better and find work." His remark was, [haughtily] "Then you can't be seen." So I came to County.

The doctors were great. Just like all the other patients, I swear by Cook County. [laughs] The only thing I wasn't sure about was where to get something to eat. I was afraid to get up and go get something, because I was afraid they were going to call my name. I *really* needed to be seen, and I didn't know who to ask where to get the food, and it was like a real long evening.

The thing that I remember most is that, as a patient, I was on the other side, so I know where they're coming from. I don't really know, but at least I can have empathy with that in terms of when somebody walks up to you and says, "I've been here eight hours," or whatever the case may be. If it's a situation where the chart may have gotten lost or something, I'll try to check and find out. It's really not something that's required, but...

Now the homeless, that's a serious problem here. Somehow, I feel that it's hopeless or helpless in terms of the homeless. I know that this is a hospital, and when they're on the street and get sick, this is the first place they come. But I would hope that the administration would have some better way—social workers, or somebody with contact with them, that could make some kind of plans or changes or whatever, so that we're not constantly putting homeless out. That's part of our job, to put them out, because this is a *hospital*. I don't have no problem with that, but on the other hand, you sit and ask yourself, Where can they go? They put them out of the mission, say, at eight o'clock in the morning, especially in the cold winter. We've been given information about contacting the Department of Human Services, and we do call them, but many times these people won't accept, won't go there. When it gets very cold out, of course we don't put them out. We try to be compassionate about it.

It varies—different officers handle it differently. Some of them believe that they're the *po*-lice, whatever that is. My idea of the *po*-lice is 90 percent social worker and 10 percent officer. You get to lock up about 10 percent of the time, and the rest of the time you're providing services. I'm probably in the minority on that: they like to refer to me as a social worker. Sometimes I resent it, and sometimes I think, Well, what the hell is wrong with that? [laughs] The bottom line is, of course, you have to take your own personal feelings out of it in order to do what you have to do. When you gotta lock up somebody, you *can't* have compassion. After all, they committed a crime, and you gotta go ahead and do that. But there are so many instances here at the hospital where that's a human being. It only takes a few seconds [snaps fingers] for somebody to get out of control—and that's patients.

I remember an incident where one of the women in Fantus was having some difficulty in walking. She was with her daughter or sister, another female—they weren't familiar with procedure. They came from Ortho, and they stopped at the desk to find out where to go for X-ray, which was right across from the desk. So they went there, and I don't know what the young lady told them, but it entailed them having to leave there and walk someplace again. But by this time the frustration level was getting very high. I could sense what they were feeling, because I probably would have felt the same thing, like, "Damn, why can't somebody tell me what's going on? Why do I have to be walking in circles?" Come *here*, and then they have to go *there* [waving arm around, frustrated] and then go over *there* and get an appointment. *What?!* And these [hitting table on each word] are sick people. I said, "Ma'am, probably what would help is, first, we get you a wheelchair." Things cooled out, and she went on her way. By the time she was going home, she said, "Thanks so much, because I almost went off on you." And I know, because I've been in a situation myself and I'm thinking, Why isn't it that I can't get better information than this?

It's frustrating. The other thing, why we're needed a lot—you've probably noticed we have officers out in the ER front triage. They've got a new system, and I don't know if it's the best thing; I personally think it would be nicer if relatives could wait with their loved ones when they bring them in. They want the patient to remain in the ER, and they want the friend or relative, whoever it might be, to sit out front until they call them—out front in the main lobby. This brings on a lot of animosity, hatred, and hostility. It's like, in the first place, administration says this is the way they want it—*I* really don't want to have to tell you to go there. This started after they opened the new ER and remodeled. The officers aren't happy about having to be assigned to front triage, because the people get very mean at times, and abusive. People are that way anyway when they're concerned about someone they love. And they really want to know, they don't want to leave the person alone.

There are about sixty-five police officers, and now we have seven or eight recent recruits who are women. As a female, I get a little annoyed at two themes I get on a regular basis: either "That's a big gun you're wearing on your side," or "Hey, honey." I've been a sergeant since December, so lately I get a lot of "Hello, Sergeant," but when I was wearing the blue shirt I got a lot of "Hey, honey." It's the street attitude. Patients, visitors…"Have you ever shot anybody?" It's a regular kind of thing—it's like one lady on Oprah said: "Men don't get it." [laughs] It's hard for them to give you just ordinary, normal respect. You ask a simple question and you want a simple answer, but you'll get a whole lot of shit in between, instead of the answer. But, generally speaking, things go very well, and there is a good amount of respect.

If we have to lock someone up, we have to put the handcuffs on them—they could do anything, or be carrying a weapon, whatever. We have to search them out there in the complex, and then bring them in here. We handcuff them to the pole, the one bolted to a wall in the main room, and then the Chicago police takes them to the lockup. If they're a patient then the officer sits on them.

The hospital's like a little city. Whatever happens on the streets of Chicago, it happens here. A male patient will come in, and he might have a girlfriend *and* a wife—they both come visit him, and then all hell breaks out. [laughs] Or the family might come, and members might be angry— you know how you have members of a family that haven't spoken to each other for years? All kinds of little messes. So there we are, in the middle of it: put them out of the hospital, or arrest them for disorderly, or whatever the case may be. We have our officers patrolling those areas, being invisible, trying to see if there's something suspicious. Of course we hope that the employees will assist us, and they do—they'll call and say, "There's a strange-looking man here," or "This shouldn't be," or "I heard a noise over here." And we have the emergency phone system, those yellow boxes, that are spread throughout the tunnels and the parking lots.

We have about fourteen buildings, and a lot of it has to be open—people and patients, visitors, are going back and forth. Our officers are constantly moving, but of course they can't see everything. Officers in the city don't see everything, so neighbors have to help each other. Staff workers report, "I had a little radio stolen," or this kind of thing—and I'm thinking, Why did you bring your radio anyway? You came to *work*. [laughs]

I think we only had two calls where they said there was a man with a gun, and that was in the School of Nursing. Of course, I didn't pull mine until I got inside the building and around where nobody could get hurt. Usually no, though, no guns. There was an incident with an officer where an individual did try to get his gun, and he *almost* got it—other officers came to his rescue. But there are crazies that come through, and hardened criminals.

It's like being a beat cop, I suppose—it's definitely a beat. [laughs] Right—because patients tend to come back. There are definitely regulars, in the sense that once they've had good results here, or for whatever reason they're here, they feel good about it and they come back again. I don't always recognize everybody. Patients will tell me, "Remember? You helped me." I was doing the job, and I don't remember them, let alone the incident, but they'll remind me. I say, "Oh, OK." [laughs] I try to remember, but I know I'm not going to. I just say, "*Oh,* it's good to see you. How you doing?"—and go on about my business.

I think there are a lot of things that could be worked out. There's a lot of new equipment that we ourselves need in this department. Have you been to other police departments? Look around, you tell me what we need. When we do a case report, we got to do copies. Do you see a Xerox machine? We go all the way to the main building, the administrator's office, to get copies! How many security cameras do you see in there? How many are *working?* We have a large complex, couldn't we use more cameras? I was recently downtown at 401 South State, and they had thirty for *one* building. In this day and age, *everybody* you know has computers. Do you see one? There's only one electric typewriter, and *it* doesn't work! We have a lot of data and information we should be able to get our hands on. As long as they're not going to give us a good salary, at least give us good equipment. If you're lacking both, why? It's not right. Most of us probably are used to working on a shoestring, we probably grew up with families who aren't rich—but we know what the rest of the world is dealing with and using, so why can't we be a little part of it?

But County, it's very, very interesting. In fact, I went on vacation and I was thinking, Geez, it'll be so good to get away from there. I had a three-week vacation: the first two weeks went well, the third week I started missing the place. [laughs] I knew I was in trouble. I really did.

Talking to People

Dennis DuPont

IS A SOCIAL WORKER *with an impish V-shaped grin, and a generally bemused manner. "I'm from the cornfields of Minnesota. My parents were farmers—my father was fourth generation on the same farm. I have a brother eleven months younger than me—he's now a diesel mechanic. My parents were kind of hoping that one of us would take the farm over, but it was just unrealistic as far as expenses, so I thought I better find something else to do."*

WHEN I WAS GOING THROUGH SCHOOL AT LOYOLA, I DID AN internship where I worked on the Neonatal Intensive Care Unit, over in Pediatrics, here at Cook County Hospital. I was pretty disgusted. That's all I did, I didn't get perspective on any of the other units. I was impressed with the doctors—they're very skilled, very knowledgeable. What I was disgusted with, mostly, was the patients: why are so many mothers, young mothers, having children? They're on public aid, and you hear all these stories: well, they're getting on public aid because they want to have an income. With no children, you're expected to go out and work, so they have babies to have an income, or they have babies because they want to have someone to love.

I'm hearing all this, and you have all these mothers who are constantly using drugs during the pregnancy, or use cocaine seventy-two hours prior to delivery, which induces delivery. So I'm hearing this, and calling DCFS constantly. I was getting pretty disgruntled about the lack of prevention, lack of resources out there to help these people. We were overwhelming the agencies. It was like an epidemic problem.

I really had no intentions to come to County and work. The politics here...I never *knew* there was so much politics involved when you're just trying to do your job. When I was an intern, and even when I first came here to work, I'd have workers who would tell me, "Don't get involved, don't offer your services to help"—as far as getting on committees to do things—"do *not* get noticed. Just stay low."

I got started in November—on Pediatrics, because that was the position that was open. Worked on Ward 46. The people reported to DCFS as abused and neglected were assigned to a separate team here at County—a team specializing in such cases. Well, I said, "No, the patient is in my ward, it's my client. *I* will go to the team, I'll let you know what's happening with that client, but I'm going to be the one responsible—I'm not

265

going to turn it over to them." I told the supervisor, "I don't want to work that way." So we got that rolling first. Then I got responsible for the ER. I guess the way that was set up was, you called a social worker whenever you needed a social worker. But many times the social worker is not available. So what I started doing is, I'd go down there four times a day—just circulate and find out what was going on.

Then I went to Ward 63, because the worker was leaving suddenly. I had two days of training to do amputee and vascular service. I got involved in the amputee clinic, and we decided to turn the ward into 100 percent coverage. The other wards, the way it's set up was the doctor makes a referral to see a social worker, the clerk calls the social worker—so not every patient was seen. A lot of patients would just go through the hospital. I came on the amputee ward and started seeing every patient on the floor. Most of them were diabetics, some of them had accidents, hypertension, whatever. So there were some complications. Now, if you have an amputee, well, of course they can't climb three flights of stairs—that's a problem, it's an adjustment problem. I got into a system where in half a day I got all the information out of the charts, I could see the patients, who is going to really need help. Everything fine with you? Great. *Boom.* I had my questions, and if they had no problems, then I'd document such. The others, I'd get my information, spend a little time, and come back the next day. Some of them were like three months on the ward, so you had more time to sit and interact, to engage and help with the adjustments.

Since April, I've been in Trauma. What I do is, I'll sit in morning rounds and then I'll start making phone calls on the things that need to be taken care of for that day. I go through Trauma and be known, be available to the residents and nurses if they have a question. And the unknowns, let me know about them now, I'll try and work on it. Unknowns are the most difficult—people coming in, no address, no IDs. We've got one now, sorta…Well, he's a known, but he's out of it—no family contact. I checked the addresses: no phone numbers, nobody near his location. We know his name, we know his address, that's it.

So today I'll send a letter to his address. I don't know who's going to respond, but I'll send a letter. He tested positive for opiates and alcohol, and was found hanging out of the car door. You can shake him, he looks at you, and then he goes back out. I don't know if it's organic-related or what. Those are the hardest. We do have an address, so this time we can track the address and maybe find a phone, like in a building or apartment complex. We can try and call a few neighbors, see if they know the person. Sometimes we can track people with a social security number, but they don't have the name of the mother, father, brothers or sisters on that social security form. Public aid is the same way: they don't have family members listed.

I try to make my way through there at least five, six times a day. A lot of the trauma patients, when they're no longer that acute, will go to R3, which is a Medical unit—like a ward. Or if there's an overload, they'll be sent to some of the other wards on the floor. So I'll make my way through R3, open up the charts, find all the new traumas, get all the information. Once I get all that done, then I start hitting the patients. People call me and say, "This person's coming in, he's intoxicated, talk to him." Well, I've learned that there's some you can start talking to, but most of the time they're not even going to remember, they're so out of it. I will try to talk to them and get some initial things taken care of, but then I come back the next day and say, "Let's start talking about serious things. You've got a problem—do you want to stop?" After I get all the psychosocial data, then I start getting into the counseling: "Do you have a problem?" "Yes." If they say no, I'll say, "Well, I'm not going to waste your time. I'll give you a list of resources—organizations offering substance abuse counseling. You've got my number, call me when you're ready. Bye." I always give them my number.

A lot of them will accept the list of resources, but most of them won't go. Once they get out of the hospital, that's it: time to go back in the community and start using again, until something else happens. One of the major problems is that there are a lot of treatment centers out there that just are overwhelmed. Many of the people who come here don't have public aid, don't have any insurance—they're very limited as to where they can go. That's a major problem. All these people that are willing to stop, but…Or you have a person who has a gunshot wound to the leg, he just got an ace bandage or something, so he needs some care—no treatment center wants him. Some centers won't even take insulin-dependent diabetics, or any patient that takes certain medications. So it's a problem. I think after three years in hospital work, I've had maybe ten patients who have actually gotten up and gone to the phone. And I'll take them to the phone.

It doesn't depress me because, eventually, down the road, someone else will go. So you keep trying. Yeah, it's depressing in numbers—but I don't know, some people just haven't hit bottom yet. I'm not going to baby you—I'll give you five, ten minutes, and those that are motivated, I'll give you a lot more time. But when I can assess somebody who's not really motivated, who's just giving me the runaround, I'll quit. I'll see them the next day, "How ya doin'?" If they say, "Hey, I want to make this phone call," great—I'll drop everything and we'll do it! It happens—rare, but I keep going, keep trying to push that. But I'm not going to waste my time if you're going to go out and start using again, and you know it. There are other people down the road that I need to order wheelchairs for, or I need to get things set up for.

A lot of patients come in here with no money, no income. There are some wheelchair vendors who are willing to do it, but you kind of got to twist their arm a little bit and give them a ton of other referrals that have insurance. We tell the patients: "Look, you've got to come up with fifty bucks, or eighty bucks. Get the money somewhere. If you have to have someone go out in the street and panhandle, if you've got some relatives. You've got to do something to show us that you're interested, that you're gonna help. We're not just gonna give it to you and say, here." There are a lot of people that do take the wheelchairs and sell them. There are a lot of patients that may need things that we just cannot...We'll maybe have to keep them here an extra day or something. Or bend a relative's arm and say, "Can you take this person? This person really needs to go somewhere."

If you have no housing, no insurance, no home...That's happened, there's nothing I can do. We call around, we do what we can. I may spend a couple hours looking around—and that means someone else is not getting the care. I know there's only a few places you can go, but I will call around again and see what we can do. Or I'll try and...I'll say, "Hey, this person, just before he came in, used alcohol or a substance." If they mention they've a history of drug use or something, I'll use that.

I had to send a patient home the other day, in his late twenties—he had a gunshot wound to the leg. He needed a place to go but he was homeless. His sister said she would bring him some clothes and that's it: she didn't want nothin' to do with him. He wanted to quit using cocaine and alcohol. I said, "When's the last time you used?" He said the last time was the day before he came in. I said, "Well, you've been here three days, so you're basically detoxed. All I can do is send you to a shelter. There are some detoxes available, but the only way to get in is to tell them you've just used." [laughs uncomfortably] I said, "I'm sorry. Either overnight shelters and then go to a day shelter"—or, I'm sorry to say, go get yourself drunk and then go. But I didn't say that. I just said, "You gotta play the game to get yourself into treatment." And that's the way it is: you've got to play the game sometimes.

Some people say you've got to lie to get the patients into a nursing home. No, we have an obligation to tell the people legitimately what's going on with the case. *Yes,* we want the patient out of here, but at the same time, we've got to find a place that's appropriate, because the patient is the one who's jeopardized. I know there's other hospitals that do that to us all the time—they dump. I don't think we have to dump back.

The main thing is, I try to get the family involved, or some relative. I don't want you to just get on a bus and go home. Get someone to come here physically, bring some clothes. And if you're homeless, you can find a relative to put you up for two, three days, or something. Sometimes they've blown it with their family, and they're not going to tell me that, but I'll call and find out the whole scoop later. I'll say, "Can you just put him up for a couple of days?" "No." "OK—thank you." I'll let them know he's going to a shelter, and they could care less. But I can't allow myself to get overempathetic and spend hours and hours knowing that I'm up against a wall. All I can do is send them to an appropriate shelter and say, "There's some people there that you need to talk to. They can help get your life back on track." I can't do follow-up with these people. I don't have the time, and most of them don't have the phones, or some person down the block has the phone. I just give them a card and say, "Call me if there's a problem."

So that's my day. I go to Trauma, and then I go to R3. Then I move to other wards on the third floor that may have some Trauma patients, and try and see them. Each time I go finish up in R3 or go on a break or something, I will cut through Trauma just to show myself, "How's things going?" At one o'clock, it's visiting hours, so I try and come around at that time to see any family that shows up. That helps me with discharge—family members, church members, somebody. I ask people, "Do you belong to a church? Go to your pastor. Have your pastor try and rake up some money from the community and help you out," buy the wheelchair or whatever. The discharge process is my role.

Dr. Mary Fabri

HAS A GENTLE, TRANQUIL *quality which comes in handy—she's a psychologist. "Once I started my internship here I thought, I am home. A lot of it had to do with values. Because it's a difficult place, not just anybody works here. There's 'lifers,' and there's people who use County as a stepping stone—it's a great entree card. When I tell people about County, I say it's seductive." She recently began to work in the Adult Psychiatry Clinic, after seven years of working in Child Oncology.*

WHEN I WALK INTO COUNTY, I DON'T SEE THE PHYSICAL SET-ting, I don't see the oldness of it. It takes until I go over to Rush or University of Illinois and look around that I think, Oh, this is different! [laughs] I don't know if it's good or bad that this feels like home to me. I mean, is it healthy? [laughs] But I hear it from the patients who come here too. It's referred to as "the County." And this sense of "my mom was born here, I was born here, my children were born here"...

There's this strong sense of the hospital being an entity unto itself. At times, it's felt almost mythical—as though the County has always been here. Looking at the front entrance, that big old structure, that's the County to me. It sort of looms over, it's not sterile and modern—it's some sort of a symbol. It's been here a long time, and so there is something that County takes on, a sense that it *will* exist. And I guess that, sometimes, whether it's a false sense or not, it's hard to believe that County could ever close. What would happen? How *could* it close? I think it's that same feeling about County, where there's a positive transference, and that transfers onto me. When I meet families or patients that are coming in for the first time, or if they're hooked into County, just by grace of County and my working here, they accept me.

My patients are mostly African American, some Hispanic, Asian, an occasional White. There's cultural differences, class differences, educational differences—and that does impact, because there's this whole sense of...Sometimes a patient will say, "Well, you probably don't know about this," and then go on to tell me. I remember having a mom say to me, "You don't know what it's like to raise a Black son." I have a son, but his opportunities are going to be totally different. I told her, "Yeah, you're absolutely right," and then used it as a way of acknowledging her—and what a hard job she has, what a good job she's been doing, and what she needs to do to continue doing a good job.

I worked in Austin High School for a year, in the school clinic that County has out there. It was very common for the kids to say to me, "You don't understand where I live." And they were absolutely right: I grew up in the suburbs. I can remember looking forward to vacation time, but at Austin High School [on the West Side] so many of the kids got depressed when it was time to be off from school for two weeks: school was a way to get out of the house. When they're on vacation, they're prisoners in their home—they're not allowed to go outside because it's not safe. You know, there are households with four TVs and four VCRs—and when I went out to the high school, I began to understand what that was about: that's how they keep the kids in the house. They each get their own TV, their own VCR, but they're not allowed to go outside. I think that's a high price to pay, but I began to understand some of how a family organizes itself, which I always felt critical of before I learned...The whole issue of poverty and living in poverty—how can someone have four TVs and three VCRs when they don't have enough money to clothe their kids? Where are their priorities? Here they're buying luxury items! But then I realized, it's not a luxury item.

I guess one of the things that strikes me so much about working at County...I'm gonna get teary. I just feel honored to work here. I feel like most of the families and the people that I come in contact with have enriched my life. My knowing them, them sharing their struggles, exploring their pain with me, allowing themselves to become vulnerable with me, this White, middle-class woman...

There's a subset of people here who want to work in public health, and they're committed to working with people who are uninsured, underinsured, the working poor. People who feel that health care is a right. One of the sensitive issues for psychologists is billing; up until a few years ago, we didn't have to do anything about that. There have been cases where bills are turned over to collection agencies and patients are harassed— and if someone is working but uninsured, they'll garnish wages. It's not supposed to happen, but it does. And a lot of it is in response to the tightening of funds coming our way.

What happens is, there are financial people here who, if someone doesn't have a medical card, they'll help them apply for one—attempt to make public aid connections. But there isn't supposed to be any turning away of people. What had to happen was, there had to be some documentations that billing was being attempted in order for us to continue getting federal and state funds. In response to that what they did is they made a daily clinic fee of $120. Someone can come to Fantus and go to six different clinics but only be charged $120 per diem. On the other hand, someone can come just to one clinic and still get charged the same.

In the Department of Psychiatry, there have been people who would come for psychological services and receive a bill and then stop coming: they felt betrayed, because they believed they could come here without concern about how to pay for it. Billing adds stress. I have a woman who is underinsured. She works in a job where the pay is minimal, she has minimal benefits through insurance—and it's almost like she can't afford to come here *because* she has a little bit of insurance: she has a $750 deductible and a 50 percent copayment. If she's going to pay that kind of money, she should be able to go anywhere—she takes three buses to get to County. It impacts on my relationship with her; she's very nervous about getting a bill. I've seen her three times, and finally the third time I took her over to a financial counselor, who soothed her somewhat. But the reality is that, at some point, we might have to deal with her getting a bill. It definitely impacts on providing psychological treatment to someone who's in need, because they're also worrying, How am I gonna pay for this? People have feelings about not being able to pay their bills, especially medical bills.

There's a lot of anxiety disorders—people are just anxious. They're not breathing properly, a lot of shallow breathers—some of what I do is teach people how to breathe, and then look at the source of the anxiety. There's so much vulnerability. But the other thing...I had this one guy who was staying in a shelter, and they told him to come here. He described a lot of suspiciousness and paranoia—but he'd been living on the *street,* so it was based on reality. There are times when someone comes in suspicious and paranoid, and it's internal; there are other times when it's based on reality. You can't generalize.

It's frustrating that there's a six-week waiting list for an appointment. Right now, we have sixteen people on the waiting list. I would say 75 percent of the people we see in a week we try and refer out to a community mental health center—but what we're finding is, everybody's funds have been cut. Some mental health centers have waiting lists just as long; some centers are only doing aftercare, when someone has had to be hospitalized. So the services in mental health are terrible right now.

I worked here seven years in Child Oncology and, yeah, I lost some patients over that time. It's a weird thing, because I met families when they were in crisis, when they were receiving the diagnosis. I always saw myself as their advocate. Physicians aren't trained for how to talk and listen to patients, unfortunately, so I did a lot of mediation. I sat in and arranged meetings with the doctors and the family. Doctors would get really frustrated: "I explained this to them before." And I'm like, "Yeah, and you're going to have to explain it again and again until they get it, because of the stress level of the news." So I've been with the family through this early diagnosis, and adjustment, and then some treatment. Then when you lose a kid...I really have worked hard to become part of their support network, so that they can turn to me when this happens.

I've gone to a lot of funerals. It probably sounds odd, but there's something very enriching about having been included in that part of someone's life. I've been to public aid funerals, which are very different from
Filipino funerals. I've been to some of the African American churches
where they have the church nurses, the women in white uniforms, who
are there to assist people—they give tissues and cups of water, they'll
escort people out. There are all kinds of different rituals. That's how I
take care of *myself*: I go and I mourn with the family. My guideline has
always been that as long as I'm still comforting and not being comforted
by the person, I haven't crossed over the boundary, so I can cry. I can hear
buzzing sometimes that, [whispers] "Someone from County came to the
funeral." In the family…it means something.

Can you look at people and see who they are and what their pain is?
Working here, you either look at people and you don't, or you look at
people and you can. I think that has to do with the listening. One of the
things I've been struck by, working in Adult, is the number of women
between the ages of fifty and seventy that are disclosing for the first time
sexual abuse—and I've only been here two and a half months! I ask
directly, "Have you ever been physically or sexually abused?" There's
this hesitation, and then they'll go, "Well, when I was a kid you just didn't
talk about these things, but yes." I think it's valuable to the person to
finally have someone ask, because the thing of it is, they didn't tell, but no
one asked either. It's not necessarily that anyone wants to process it or go
over it—most of them don't—but it's not a burden any more to carry
those secrets around.

A lot of times, people will be referred to Psych from Medicine, and
they don't like their doctor. People have told stories in ASC about being
told never to come back again. They're referred up here, and there's
nothing wrong with them psychiatrically, but I think the amount of work
physicians are doing, some of their attitudes, how happy or unhappy
they are, cultural differences…A lot of our residents are adjusting themselves, to this country and customs—let alone Cook County! It's a complicated mix. There's this woman who said that the doctor in ASC told
her never to come back again—she had chronic headaches. It turned out,
in my getting a thorough history from her, that she'd had a head injury
ten years ago—she had been beat up. She'd had an angiogram done that
had been abnormal, and a CT scan was recommended. He didn't get any
of this information, he just saw her as another chronic-headache person
who had come to the ASC twice. I'm not saying it's his fault, but with the
volume of people—it's next, next, next, next, next! The time it takes
sometimes to get information from people…I can remember when I
worked in Peds, this kid was really sad and crying, so I was called in to
consult. Well, of course he was sad and crying, it was his first time ever
being separated from his family. All it really would have taken to figure

that out would have been to sit and talk to the kid. But doctors don't see that as their role at all, which is a problem with medical school training.

Another thing I've learned from working here is that families are really committed to getting better if given the opportunity. Especially in Child, there would be families who would bring their kids in every week for a long time, working on psychological problems. People assume, or what we hear about in the media, are all these neglectful parents who don't take care of their children—and they certainly do exist. But I think the other sign of the coin is there are a lot of families who *do* take care, who *are* committed to better mental health.

I deal with medical residents and psychology trainees—interns. I think one of the differences is that the training groups have become more international, with foreign medical school graduates. I've seen it as a resource, because the population is so diverse. I can remember working with a family from Bangladesh who were Muslim: they believed doctors are here as messengers of God, and the mother kept going down to kiss my feet. It just made me crazy! I found a resident who was Muslim, who could help me deal with this family. So I've always found the residents to be helpful as cultural resources: How do I understand this behavior?

One of the things I like about working here is that it consistently, personally challenges me to look at myself and my attitudes and the subtleties of how I ask questions of people. Like, I hate to ask it, but you have to: "Do all the children have the same father?" There would be times where I wouldn't ask it as question but would just state it almost. I would hear myself making the assumption that they don't, and knowing that I'd be communicating it.

Every two or three years, I look for another job. At one point, I was looking to relocate to the Pacific Northwest—and I was amazed, this one hospital flew me out, all expenses. They said they wanted to meet someone who worked at County. [laughing] Like I was an endangered species! If I go to conferences, I'm viewed with a lot of respect. I think a lot of people view professionals here as working on the front lines. I, personally, don't. The front line is being in the community.

The people that I associate with are of like mind. When I venture out into visiting my family or in a setting where I'm with people that I typically don't associate with, I'm shocked at the attitudes—that generally people think very differently than I do. I can remember one time my father saying, "Well, how long are you gonna work with those insolent people." I said, "Don't you mean indigent, dad?" And he said, "No!" If I'm in a social situation it's, "Oh, you work at County, what's that like?" I think, What do you mean?

On the Wards

Lillie Jones

RETIRED FROM THE *Dietary Department in '91, after nearly three decades at the hospital. She's energetic, friendly, and feisty. "Don't tell nobody how old I am. [laughs] Over sixty-five—just say that."*

I'M FROM TENNESSEE, AND I CAME TO CHICAGO IN 1940. I needed a job, and I went to my alderman. I had been working with politicians—this was 1963. First, they sent me downtown to be fingerprinted and registered, and then they sent me to County Hospital. They had a job opening in the Dietary Department, and I got hired. In exchange, I had to go to the Democratic office and pay my dues once a month. You'd pay your dues, and they would mark your book. They'd say they had expenses, for things like parties, trips—and that they wanted you to contribute something. I went to *so* many political meetings. If there was a dinner you had tickets, and you *sold* those tickets or you *ate* those tickets— either way, you paid for them.

County Hospital, at that time, was covered with political workers in almost every department except nursing. If you didn't give some money, you'd get fired. They had a word for it: "viced." They'd pull you off the floor. If you didn't pay your dues, you don't attend meetings, you're viced. When you work at County, you're tired when you come home. Then I'd come home and I'd work for a precinct captain. You'd have to go door to door and you had to make a report. They'd call me, say, "Lill, we got a meeting…" And I'd go. So you had two jobs, so to speak.

I was in politics until '67, when I resigned—from politics *and* County. At that time, the County Board president was [Richard] Ogilvie and he wanted to become governor. He said, "If you vote for me, I will change the system at County Hospital, and you can go in through civil service." So that's what happened! I took the civil service exam and went back to County. This was still '67. It was hard work. If something don't happen at County Hospital, it never happens anyplace in the world. It's a place like no other place in the world.

I served food all over the hospital. There was so many patients to be served. A hundred and forty on some wards, 175 on others. It was hard work. The food was awful when I started. Garbage. We never used anything except spoons to serve the patients. Casseroles, things like that. They did not have knives and forks. In the later years, the food improved, I think, because we raised Cain. We're the ones who were exposed to the patient, and everybody who came to County Hospital wasn't so poor they could not eat: they knew food and they knew garbage—they knew the difference and they'd get angry with us. We, in turn, would get angry with the director and say, "Hey, can't we improve this food some?" When you stick a tray under somebody's nose and they say, "What is *this?* I don't want this! Give me some food!" I felt terrible for them. But it improved because we kept on pushing for better food.

Most employees I met was just laid back as though they were helpless; they didn't push for too much. There was a group of us who, in 1969, went out on strike—the first strike County Hospital ever had. [grins proudly] There used to be 320 employees in the Dietary employment, and ninety of us went out on strike because we did not appreciate the working conditions. The pay was lousy—we hadn't had a raise in three years—and they put too much work on the employees. And we had some supervisors who did not know how to talk to employees: instead of asking you to do something, it was, "You better or you're going to get fired." Local 46 was the union of the hospital at that point. We wasn't satisfied with what Local 46 was doing for us—they was like a company union. We objected and decided we're going to another union, which was AFSCME: so we went out on strike, and they gave us hell. But we were rebels and we held out—we were out four months.

The rest of the 320 were afraid to go. The administration was saying it was illegal for us to strike or protest. [laughs] They tried to fire us. Come payday, they sent word that they were going to call the city police to keep us from going in. The County called a set of cops and our union—this was AFSCME now—called police, and there were state police—cops everywhere you could look. It was a mess, but we got paid! [laughs] We had to go to federal court, and we got a Republican judge. Local 46 said it was illegal, that AFSCME was stealing employees or whatever. The judge said we had a right to strike, a right to protest. There was ninety of us—all women and *one* man. The rest of the men was scared to death and, honey, we must have had a good hundred men in Dietary! That was the first strike in the history of County, and ever since that time *everybody's* been protesting.

I talked to patients when I brought them the food. Some patients would be happy with the hospital; some patients said they wouldn't go anyplace else except County Hospital. I must say, County Hospital has the best doctors. If there's something wrong with you, and you cannot find out anyplace else what the trouble is, go to County and they will surely find out.

In my job, you had to have compassion for the patient—you put yourself in that patient's place. You're in the hospital, you can't get anything except what I give you: am I gonna give you some crap?! You know what I'm saying? I felt so sorry for them, I'd say, "Listen, you guys *got to* send me some different food for these people. These people look at this stuff like it's poison, and it *tastes* like it's poison!" The biggest thing patients would complain about was the food: that was the thing most people focused their mind on.

I remember once we had a lady on a low-salt diet, she was a new patient. When I first worked at the hospital, we did not serve salt packages. We had salt in soufflé cups, and we'd put them on the tray. So this lady said to me, "I would like some salt"—I said, "You're on a low-salt diet." She said, "I don't give a so-and-so what I'm on, I *want* some salt." She got up out of that bed and I stepped back and let her take her salt. I thought, County don't pay me enough to get ripped up. And employees have gotten attacked by patients, because the patients want certain kinds of food and they won't give it to them—the patient will knock your block off. And *I* didn't intend to get hit! The next morning somebody said to me, "Lillie, you know that new patient they brought in yesterday? She had a .38 automatic in her clothes!" I said, "I'm glad I didn't object to her getting that salt." [laughs] But several of the employees have gotten conked on the head because they wouldn't give them food. I always said, "Don't fight over it, it's not worth you getting killed." See, if a patient is so upset, they're hungry, just give them what they want. Hunger makes people angry.

I went to County as a patient before I ever went to work there. This must have been 1960, and it was not so clean. They had roaches and rats crawling over your feet. I have to give County Hospital credit: they have cleaned it up tremendously since, in the thirty years. 'Bout time! [laughs] So much has changed there. It was all that blue and that green and that awful color in the lobby—battleship gray.

When Dr. Haughton came, he changed that—he said he'd never seen so many strange colors in his life. Haughton improved it. I think if he had stayed, it would have been a different ballgame altogether. Some people did not appreciate what he was doing, but I remember when he came on OB, we had so many patients, we had patients out in the hall. He came up and he said, "Get these patients out of the center, out of the hall! They're not cattle." Thank God. And they did it, but the County Board didn't appreciate it. I went to one of those meetings they had downtown—they was trying to get rid of Dr. Haughton. They told more lies down there. And they said he didn't want to listen. I guess he was a little bit stubborn, but, hey, they had *Karl Meyer* there for so many years, and he didn't do a thing! [laughs]

County Hospital will always be political, I think, because the County Board runs it. That goes for any County hospital. Politics, whether they like it or not. And the citizens of this city will not pay for the upkeep of a County Hospital. I don't believe all the talk about a new hospital—I'd have to really see it to believe it. Down through the years, every time we turn around, we're going to get a new hospital. I don't believe they're gonna do it until that hospital falls down.

Loretta Lim

IS FROM THE SOUTH SIDE *and has a touch of the wry outsider about her. She works part-time at the hospital. "I came to County when I was seventeen for nurse's training. I wanted excitement, and I wanted to be where it was happening. Now I'm older than seventeen, now I'm forty-two. Since I was seventeen, I've been at County, with a couple of little R&Rs: maternity leave or personal leave for six months or a year."*

THE JOB I HAVE NOW IS SCREENING WOMEN FOR CERVICAL and breast cancer. I do breast exams, pap smears, and give them lots of information about their bodies—on the use of hormones or the *not* use, on self-exam of breast, on the misleading information about mammograms, about cervical cancer. I've been doing this for five years. I get to do research on the side, and it even helps my interests, for my future hot-flash days.

It's a totally nurse-run clinic with terrific medical support. It's very unusual, because the speciality of nursing, the profession, doesn't encourage taking individuals and finding their best points and having them excel in that. You have to fit their mold: it's historically that way, back to where nursing came from, whether because it was an all-female profession, whatever. And then County has a union, which I was always very active in. That's definitely a reason why I'm here still.

When I was most active was in the eighties when I worked in the trenches. I worked in the wards, which was total hell. In general, nursing, whether it's University of Chicago or County, it's extremely difficult, because on the one hand you're supposed to take care of all these things you're knowledgeable in, and on the other, you have few resources to do it. So you're at a disadvantage, because of this knowledge and this license. You're responsible for this patient from head to toe—but they're full of problems, unsolvable problems—and if you're empathetic and caring, you'll be burnt-out. And then there's always this switch back and forth with "let's have nurses do it all" and "let's have nurses' assistants help more." Every two years, there's a change in policy of "let's have it all RNs because we want it really professionally done," they give us a lot of RNs. Then we get raises or something—something happens—and they're back to scaling down the RNs and upping the nonprofessional help.

It's a nursing department that's got to fill slots and got to have coverage, and some people do enormous overtime. I would say the majority are overtired. You can earn $80,000 as a nurse, because you do enormous overtime, but I don't know that that's good for the patients or the woman herself or the man, I don't know if it's good. I was exhausted after eight hours. You don't sit down: you're not *just there* with a paraplegic that has a wound, you're there with a paraplegic that has social problems up the yang. You know, you have a different clientele.

My shift was till eleven—evening, we called it. Lots of action in the evening. Visiting hours are in the evening, so there would be crowded wards. Already they were crowded with patients, and then there'd be visiting. There really wasn't much control as to how many people could visit, so you had another duty of being a security officer. You have to really talk yourself into the gratification—so I don't do the trenches. It was hard to leave them, because I had this notion that, "Oh, well if I go…if all of us go…" But I was burned-out, and my friends would say, "You gotta get out of there." There was a patient, a paraplegic, who stabbed himself one night just so I would get him some narcotics. He had no legs—they had been amputated—but he had stumps, though he couldn't feel anything. He used the fork from dinner, stabbed his stumps and made a lot of blood, because he didn't have an order for Demerol—but, I'd be damned, I had to get it for him! I said, "Anything you want." Which is against all the rules, but that was an example I'll remember, how he did that on the ward, which means twenty-five spectators. Ruins your whole night. You can't take care of the other twenty-five, because you're busy writing up these incidents. You have to write it all. It wore on me.

The Cook County Jail wore on me. I worked there from '77 to almost '80. I was in the women's jail: all the inmates had to have a physical and a pap, and on various occasions you had to go up and check what they might have hidden in their body parts. The only help I had were inmates that had done the worst crimes. You couldn't have an inmate be trained to be my nurse's assistant if they were going to be released—so I had to have somebody in for murder. Those were the only people that I could have to train! Someone had to hold the slides. Somebody had to be there because if somebody went wild—I'm alone in this back part and there's no guards with me—and anybody could be upset on any given evening. I had two women who worked with me. Both had killed these men that bothered them. They were the funniest women but, you know, able to be very violent too. It was just out of a book.

I was there when Gacy was there. I was assigned to Psych over there a few times. It would be evening, and it would be news time. We'd sit on a bench: me, some mass murderer on one side of me, and him on my other side! The whole time he was in that jail, they were still tearing up his house. He'd look at the news and say, "I'm going to sue them." And the inmate next to me would say, "Hey, nurse, you think he crazy?" And the one *asking* me had butchered these kids in his garbage truck! So I'd say, "I don't know...What do you think?" That was the...rapport. I was drawn to the jail job and feeling like there was something helpful coming out of it, but I didn't befriend too many of the women, because it was extremely risky. Their lifestyle and mine had nothing in common. But the eight hours I was there, there was camaraderie with some.

I can't imagine that I'd ever want to work there now. But I was an idealist and I liked drama, and I also did believe in...Well, such a high percentage of people were just there for minor stuff, so you could feel that you were serving the needy. [sing-song] Always "serving the needy" kind of thing, you know how that goes. But at a private hospital, it was never as clear to me that I was needed. I tried a private hospital one year, to see the difference, and I came back here after I got what I wanted from the private. I learned a lot: they had very good training programs for cardiac and intensive care. It was clear that I had work to do, but there were support systems in the nursing profession and in the families of the private sector. I mean, the thing about somebody needing an ear—they had phones, TVs, and family. And at County there's no phones, no TVs, and little family, so you have to be the fill-in for twenty years of hard living.

Norma Singer

ALTHOUGH THE DAY *we meet she seems bruised by the difficulties of working at County, her passion for her work and for the hospital itself are apparent. "I felt early on in childhood that the Lord was propelling me toward nursing. I remember by seventh grade that it was very solidified in my mind that I was going to be a nurse." Her first jobs were in private hospitals.*

I GOT KIND OF TURNED OFF ON PRIVATE HOSPITALS. THERE'S a lot of game-playing and ego-massaging with everybody—supervisors, co-workers, doctors, patients, families.

I went to County in 1970, and the first week or two I thought, Oh, what have I done? You know, because you don't have equipment, you don't have the niceties at all. You go to County, and it's like Civil War times. When I started there, we might use a basin for two or three kids, to wash them. The beds were like you see in old pictures: thin, sagging mattresses. Broken, *truly* broken equipment. Doctors you meet from nice name-brand schools rotate through and they ask, "Why do you work here?" I say I like the freedom, to do things for patients and really be where you're needed. For them mostly it's passing through.

There were things that were hard to adjust to. In a place like County, where the politicians ran it and jobs were rewarded different ways, there's a lot of vying, I guess you would say. Like the professional physicians, nurses, you stack them up against the transporters and the clerks, and there's an ongoing battle all the time. A doctor writes an order or a nurse says, "This needs to be done right away." Well, you know, the transporter went to supper. "I'm sorry, we gotta have someone"—and they just look at you and roll their eyes. Whereas, in a private hospital, you pick up a phone and there's no question: someone will appear to do your bidding. At County, you eventually learn you have to win people over, you have to use your personality to inspire a little loyalty or something.

The nursing staff now is mostly Asian—Korean, Filipino, Thai. That can be a big problem, because they're trained differently. We are trained to be more individually accountable and to think of ways to solve the patient's problems on our own. Asians are very rule-oriented, everything is traditional and going by the book. And, you know, sickness doesn't go by the book. Sometimes they're very didactic about things, so that causes problems—at least it has for me. There's tension between Asians and

Blacks, more I think than between Blacks and Whites. I've gone to wards where it's, "Oh, thank God, there's a White 'American' nurse that's going to work with us tonight! We're sick of those foreigners." Because the foreigners are seen as rigid and, I hate to say it, class-conscious. I think they treat the patients differently, and sometimes rudely.

I had a woman patient, she had surgery to fix her leg; she had broken and shattered a bone, and she was in severe post-op pain. Her sister came out, tears running down, and said, "Can you help? She's in so much pain." And when we talked, she told me, "My sister has tried to commit suicide in the past. She has a severe drug and alcohol problem which she's not always been honest about. I don't know if you guys have that in the record, but what you're giving her is not helping her. Can you do something?" I went in, and I could see she was in pain, so I just went and moved her medicine up, gave it to her earlier. I called the doctor and said, "There's other drugs for alcohol abusers, and we should really give her those, because what she's getting now isn't helping her." Sometimes the lack of alcohol affects their nerve endings—tranquilizers can help the pain medication to work better. He agreed, "Sure, fine," so we did— well, the patient did fine, and she and I had excellent rapport.

But later on my supervisors became upset about my handling of the situation. I was pulled in a conference and asked, "Why did you give this medicine more often?" I said, "Because she needed it." Then I was told, "But this isn't the way we do it." I said, "But you can't reduce suffering to a protocol." But my superiors were very displeased, and I got into mega trouble. Rather than saying, "Well, the patient got the care she needed"... This is my point: they don't say, "OK, this proves that there's a problem, now I'm going to take it forward and work it out—we'll change something so that everybody gets really good care." It's "No, no, you're wrong—the doctor said every four hours, you cannot give it every three." People are doubled over with pain, and we're looking at our clock going, "It's not time, you can't have pain medication." And that's outdated.

Here's the biggest drawback at a place like County: there's too big a difference in how public patients are treated and private. There should be no difference. You go into County, and we tend to treat everyone the same: as if everyone's a drug addict, they *all* want to get that Demerol. The first perception when a Black person comes in: "Oh, you're homeless, you're a drug addict." It is not always the case—it's the case a lot of times, but a lot of times they're middle-aged Black people, they're just like anybody else. They got a gall bladder attack, whatever it is, they come in and their first or second days are rough. I say you have to treat them like you would a rich man at Pres[byterian] who got his gall bladder out.

As far as I can see, everything is already in place at County to be...You can do just as good and cheaper—because it's not carpeted, not steak dinners, not color TV—but you can get people in and out, you can heal them for a minimum dollar. But you need research information too, and the speciality units have it. But everybody looks at the ward like it's the trenches, the foxholes. My whole point about pain medication is, patients are not getting what they need on the ward, which I say costs the taxpayer money: patients stay longer. When County had a School of Nursing, you got new ideas a lot. I heard a lot of hospitals complain about this: when nursing schools closed, some of those hospitals felt that everything suffered, because there was no longer input about what's going on. You go in a place like County, and it's like you're in nursing school in nineteen-nevermind.

And there's such a volume of work to be done, it's like everybody focuses on this work thing: put in your hours and go home. Sometimes in rounds, some nurse would give you a report and you stop and say, "What?! He's been like that all day?! Well, did you call? Did you do this? Did you do that?" "Oh, the doctor is in surgery." Well, "But did you *do* something?" "The doctor will come and decide." And sometimes this stuff has to be done on the phone. It's STAT—immediate, urgent, it's got to be done *now*. Everybody throws their hands up like, "That's County." But it's *not* County, it's that nursing has regressed.

The real issue is, there's such a volume of work, it cannot be done in eight hours. We're doing as much as we can as fast as we can, and *still* things don't get done. At the in-service meetings, the poor nurses are sitting there glassy-eyed, beaten down, not even opening their mouths. I've said, "Wait a minute. Every time we walk into the nurses' station, all night long, there are orders. They're being done as fast as they can. Do you think they're being ignored on purpose?"

Last weekend I was the *only* RN who showed up on my floor from three to eleven. The other nurses called in sick, so they had to pull help for me. Twenty-nine patients, a lot of IVs, some sick, some not so sick—but *everybody's* there for a reason. It's eighty-five degrees, the patients are sweating like pigs, there's no air conditioning. The patients have had surgery or whatever they've had. I have no one to pass water to the patients. I said to this one ancillary person, "Did somebody pass water?" "I did that at two o'clock"—shift-change time. It's eight o'clock now—six hours later! That water is long gone. The other one said, "No, I'm not doing it, my feet hurt." I go home thinking, *My God*, a glass of water. This is 1993, Chicago, Illinois. Now *no one* can tell me it's not getting worse, when you have that attitude.

When I came there they had all kinds of ancillary people. But now there's this big thing: "Well, we're not going to have ancillary people, we're not going to have PCAs [Patient Care Attendants]. Well, who *are* you going to have? You have patients bedridden, some woman with a cast on her leg—how is *she* going to get a glass of water? I was really, really down after that. Because there was no excuse. And I lay it totally at the door of nursing, I don't blame anybody else except nursing. That is our dirty little secret at that hospital. As far as I'm concerned, they're too caught up in the politics—they're not moving nursing along. Although, I have to say that the staff nurses are the *glue* that holds that place together—even if some of us are bitches, and sometimes to the visitors.

One woman one night was distraught because her son had to have his jaw wired. When he came back to her, he was grotesque—his face was all swollen and puffy. She was in tears, she was petrified. She said, "They've screwed up, they made a mistake, something's wrong." This one nurse said, "I don't have time to talk to you. We'll call the doctor." I went up to the lady and I said, "What do you need?" She started crying again. I told her, "That's very normal, it will all go down." "It will? Oh, OK." That's all she needed. It's just depressing to me—*that's* the part where you second-guess why you're working there. Not because of the patients, not because of the broken equipment, not because there's no air conditioning, but because you haven't enough peers working alongside you.

I was running an errand one night, and I heard this patient yelling at the supervisor, saying, "That nurse will not touch me again. She will not come in here. She is not to have anything to do with me." Later, one of my patients said, "You're easy to get along with, but there are some bitches on this floor. Some of those nurses are just so mean, I won't let them touch me." Because they're being touched roughly and brusquely and treated like...

Some of these patients, you look at the body and you can read their life: scars and scars and scars. It doesn't mean they're less than human. This one girl—a lot of needle marks, it was obvious. But she's a nice person, and there's something winsome about her that I like. She and I click fine, no problem. So I get it all: she spills it all out, how she didn't like the way the nurse put her IV in, she was rough with her, and it didn't work right. It was hurting her, and it started swelling right away, but the nurse just ignored it, didn't care, said, "I don't have time." So I come on duty and I get this deluge of bitterness, and *I'm* feeling bitter too: I'm aligned with the patient. My patients come up and say, "Thank God you were here, oh you're an angel for putting up with this and blah, blah, blah." And I'm saying to myself, "I don't want to be singled out—I want *everybody* to be this way." Why isn't everybody?

I grew up in a pretty White area, WASPy. Now, when I go back to visit it's such a shock. All White doesn't look right to me anymore. But you know, when you're at County...I came in through Peds, and kids always win you over. Then I went to the Operating Room, and it's all speciality. You really form bonds at County, you really get to know people, and you don't see color anymore. I don't.

I would not fit in the private sector. You're just ruined forever for the private sector once you've been in public, because you get such a slice of life—you get real life. You don't get rich people whining and having facelifts, and "rub my back" and "pull my shade," you don't get that. You get people that are so grateful: they're so sick, and they're so grateful to get well.

I know there are rich people that are very, very sick, and very, very grateful for their care. I know that. So what's the difference? I don't know. I think either you fit at County or you don't. My good friends are at County, and that's probably why I'm still there. I couldn't leave now, no matter how bad it was. It's a family you're bonded to. I'm a County person.

Esther Villanueva

First came to the United States as an exchange student from the Philippines. Since 1972 she has worked at the hospital. "The American style, it takes time for the foreigner to get used to it. It's not that we cannot understand English, but the way, how you talk, takes time for me."

I CAME HERE IN 1972. AT THAT TIME, IT'S VERY NICE, YOU LOVE to come to work. There wasn't too much pressure that you didn't do this, you didn't do that. There's not too much people always complaining, at that time. It's recently that they're always watching, all the inspectors, JCAHO [Joint Commission on Accreditation of Health Care Organizations], the Board of Health keep coming over here, inspectors, and how clean the hospital is, the ward. They keep talking about how we document that, and this and this, in order to be paid by the government. So they are always worried about if we will not pass the JCAHO we will lose this hospital, and then we will not have money to pay us. That's all the main concern, that's what they are talking about.

If we do not document…because those inspectors they check the charts, how good is the documentation. Like we document the patients about their medications, how are they being treated, and how their dressings is, sterile, and so on and so on. Every month they're checking. They panic and they get you. They come on the ward and they go, "Get ready!" You should be ready with your nursing care plans, your documentations, the narcotics should be in order, it should be tallying with what time did you get the medication, what time the pain shot? Did you teach the patient the correct way, and it's documented? Did you teach the patient and he respond and he demonstrated about the dressings? If something is not in order, it's always the charge nurse they call, and that's a lot of pressure and stress. Plus, if we have too many patients, they don't have help, because those who retired, they did not replace them anymore. We're short all the time, and you work so hard. Filipinos are more, how do you say, we can work, work, work, you know?

The patients before—we're talking the seventies—they were not as bad as like these days. Now they act different. It has something to do…[searches for words] The patient that comes are people from the streets. Most patients on our ward are like gangbang. They fight, and gunshots and fracture because they fight in the streets. They're tough!

The men nowadays are more rude, they don't respect you, they threat you. And before, it was not like that. Like gangbang, OK, if he goes to surgery and if he is a drug abuser, of course when he comes back he will be asking for a shot in a minute. And even if you give him the shot now, after a few hours he'll say the shot did not help him at all. He'll be ringing, ringing, ringing until he gonna get another shot. But it will not be given, because it's not yet due.

Things aren't always simply consistent. Even if we tell the patient that they will come at this time and such and such, the patients are doing their own ways anyway—they do their own ways, no bother what you gonna tell them. More of the patients, they don't respect you, they don't treat you nice. They shout at you and they curse you out. Like if you tell them that it's not time for their pain pill, "It's time! it's time!" even if it is *not* time. We have a patient there last week, he cursed you out. Even if you explain it right now that it's not time to take it, he will be telling another nurse that he need a pain pill, and another nurse and another, and you told him already that it is not time. No respect. Not like you are another human being just like them. They curse you out, all kinds of names. If they are mad at you, they say "motherfucker" and so on and so on. It didn't used to happen. It's not all of them—sometimes we have nice patients.

The culture is very different, especially the Blacks. It's hard to get along. They're very demanding, and when they're demanding they want it right away. They shout, they get temper right away. Most of the employees around here, they shout, they speak loud. I have big voice too, but it's just like they make *that* kind of voice. If you don't know them, if you are a sensitive person, you couldn't take it. When you are new here, most of the Blacks who are here have been here long—especially the housekeeping and the PCAs—and if you are new, they talk rough. The tone is rough. Maybe it's because they are more vocal—we are not really vocal. We are submissive; and we want to do our work first before talking, talking, talking.

They put too much pressure: they want you do all the work, especially on weekend there is no help, and they will tell you, "Do the best you can." Everybody is saying if you go to private hospital, it's worse. The environment will be different, but in private hospital, private patients they are more demanding—like you're servants, you know what I mean? In here, they're demanding too, but what I like on my ward is we have all men, OK? They can do almost everything for themselves. They are not as worse as the women. Women, when they have broken hip, broken leg, they're like a baby, and the men, no. It's easier to take care. They don't need as much.

People say the Filipino doesn't have much compassion for the patients? I don't know about that—I don't think that's true. In fact, if you are more concerned...I don't know, this is me. If you are very compassionate to them, they don't understand that. Like if they're insisting to go and sign out against medical advice, and you are talking to them: "Why are you signing AMA? You should stay. We are very concerned because of your leg." You think they will listen to you? No. If he's nice— a nice guy, not a problem guy—of course you have compassion, that natural instinct. You have to be concerned.

I don't know about on another ward, but on my ward we're dealing with many people, their lives are tough, and their manners. If you are born with a mother who deserted you and this and this, of course you have a different attitude, you have problems. Sometimes we talk to the patients. Sometimes they are very nice, sometimes not. They're moody too.

Live and Let Live

Vince Janczy

ORPHANED AT THE AGE *of three, he grew up at Maryville Academy in Des Plaines, Illinois. He studied at the Alexian Brothers' School of Nursing and has been a nurse at County since 1975. "I walk in my office, and I see people selling my nursing staff jewelry. I walked in on one of my nurses, she was trying on a new dress. [laughs] I said, 'My God, what store is this?' People sell food, peanuts. It's the greatest show on earth. I enjoy the humor of it all."*

HOW I GOT TO COUNTY WAS I SAW A LITTLE AD IN THE NEWS-paper wanting an OR instructor at Cook County Hospital. There's an old saying there, "God exalts none but the humble." But then I add on, "County will humble the exalted." You come in there with a blaze of fire and all this other stuff, and they're going to open up the back door and you're going to fly right out. I've seen many of them come and many of them go. People come in there thinking that they're going to change everything. County don't change.

My first day up at the Operating Room I was overwhelmed. I thought, what did I get myself into? Coming from a place where they had like ten operating rooms, all of a sudden I walk in and there are eighteen operating rooms. And I was going to be the instructor for the other nurses! These folks that were there since the time of Methuselah. [laughs]

This is the way I look upon surgeons: they all think they're the fourth person of the blessed Trinity, but until I see any of them walk on water, they put their pants on the same way I do. OK? They have their role to play in the Operating Room, and we also have our role. The collegial intimacy, you might say—it becomes so strong and so meaningful. It's an emotional high. When you're holding the retractor, or helping clamp bleeders, or helping to stitch up that patient, the interdependency is so strong that you really work not as two separate people but as one. That's where I learned about surgeons, how to work well with surgeons, be sensitive to their needs and all that. If the surgeon and the anesthesiologist ask for something, you accept that like God telling you, in this sense: they would not say it unless it was important. The most important function is this: keep your ears open to what they are saying and your eyes on the field. Then you learn to anticipate their needs, and then the minute they're asking for something it's already there—because you know.

We would converse, but the prep time and the time during the operation is serious business. Very little humor going on during that time. The levity comes at the time of closure, when you know you're on safe ground. I remember one time, we were doing transsexual surgery at Cook County...This was back around 1978. I was the OR instructor at that time, and I thought I'd have a little fun with the students that were there. In one room we had a male turning into a female, in the other room we had a female going into a male. A student came up to me, real meek, and said, "Mr. Janczy, what do they do here?" I said, "Well, what they're doing is they're taking the organs from *him* and putting them in *her*, and they're taking her organs and putting them in him." She believed me! [laughs] And do you know what? I let her. Because she was so naive, I thought I'd have a little fun.

The operation made me feel uncomfortable, because I thought it was a violation of the laws of God, a violation of the laws of nature. But I think one of the most important tenets in nursing—and it's very important to keep this in mind, and I see this happen too frequently—is that nurses will judge their patients. If you start judging your patients, that's the time to get the hell out of the profession. I said I do not believe in abortion, but I am not here to judge people. That is something that is between them and their God and their conscience. When you take the Nightingale pledge, we say we shall not harm. And my personal theological belief is that it's the destruction of a human being. There are a lot of other nurses who feel that way, but there's also a lot of them that don't care.

Cook County Hospital is a good place to study about interculture, interracial relationships and all this stuff. One of my nurses is a Buddhist, I got one that's a Lutheran, the other's a Catholic. We work together as a team, and it's marvelous. I feel such a strong attachment and dedication to County. I think what you have to understand is when you see patients the way they are...I've had many of them come in that Operating Room that would never leave alive in any other hospital, and they leave alive in our OR. That's satisfaction.

Now, I work in the clinic, and you see illnesses and diseases and surgical problems that you don't see just anywhere. If you ever saw the movie *St.Vincent DePaul*, you see how these people look—and that's what we see. The only difference is, in the movie, you don't get the smell. Like there are times where I've had to have the nurses move out of a room because the patient smelled so bad that we had to fumigate the room before we could bring them back in. We get a lot of homeless people there. If I see a homeless person standing around in the clinic or something like that, I make it a point never to disturb them. I figure they're there for shelter. I'd be working on a weekend, and a guy would be laying on the radiator. One of our police officers would say, "I'll tell him to go," and I'd say, "No—while I'm on duty, let him lay there." The guy is there because he has nowhere else to go. I've walked into the washroom there on a Sunday morning, and there's a homeless guy cleaning or shaving. I'd just let it go. They would not be there unless they needed someplace to go, and I'm not going to deprive any human being their right to keep warm.

I can't say as an absolute rule that male nurses were promoted to administrative positions more quickly than women. I have seen some advance, but I think for a lot of the men, they've had to work harder. You got to remember something: nursing is 94 percent women and 6 percent men. So I think for men nurses, they've had to work harder to get into those positions. I don't think you can do it on having an attitude. There are a lot of men nurses that are gay. A lot of people look upon male nursing as a sissy thing, you know, a track for either homosexual groups or people like the artsy type. Most of the men that I knew that were in nursing, even if they were gay, I found them to be very sincere in their work, very loyal, very dedicated, very caring people. They really care about their patients—outstanding nurses. I have learned to accept people for who they are and not what they are. I'm not here to judge them. Some of the men that I've known that have died of AIDS, I really felt bad. It's such a shame because there's so much talent that's going down the drain. So many good men, and women now, that are dying because of this disease.

I ran the AIDS clinic for six months last winter. I had my nursing staff wear gloves when they were taking temperatures, and patients did get really adamant, including the chairman of the Department of Women and Children, Mardge Cohen. She got on my case about that: because I was wearing gloves, she said I was insensitive—and I can appreciate where she was coming from. I told her, "I'm following the procedures established by the County of Cook." There was a patient advocate who practically punched me in the head. I said, "If my nurses come down HIV-positive because of negligence, not following procedure, it could affect their ability to collect compensation, number one. Number two, I can get sued for not doing my job right. Number three, I don't want to weigh that on my soul." We had a knock-down battle, but when I pointed out the liability, I think that rang a bell. I was not doing this out of malice, I was doing it as a representative of the administration of County. I was looking at the big picture. On the other hand, I was the most vocal about the cold problems in their clinic during the winter: it was terribly drafty, and I was the one most vocal and doing the most about it, trying to get it fixed. So, on the one hand, they were beating me up, and on the other hand, they were shaking my hand.

I'm in charge of the same-day surgery preadmission. We are the bridge between the outpatient clinic and the hospital. Ever since they started this mandatory financial registration thing, we get a lot of people who give the wrong information because they don't want to get billed. What happens many times, when they have their financial interviews or in their clinic for registration, a lot of patients will give the wrong numbers—

they'll give the wrong addresses, wrong telephone numbers, wrong social security numbers. I get telephone numbers for the Chicago Park District, St. Andrew's Parish, a Chevrolet dealer, all this kind of stuff. If a patient cannot afford, then we send them to the finance office and work out a scale—and if the patient cannot afford *that*, so what? They're taken care of. We're not trying to crucify a patient because they can't pay. Whether they can pay or not, they'll get taken care of.

A lot of times, nursing people say it's a profession. Nursing really is a vocation: you got to be called to that kind of work. It's not something that you can just walk into as an eight-to-five job and do it well. You look at nursing today, and it's like a body mechanic shop: come in the hospital, get your head replaced, and out you go. I knew the minute they started calling patients "clients" that they were looking at it as a business, and they were *losing* that humanistic spirit. They were taking the humanity out of the profession.

If you look at the nursing management books today, it's not the type of textbooks that I learned from. The difference is that you could see more of the humanity in the care of the patient—the psychological, the spiritual, the physical, emotional. The caring, real involvement in doing the very best for that patient's comfort and his needs. The Department of Nursing is missing a point on some very fundamental things. What they have to understand is that the more paperwork you give to your nursing staff to fulfill the requirements of accrediting bodies or whatever, the more you distract them from what they should be focusing on—the patient. The poor schlock that's here to be taken care of. You don't find nursing care in a paper.

When I first got to County there was something about it...Once you get bit by the bug—it *never* leaves you. When we got our new OR director, before I left the OR, one time he really got on my case. He told me, "Mr. Janczy, if you don't like the way things are being done, you know you can look for other alternatives." My response to him was, "Let me tell you something: you are my seventh director since I've been here at County, and you will not be my last." And of course, I'm already on my ninth! He's gone, and [sings it out] Vinny's still here.

ER and ICU

Georgine Kemp

SWEET AND TOUGH all at once, she is glowing the day we speak. She's recently taken the unusual step of demoting herself from nurse coordinator to charge nurse, and is enjoying her new job. We sit in a glass-walled room in the ER area. Practically every one of the people streaming past waves at her. She always waves back. Laughing, she says, "Everybody at County knows me, and I don't know the half of them."

I GREW UP IN MEMPHIS, TENNESSEE, BUT I'VE BEEN HERE MANY years. I was an LPN for fifteen years, and then I went back to school and got my RN. I been at the County since '81. What drew me here was, I had an uncle who ended up having brain surgery, and I watched the nurses at County—and I was impressed. I didn't get hired right away. After about seven months, they called me and said that the only opening that they had was Emergency Room.

I wanted the ER experience, and the first six months—I have *never* had so much experience! [laughs] The thing that really blew me away was the load of patients that they had coming to the Emergency Room—that was in the old ER, and it was small. It used to be that the stretchers were in the hall from one end to the other, no privacy. We'd take them into rooms by severity of their illness. It used to bother me when patients were in the hallways and you got these patients on these stretchers. Some of them, they're short of breath and they can't lay flat, so you have to raise the head of the bed up. Then you get a gunshot wound coming in, and in the old ER they had to run straight down the hall past where the patients were. They had to go almost to the front of the hospital to get to the Trauma elevator. Since they built the new ER, they don't come inside the hospital—they have a little tunnel.

But I miss the old ER. If you are a nurse, you have some special skills. You have quite a lot of special skills, OK? In the old ER, if we had a seizure patient that come in, we knew what the standard orders were: before the doctor even saw him we would start saline IVs, draw blood on the patient. They made new guidelines when they moved to the new ER, they tried to make it better. I think they were trying to do it like the private hospitals—but this is County, you *can't* do it like the private hospitals. The way it is now, we can't do anything unless the doctor writes the order on the board, the big one in the center of the ER. The board is very fascinating. A transporter yesterday had a patient that needed to go to X-ray. He had the X-ray slip and he said, "Now where is the patient?" I said, "The patient is in the hall." He said, "How do you know that? I said, "Look at the board." He said, "But how do you read the board?" I tried to explain it to him, but he said, "That's OK." [laughs] There's a science to that board.

Being a CN-2, a charge nurse like I am, you have to constantly watch your stations, plus you have to watch that board. A doctor may have a patient that's going to X-ray. You probably were doing something else and didn't know the patient went to X-ray, so you come back and you look on the board and you see that it has "Station 14." And so you look in 14, but that's not the same patient that was in there when you left. So now you look on the board. What happened? The doctor or the nurse forgot to put it down. Sometimes you go crazy: "I *know* I left this patient here!" So you call the doctor: "Where is the patient?" "Oh, I forgot—I sent the patient to X-ray." "What time did you send the patient?" "I can't remember." So I got to guess at the time. When that patient comes back from X-ray—and you're still watching the hall, because you got to watch for new people that's coming in, old patients that went to X-ray—and you see the transporter. "Who is this you're bringing back?" He'll tell you and then you have to erase X-ray and put hall again.

I was the nurse coordinator, and I demoted myself to CN-2, which is a charge nurse. I was nurse coordinator from '91 up until September of '93, but it's stressful: you have to take care of all the problems in the area, not only staff. You have staff, you have patients, you have patients' relatives, you have visitors, you have doctors…*You* are the person who has to take up everything that goes on in this area. Something comes up missing, the coordinator has to take care of it. People call in sick, the coordinator has to find people to replace her. People still can't get used to the idea that I'm not the coordinator. Someone came to me yesterday and said we had a patient over in X-ray, he had his own wheelchair and it was missing. I said, "I'm so sorry, but I'm not that person."

People that's been here for a long time, they know the system. You don't have a problem with your attendings and people that's been here for a while. You get these new residents who come in every July, and all the nurses get really uptight around June: they say, "Oh God, we got all these new residents coming in, and now we got to teach them all over again." *We* do more training than the doctors do. You have residents that come in and they say the nurses cannot tell them what to do, anything. I always explain to them, "Maybe in a private hospital, but this is County Hospital and the nurses usually are right about what goes on in the area." The residents should have had their orientation before they come down to the Emergency Room, but you've got some that's real high-strung, hot-headed, or whatever. The attending will tell them, in front of the nurse: "The nurses have been here for a long time, and if they tell you something they *know* it's right." The nurses can take care of these patients in here almost as well as the doctor can. The doctor examines the patient, then they go to the next patient: *you* are the one who is doing vital signs, doing their medication, IVs, whatever—and you can look at the patient and tell when he's changed. You are the one that has to go to the doctor and tell them…Some nurses go over there and actually pull the doctors over.

I don't like to see a lot of patients in the hall, because it makes you nervous: you don't know how ill these people are on these stretchers who can't get a station because we don't have any left. You constantly have to go back and forth, back and forth, doing your assessment, talking to them to see how they're doing. People know when they work on my team, they say, "Oh God, is this Kemp's team? This hall is gonna be clean." They know it! I clean it out. I tell the doctors, "You got to make them dispositions. If you have patients waiting for beds, then you gotta call these other wards and see if they have beds. You gotta get these patients out of this hall." And usually they start calling. You have to stay on them, but it works out fine. When I leave, it's empty. [laughs]

We have a lot of nurses that transfer out because of the stress. You might get yelled and screamed at. I don't usually yell and scream at people. If I ask them to do something and they give me word for word why they should not, then I don't argue with them in the patient care area. What I tell them is, "Let's go to the dirty utility room and talk." I take them in there and say, "It smells funny, don't it?" They say, "Yeah." I say, "Because it's dirty, and that's what we're doing. We're getting down and dirty." [laughs]

Some of the patients, they curse me out and oh God…The nurses down here, doctors…Everybody's been called all kind of names. We get the alcoholics in here, we have patients in restraints. They be saying what they gonna do as soon as they get out of the restraints. They call you *bad* names—I've had them call me "you old dirty Black bitch." I just look at them and I go over to the stretcher and I say, [serious] "Who told you my name?" They say, "What?" I say, "Who told you my name?" They say, "I called you a dirty…" I say, "Yeah, that's my name, but who told you?" They start laughing, and from them on I don't have any more problems with them. When they see me now they say, "You know, when we first started coming here, you know, you were just a fool." I say, "Yeah, I was, but you like coming to County, don't you?" [laughs] They're what we call repeaters.

We have people that sit in the front day in and day out—some of them have no homes, no place to go. We have some people who register in front triage, they know the system: once you register, Cook County Police cannot throw you out of the area, because you have registered. So they register and they leave. We call them three times. After you call them three times, then you break the chart down—and then they come back and register *again*. They know that you have to call them three times, and they know as long as they have a chart up in that box, Cook County Police cannot put them out of the hospital.

I just love working here. [laughing] I like the excitement. I mean, it gives you energy. My thing was, when I came to County, I was going to work six months, like everybody else—get the experience, then go to another hospital. People say, "What you gonna do, stay down here till you retire?" I say, "Yeah, if I broke down here, they'd have to carry me out. Other than that, I'm gonna be here." I love it here, why go anyplace else?

Dr. Cory Franklin

DIRECTOR, INTENSIVE CARE *Unit. By appearance, he could be a sportswriter—rumpled in Oscar Madison style—and indeed, he once considered sportswriting as a career. His office door is covered in sports clippings. "Those are about baseball, but they're about more than baseball..." Dr. Murray Franklin is his father.*

My DAD WAS A PHYSICIAN AT COUNTY FOR MANY YEARS, primarily in the forties and early fifties—so we go back with County Hospital a long time. I'm in Internal Medicine, and my subspeciality is Intensive Care.

When I got out of Northwestern, I came to County. The medical schools, to a certain extent, hold County in contempt. A lot of the doctors at the medical schools with great reputations wouldn't do very well here, I think, because the problems are difficult. How well you do can be seen here: you can hide a lot of things at the medical schools. It's harder to hide that type of stuff here, and people don't care as much about your reputation here. The patients want to know, do you do a good job? It goes back to a more elemental physician-patient relationship, and a lot of that gets obscured at the universities today. I remember when I was at Northwestern, I was actively discouraged from coming here. When I was doing my residency, I went back and did a couple months at Northwestern, because they had good training in a certain area at the time— ventilator management. I would wear my County jacket over there, which I rarely wear over here: if you told people you were from County, it was like an aunt died—"Oh, I'm sorry."

In Medical Intensive Care, we get very sick patients who are not Trauma or not Surgery, and, in general, not heart attacks. In general, we get bad pneumonias, infections, strokes, problems with blood pressure. We get about 120 AIDS patients a year in the Intensive Care Unit, which is probably as many AIDS patients as any ICU in the country. They might be here for a day, might be here for a month. We were one of the first places in the country that established that AIDS patients can do well in Intensive Care, just like other patients.

The first couple years of the AIDS epidemic, people were very pessimistic about putting AIDS patients in Intensive Care; indeed, even today some hospitals are extremely pessimistic about it. They just think the patients are terminal. And what you learn after a while is that HIV infection is a chronic disease: yes, it doesn't have a cure, but it has exacerbations and remissions just like anything else.

Back in '86 we lost our first, roughly, ten AIDS patients who were in Intensive Care. One of the AIDS social workers—a very concerned woman—said maybe we shouldn't be putting these people in Intensive Care. She felt that we should do a hospice-type thing. Her argument was based on compassion: she didn't want to see all these people suffer. And it was a seductive thing to say, "Well, maybe we *should* do that." But it was unprecedented, in my experience, to have a specific disease where you say that just because they have this disease, you don't put them in Intensive Care. I said to her, "Give me another eighteen months. And maybe it's a good thing to do, but I just don't know yet." About three months later we had a survivor. Well, the moment you have one survivor, you now turn it into a much more complicated ethical question.

What happened was that, within a year, we began to see more and more survivors. We began to develop certain patterns, we were learning how to do things. In the late eighties, we published our first paper on it, saying the mortality of this disease in the ICU is not 80 to 90 percent, it's actually 50 to 60 percent. That's different. We were vilified: every reviewer said, "You gotta be making this up, this isn't our experience, this is terrible," blah, blah, blah. But what was a big issue five or six years ago is not even a question today: nobody thinks twice about admitting an AIDS patient to the unit today. That is a radical change from a long time ago. The interesting thing about AIDS—and again, something I learned at County—is that the field can change very quickly. At least in Intensive Care, with AIDS, I'm confident to say we're among the leaders in the field.

I teach residents here, and teach medical ethics at a couple of the medical schools. Ethics was my interest when I got into intensive care. For a long time, when I was in medical school even, maybe we heard the term once—and this is less than twenty years ago. I think three quarters or more of medical schools in the country now have specific courses on medical ethics. It's very important, teaching people why we do what we do, the benefits of what we do, thinking about whether we should be doing things or not.

I have one class on the Tuskegee syphilis experiment. Most of the students don't know about it, and some of them have unusual ideas about what actually happened. What happened was, the U.S. Public Health Service in the thirties decided that they would observe the natural history of syphilis in rural Black farmers in Alabama. So they enticed the people, with free medical care and things like that, to get followed up in their system. At the time, there wasn't really a good treatment for syphilis—but even when good treatments became available, they didn't give them those treatments. The experiment went on for years and years and years—up until the seventies—and nobody ever thought to say, "This is not a good experiment." Nobody thought to say, "This is immoral."

I put it in the context of the Nazi experiments at Dachau, saying, "This is what the Nazis did and this is terrible—but even our own government was doing things that can't be justified and weren't right." My sense is, doing a lot of reading on it, that I don't know that it was out-and-out evil. It might have been banal and benign evil, and I have a feeling that, in their own mind, they were doing what they thought was good, most of the physicians. But you have to explain to the students that even though you may feel that what you're doing is good—which is a very natural impulse—it may sometimes lead to an unspeakable evil.

I also do work on fraud. A lot of the students worked in laboratories, mostly hospitals and universities. You'd be surprised how many of them write in their papers: "I was asked to commit fraud," or "I was asked to alter statistics"—asked to fudge results or to redo statistics in a way that wasn't completely straight, things like that. A lot of the conventional wisdom in academic medicine today is that this fraud is some sort of aberration; but this is the type of thing that leads you to believe that it's not simply an aberration.

It's very unusual that I give them my opinion on an issue, because I don't think that's what you should do in medical ethics. The one time I did tell them how I feel is with Jack Kevorkian, you know, "the suicide doctor." It's a complex issue that's presented in a simple form: if somebody wants to die, they should be allowed to do that. But, in actuality, there are three questions: First, can suicide ever be considered a moral act? Well, you could get a whole library on that issue. Second, is assisting someone else in committing suicide ever a moral act? There's not whole libraries on it, but there's whole shelves on it. The third question—and the real question in the Kevorkian issue—is this: Is it appropriate for society to legitimize assisted suicide by decriminalizing it? That question can only be addressed if you feel the answer to the first two is yes. But you get Roman Catholics, whole groups of people, who feel that the answer to the first two is no. When you tackle the third question, I think it's very, very hard to say. And what people tend to do is to fall back on the autonomy argument. But I think when you look at the limitations of the third argument, there are some very limiting factors.

If I had to say one thing about health care reform, it's that whatever system the administration and the Congress put into effect, the people that put it into effect should have to live by those rules. As long as they have to play by the rules they make, then I'll be happy. I think it's a good thing that they're orienting more toward primary care. God knows, the entire community—whether it's indigents or the middle class—everybody needs more primary care. But there's a part of me that says it's a bad idea to pit primary care against high-tech medicine.

There's a lot of stuff we need to do to revamp high-tech medicine, but those things should complement each other rather than be competing with each other. The fire department can't always be considered as cost effective: they may put out one fire a month, but you're not going to scrap the fire department and simply say, "We're going to teach better fire prevention to people." So the push toward preventive care is a good thing, but people make this an either-or situation, and I think that's a short-sighted approach.

Coral Stevenson

"I ALWAYS WORKED *nights. I don't like it, but I had no choice. I had a daughter, but her father and I were separated, and I had no babysitter. So it was a decision that was made for me: I would take my daughter to my parents' house, and they would keep her. I would rush home in the daytime and get her ready to go to school, and then I would have time to spend with her in the afternoon, to help her with her homework. My daughter is grown, but I guess I'm so used to it... I keep telling myself I can go to days now, but it's a hard transformation.*"

I WORKED ON THE ADMITTING WARD FOR ABOUT A YEAR. IT was very hectic. There were men and women all together. The lights were on all night because we were constantly getting patients, constantly sending patients out. What we did was, we got the patient in and got them stabilized, until they could be transferred somewhere else. It was like an assembly line, and we never knew exactly what condition they were in. We may have thought that this patient was stable, but all of a sudden we were coding the patient. Coding is when the patient is in cardiac arrest. We had a patient, he was about twenty-five years old, he came in with heart problems—he was a cocaine addict. He was talking to us that night, and all of a sudden we heard him go [expels breath] and that was it. He was on monitors and we were right there. We worked on him as hard as we could, but he didn't make it.

A patient would come in, and get upset and angry because, "My doctor told me that I could go home after he did this," or "I shouldn't be here in the first place." We'd get the patient who was going into DTs, and we'd put them in leather restraints, but they always come out. We had one patient, when we admitted him we put him in leather restraints. He made a comment to me that he wanted his drink. I said, "Well, what drink is it?" He said, "Mad Dog." The doctors examined him, and the man said, "Let me out, let me out!" The doctor made a comment, "Take them off." The man called the doctor over, and he said, "Here they are"—he had taken those leather restraints off! You need a key to get out of them, right? He handed them to the doctor, and I said, "Well, you see, you told him to."

This is something I find funny, but for some reason or other, they would always throw their clothes off. This other man pulled his gown off and ran down the back stairs with nothing on—security had to come. It was a pretty common...Maybe it was just the nights that I was there. [laughs] I find, when they get out they get out of everything, and then they take off. When they take off, they're very hard to catch. It's not a boring place to work, believe me.

After a year, I transferred over to NICU, Neonatal Intensive Care, which is what I always wanted to go into. I've heard a lot said about County nurses: some say that County nurses are the best nurses, some say I wouldn't work at County. One thing I can tell you is, if you work at County, you've got to know what you're doing. It's like, if the doctors make a mistake, that's you. If you don't have the know-how to know that something is wrong, then it's not the doctor that's going to be at fault, it's *you*. I'm not saying that we know as much as a doctor does, because we don't—but we have to know what we're doing. Sometimes we get very, very sick babies, newborns, and one mistake, one very little mistake, and you could lose that baby. Sometimes we have to stand on our head, pull our hair, and actually perform to get the doctor.

I'll get kind of nasty. I said to one doctor, "There's something wrong with the baby: he's not doing this, he's not doing that." He said, "I don't see it." I said, "I guess you *wouldn't* see it if you just walked up here a couple of seconds ago. He's not going to perform for you on the spot, but I've been with him all night, and I know what he's doing. Do something." One particular baby, I guess because he was dying, they felt there wasn't very much they could do for him. And you can't let a person just die. I told one doctor, and he said tell the other doctor—so I told the other doctor, but it was like they were passing the buck. It's like, "Will someone do something?!" [intense] "I know the baby's dying! Give him something, do something for this baby!"

When I got through hollering and going through my dramatics, they came. They looked at the baby, and they did something for him. He lived—he did live. It was a combination of everybody there that saved his life, it's just that I got him some attention that night. But I can understand, they were busy. In my mind and eyes, this was the only patient on the unit and this patient needed help. Babies can't speak for themselves. We're a patient advocate: we have to be the one who do the talking for them and get them the help that they need. We see what's going on. One doctor wanted to sleep and I told him, "You're gonna have to wake *up!* We're here to take care of these patients. We can't let them just go because you want to get some sleep."

One particular time, we had another baby who was coding—that's a code blue. He was in respiratory distress. Everybody was standing around, and I told them they were going to have to stop standing around. We had brought the crash cart, and we were doing what we're supposed to do, but they were all standing around talking to each other. I asked them, "Just what do you think you all are doing? What about this baby, the baby is dying. I didn't see any order in his charts that he was 'do not resuscitate.'" I said, "If you all don't do something I'm going to call the administrator and see if we can just get you to do something." And I guess...[long pause] I have to be careful what I say, but it's true that the foreign grads tend to snap to when you mention authority to them, and that's how I got them to turn around. And that baby went home also.

They were foreign doctors and nurses, and he was a Black baby. We do wonder if that has a lot to do with it, as to some of the things they do and the way some of the babies are being treated. I'm not saying that they don't have the knowledge, because they do, they definitely have the skills. It's just that a few of them, you sometimes wonder about their compassion. The majority are caring: they treat the babies as if they were their own, they bring them toys and things from home—and when a baby dies they cry. But discrimination is there, it's felt. A friend of mine was an administrator, a coordinator: she admitted that more opportunities would be given to the Filipinos than to Black nurses, but yet the Filipinos couldn't understand what the hostility was. This is everywhere, not just County. The foreign-trained nurses follow the rules strictly to the letter, they won't question a doctor, they don't believe in arguing. One lady had her own insulin—she was allergic to all other kinds, and she was trying to tell the nurse that. The nurse said, "You have to take this, the doctor said..." The patient said, "But I'm trying to tell you..." I said, "*Wait!* Did you hear what she's saying?" It was then that the nurse stopped. They say it's a language problem, but it's not: they believe in following the doctor to the letter, and sometimes you have to listen to what's up here [points to head] and what you know and what you see— and realize that the doctors can be wrong.

I'm in the union, and the way I see it is, we have a job—which is nursing—and we do it. Everybody pulls together in the long run. I don't think there would be the problem of tension between races if there wasn't some driving force behind it. I guess I'm looking at it from the point of view of being a union representative. If we would concentrate on what was more important than those little matters, they wouldn't matter at all. We being the nurses, all races together, we should fight for what's important: for a better raise, better working conditions, more autonomy.

At night in the NICU, we do just about everything they do in the day shift, but we have a hard time convincing the day shift of it. They think all we do is sleep. The only difference is, we don't have the doctors at the bedside, we have to call them. The majority of the time we stabilize the babies on our own. The majority of the babies are premature, but some of them are post-term babies: they've gone forty-one, forty-two weeks. Mexican...[hits table] There I go again, I'm sorry. I'm stereotyping, and I don't want to do that. The Hispanics sometimes have babies who weigh fourteen pounds, eighteen pounds—those are *sick* babies. The PFC [Persistent Fetal Circulation] babies are sick too. We have big babies born to diabetic mothers. And then we have a lot of drug addict babies which are, in my opinion, the worst. Those are the long-term care babies, where some of them don't make it—and if they do, then their long-term goal is not very good.

It's hard working with those babies, because I don't know how they feel. It's like, maybe they want to be touched but they don't want to be touched. [squirms as she talks] They're always crying, always irritable. You can't touch them, you can't do anything. They don't give you eye contact. They're totally unconsolable. They can really burn you out, because there's nothing that you can do for them. Every now and then, I have to take a break and ask that I not be given those babies for a while.

Some of the babies have physical deformities and, because of that, the moms just don't want them. That's hard to take, when you find a baby that was brought into the world and someone doesn't want him. And he's that small and sick. We have had babies who have had other problems. You get attached to all of them, even if they're there for a short time. I feel as if I'm really helping somebody on the shift, even if they can't say "thank you." You know, they grab your little finger and...[she squeezes air and smiles]

Burn

Dr. Marella Hanumadass

Associate director, Burn Unit. Dr. Dass, as he is known, sits meticulously changing the shapes of three paperclips as we talk. His reserve is belied by an occasional loopy giggle and the kindness in his eyes.

I was born and brought up in India, and I went to medical school there. I developed a special interest in caring for burn patients and came to Chicago as a fellow in the Burn Unit in 1975. In June of '77, I became associate director.

The unit was started in the forties, and this was the only civilian unit, maybe in the country. The real Burn Unit, as it exists now, was started by John Boswick in mid-sixties, and it is continuously in existence since then. Even at that time, there were only twelve units in the country, so naturally this was one of the big units, and the only center for the Midwest. Now we have about 120.

When I came here, Dr. Matsuda just started as director, so I helped him develop the protocols for treatment of burns. We thought there's got to be a better way of treating these patients. The patients are going to hydrotherapy, tubbing and dressing changes three times a day, even in the middle of the night. Applying antibiotic creams, waiting for the dead tissue to separate. And then, if they survive long enough, they go to surgery for grafting. So here we are, surgeons, and if somebody has a big laceration or an injury, we take them to surgery and sew them up. I think burns should be treated the same way. Gradually, we started taking them to surgery, and under anesthesia we excise the dead tissue from the wounds and started grafting. This was new, and it saved a lot of nursing time, a lot of pain for the patient, length of hospital stay. For example, a 25 or 30 percent–burned patient used to stay forty days; in the first two years, we cut that down to seventeen days. Of course, surgery alone is not going to help. Nutrition is the other thing: They need extra calories, extra proteins. We can excise and graft, but unless they have enough strength to heal and also fight infection, they're not going to make it.

One of the salutary results of this early surgery is not only that we were able to save patients' lives, but we found, to our surprise, that the deformities and the contractures the patients used to develop have gone down remarkably. Because we're doing early surgery, early mobility, early getting out of bed, rehabilitation could be started really early. My first two years here, we used to do at least fifty to seventy cases of reconstructive surgery, and that has gone down to less than twenty now. A lot of reconstructive cases we do are from other hospitals: they refer to us for reconstruction.

The other major, major contributing factor is the concept of team approach. It is not enough that the surgeon does his job, the nurse does his job. We need the ancillary services—occupational therapist, physical therapist, dietician, pharmacy, social worker, psychologist, schoolteacher. We feel everybody plays an important role in healing process, not only physically but mentally—so they can adapt themselves. There is no way honestly I can say I can make the burned patient like a preburn person. All wounds will heal with scars. Some patients make better scars than others; some people make worse scars; some people develop contractures. The goal is not just saving the patient, but making their life as close to normal—so that they can have a normal family life, normal social life—but with the deformities and the scarring, with the change in their lifestyle.

A lot of people ask, "How can you stay for so long treating this misery?" Not many surgeons like treating burn patients, not many nurses like burn patients, to be frank with you. We see a lot of misery, a lot of pain, a lot of suffering, but we also see the results. The other day I had a patient I treated when she was three years. Now she is young lady, eighteen years old, finished high school. When I saw her, it was so delightful to see. I've seen others: one was eleven or twelve years old when he got burned—he's now young man, and he wants to come back as a volunteer and talk to the patients, help the youngsters. Some of these things make you feel good about it, and to feel that what we're doing is, after all, not a fruitless or worthless thing.

We see all kinds of things, including abuse. Not only children, we see adults. People get mad and throwing hot water, hot liquids at each other, throwing chemicals on the face. We try to keep out our personal feelings about how it happened, we treat them as a patient. We approach the family of a burn victim—even if there's a suspicion that they are responsible for that—we try to keep our anger and our personal feelings away. Sometimes we treat arsonists, people who are suspected of causing a building burn. Still, they are patients to us. That's very important. For the young residents coming, and some of the staff, they get angry and emotional. I sit with them and talk to them about it, counsel them through it. Because, as humans, we can only take so much. It's not taught in the medical school how to separate this personal feeling from the professional responsibility. One has to learn by experience how to protect yourself.

Child abuse is a very complex problem. I don't know who to blame: it's the society, the time, the family setup or lack of family setup, all these contribute. And sometimes it becomes very difficult, whether it's out of abuse or out of neglect. For example, if any child, one years old, two years old, get hurt or burned, it's always a neglect. They're supposed to be supervised. But, as parents, we see the kids fall off the chair or a couch, and they get bruised; they fall off the bicycle or the stairs. It's very difficult to draw the line. But some of them, it's obvious that they are neglected or badly abused. And the abuse could be as a punishment, or to get out frustration directly, or to cover up something else. We have a Child Protective Team of experts—both pediatricians, psychologist, nurse, and social workers—that can detect these things.

Some patients with burns, they don't know what happened. They don't know what happened to them in ICU, the procedures we do. Some of the medical procedures themselves are very, very painful. Fortunately, most of them, they don't remember the first few weeks or months, what happened. But some people, it comes back to them, and they will tell: some people have nightmares, they dream about these fires. So that's why they need psychological help, counseling.

With the families, we try to be as honest as possible. It's very important—even though there's some amount of denial on the part of the family—we have to tell how serious the situation is. For example, a toddler slipping and falling into a hot tub of water, he is burned, and his survival is very slim. It's very difficult for us to tell that. The parents think that he fell into hot water, he'll be in the hospital, put some antibiotic cream, he'll be all right. Burn patients, immediately after burn, even though they are in pain and screaming, they're all right, body function–wise. But, as the time goes by, they get sicker and sicker. It is difficult for a lay person, especially a family member, to comprehend that. We have to tell all these things: he'll be all right today and we're going to start IVs and give fluids, but two weeks, three weeks from now...We tell what can be done, and we have to take one day at a time.

First the damaged skin has to come out, and that has to heal. If it's a third-degree burn, we take them to surgery and excise them and put skin graft. But second-degree burns, they take time to heal. And during this process nutrition, infection, other organ dysfunction, all this come into play—so that's why it takes so long for recovery. The burn is not just skin deep. The skin is the largest organ in the body: it is not a wrap, it's not just insulation, it's a functioning organ. And when that organ dysfunctions, also internal systems are affected. When you're upset, when a very close member of your family has been burned...And some of our patients and family members are not that bright, you see. Even for an educated person, if the patient is his own personal family member, it's very difficult to comprehend. That's why we repeatedly ask, "Do you understand what I'm saying? Do you understand what I'm saying?"

The burn patient, they're all wrapped, bandaged. Even when the face is burned, the eyes are closed—they cannot see or they cannot hear because of the medications—we encourage the family to come and visit. We think that they cannot hear or listen, but suppose your family comes, they may not be able to respond, but they can feel it. We let them touch the patients: there are a lot of communication methods, it's not just voice or eye contact. I personally feel that's very important, for both the family as well as the patient. Most of them, they visit. But the problem I see is the other way—sometimes the parent, the mother, they don't visit. Either it's too much for them or they feel guilty. Or it was an intentional thing, that's what they wanted. So there are various factors, and that's more of a problem. Our social worker calls them. Whenever the visitors come, they have to sign. Once in a few days we check which patient the visitors are coming, the friends or relatives, or for whom are not coming. We keep track of that.

I've seen some real nice, caring families, but I don't say that the majority of people are like that. I still remember, in the early part of my working at County, we had a child. It was in the middle of December, and the parents were asking about whether the child can come home for Christmas. I said, "I'm not sure, we'll try our best." We all got excited when we were able to send this kid home for Christmas. And the parents came and requested me, "Doctor, can you keep one more week, because Christmas we're going on vacation." And that means that they want us to babysit at the County Hospital. That's one time I got really—at least internally—upset with the family.

Do I ever have patients in such bad shape that I think it might be better if they died? Hmmm…[long pause] Well, let me answer that question in a different way. Again, I'm often, as a professional, not personal…Personal reaction–wise I would have different reactions. Personally, a couple of times I have felt, What am I doing, to prolong the misery? But at the same time we *never* withdraw treatment. The reason I'm saying is, some people practice that. In the sense, if there is no hope at all, then they feel it's morally and ethically justified not to prolong the misery. I think the health system in this country, they're moving in that direction. But again, it's a personal choice. We never withdraw, give any less treatment, to a person for whom we think there's no hope at all. If I prolong somebody's life, the family can come and spend time with them…I think that is good enough for me.

At County, you'll talk to some of the patients, they'll tell you: "My doctor." They think that you're their personal doctor. And sometimes when the residents change, new residents come, they get upset. This "my doctor" concept is there even at County: "My doctor, my hospital." Sometimes the patients in the clinic, I don't see them. Residents see them, and when they come back, they'll remember the name, "I want to see Dr. So-and-so." And somebody says, "He's not here. But hey, his boss is here." "Oh no, he's not my doctor." And I feel very good about it, because that resident gave that impression, and that's what we want to see.

You know, when I came to the County, I was not sure whether I was staying more than a year. I had a fellowship, I came for training, and then I was pleasantly surprised that I was asked to continue. Even then I thought that I would spend a year or two, but here I am. A County person.

Lloyd Rockmore

COLORFUL DOESN'T BEGIN *to describe him. He's part Mad Hatter, part sly-grinning anarchistic Groucho Marx. "I have ten more years to go. I told them I'd give them thirty-two and that's it. I mean, there's no reason for me to go anywhere else, I'd still have to work. I haven't won the lotto yet—I won't do that till tomorrow. [laughs] I sort of love it here, [whispers] but I'm not going to tell them."*

I'M A CHICAGOAN, BORN ON WARD 54, HERE AT COUNTY. IN the service, I'd been trained as a corpsman—and a buddy of mine and I got to thinking this is not a bad field to get into, so we decided to go to school and become nurses. I wanted something that was going to be secure and would have upward mobility at the same time.

I went to Malcolm X College and got an associate degree. And because I don't have a degree, a BSN, that's how I got kicked off the Burn Unit. When I started at County, I was working on Ward 63—my first love, Med-Surge [Medical Surgery]. I've been at County for twenty-two years, and I've been a supervisor for twenty. But patient care is really what I like—that's why I got into medicine.

No, it's not that I like talking to people—I can't stand talking to them, they get on my nerves! [laughs] They don't want to listen. What I eventually end up saying is, "Look, I'm well, I go home at the end of eight, you'll still be here. Now, *I'm* trying to help *you*—there's nothing you can do for me!" So it's a little dialogue like that that we go through. And I am helping them.

In '75, there were problems on Ward 56, the Burn Unit. I asked if I could have nurse coordinator, and they said no, they were looking for someone with some degrees behind them. But I ran it interim from November 3rd until, I think, about the 26th of February, and then they decided, OK, let him have it. I worked it for thirteen years and four months. As nurse coordinator, I tried to pull us together, do things that no other coordinator was doing. We had weekly combined staff meetings, in-service meetings. In-service is different training that they would need to improve their patient care. We were...I called us "family." There was no distinction between RN, LPN, PCA: we all worked together. Believe it or not, the PCAs had been trained by John Boswick, who started the Burn Unit. They knew a lot more about burn care than what we did, from way back in the old days.

317

The nurses I got together did what they were supposed to do and got along fairly well. In fact, one of my nurses just expired from CA [cancer], and that was kind of upsetting. It's hard to work in the Hydrotherapy Room, the treatment room, where you're tubbing your patients. They're screaming, and it's hot, they're kicking and fighting. And she volunteered, because I asked everyone: "Who would like to work in the treatment room on a regular basis? Who would like to work in ICU on a regular basis? Who would like to be in the OR?" If you work where you want to work, you do a better job.

The Hydrotherapy Room is the worst—because while we're trying to help you, we're inflicting pain and discomfort, but there's no other way to change the dressing. You soak the patient in the tub, or they take a shower. If they can take a shower, then they can get the dressing wet enough to remove it themselves. But when you are putting them in the tub—and I want them out the tub in less than twenty minutes—then that means it's not going to soak real well, and as you pull it off, *whooo!* That's the drain from the wound that has stuck onto the gauze, and it's difficult to get it off. You're inflicting pain and discomfort, and you're saying to yourself and to the patient, "I'm trying to help you, I'm doing this for you." It's hot back there, because we've got the doors closed—you've got the shower, you've got the two little tubs, you've got the big tub, you've got everybody talking, you've got people screaming. This one screams, that upsets these two, these two get upset, that one…It's a mess. And that nurse, she *ran* that bad boy, she really ran it. It was beautiful.

Sometimes you've got this yellowish-greenish-looking stuff there, and you have to scrape it off. You *cannot* wait for it to fall off, it *must* be scraped off. And that's…it's bad. Oh, we had so many of us running and crying…especially when the babies came. And they give you some sorry excuse about how the baby fell in the water. Well, *no* child puts both feet in the tub. They don't jump in the tub, and if we see that both feet, both ankles, both calves—'cause we always look for those little ring marks. And we can tell what's happened. It hurts us, when we see a baby burned in the pubic area—because you *know* the baby's been raped, and they burned them to cover it up! The doctor may have missed it, but in doing the dressing changes the nurse, with her tender loving care, would notice all these things. It hurt a lot of the nurses to see some of these things. And then when folks didn't have anything to do, and they would burn the kids with cigarettes and stuff. See, you can't tell me the baby walked *into* a lit cigarette…and burned the cornea?! You can't tell me that—the eye of the baby is not burned, but the cornea is? But you gonna tell me the baby walked *into* the cigarette?! "I was holding the cigarette and…" I mean, it's really weird some of the stuff you hear. That's one of the reasons why I didn't want to be around the families, because they lie. And I've never lied once in my life. [throws his head back and roars with laughter]

We've had patients in real bad shape. I would try to convey this to the family with their "I want to go in, I want to go in," by saying, "Remember them as they were, because what you're going to see when you go in this room is not pretty." I don't know what they think they're going to see, because the patients, they just get big as I don't know what with the fluid leaving their vessels and...It's really a horrible sight. They'd want to go in anyway. But then they come out screaming and fainting and going on. I remember, one time, one ran down the hall and went into the bathroom and fainted. Well, it wouldn't have been bad if she'd been your size—we could have pushed and gotten the door open, all right. But she was *big*—and when she fell up against the door, there was just no way we...[laughing]

But things like that, people screaming. And you never know what's going on in the patient's mind. Even though they have listed "comatose" or "semicomatose," that's the reason why you *don't* say anything around them that you don't want them to really hear. And don't act stupid, because it's there, it's there. One day, when they come out of it, they'll let you know: "You know, one day when you came to visit me you said such-and-such."

The thing about burns is this: as you improve the pain, discomfort intensifies. All the nerve endings come back into play, and then you're on your way to recovery. In Med-Surge getting better means pain reduction; but with *burns* getting better means pain, really, a lot of pain. Adults would be in the fires—and where someone either accidentally playing with the lighters, or went to sleep with the cigarette in the bed...Or when they're hooked up—you know, when the folks come in and turn off the electricity and then they go out and reconnect it. But you also had your share of folks who got angry with each other. "I'm gonna fix you just as soon as you go to sleep." We had our share of hot water and hot grease, stuff like that. Believe it or not, it looked like it drew the people closer together. Unless it happened a second time, or a third—and I've seen it happen two and three times. It's like, "I've caused you a lot of pain and I really didn't mean it"— and in most cases it sort of like drew them together. If it happened again, it was just something that they did on a regular basis. [laughs]

Then you always had the people that pour the gas in the carburetor to start the car. And you had the *real* intelligent ones, that had been paid to start a fire. They're not good at being arsonists—they have not checked a way out. They get caught up at the front door and can't get out. The back door is locked or has gates in it and they can't get out. And then you have the real *highly* intelligent ones that are stealing gas out of cars: they want to check to see if the gas tank is empty and light a match! "Is all the gas out of the tank?" "I dunno, lemme check." And you got the people that set themselves on fire: like, let's say, folks that are in prison that have squealed on someone else—and that's a no-no—

so they set themselves on fire to keep from being placed in the general population.

This is a great place. You work here, you can work anywhere in the world. [laughs] You see everything—and every excuse for what happened. We really worked together well. Plus, I protected my group, and I didn't let people mess with them. At the American Burn Association, my first paper that I gave was in '78, and in conclusion I said, "The patient comes first, my staff second, and hospital administration, maybe." [laughs] Because that's the way it was. I knew what was best for the patient. I knew what was best for my co-workers—which is something else they didn't like, they didn't like me calling them co-workers, because I'm the supervisor. But we're all in this together: if they needed help at the bedside, I would help them. I think that's one of the reasons that started my demise—that along with not having a degree, because they wanted all degree nurses.

I was at the American Burn Association conference in '89. Came back, the office was clear. I'd been given a lateral move from nurse coordinator of Burn Unit to Tour Supervisor on the three-to-eleven shift of Critical Care. At the time, I was highly perturbed. Now...[chuckles] I don't care. When I was in Critical Care—I guess because I was stirring up the water, always bad-mouthing things and stuff, because I was still in that I'll-pay-you-back phase—it was decided, "Why don't we make him a clinical equipment instructor?" That lasted until I broke my arm roller-skating.

Even my director of nursing now has written me up. I got a file this big. [spreads arms wide] See, I don't believe in...why be normal? Things I did, those were things to help the unit or to help the patient, and if it was against policy I got written up. So I stayed in trouble. An example: Well, I think it's against IDPH [Illinois Department of Public Health] policy, as well as hospital, as well as anybody's policy, to throw trash down the stairs. [laughs] I kept asking them to clean out this little cubbyhole, where the trash was coming out into the hallway. So let's keep this clear, right? I staged these pictures that I took of all the bags coming out the door. So, one day—well, not one day, it happened several times [chuckles]—I just threw all the trash down the stairs. That's the way I am: you either do it my way, or you're in trouble. But one time, I didn't do it that way, I took it all down on the elevator and stacked it in front of the environmental supervisor's door—and he couldn't get out. He finally opened the door, and all the trash fell in on him. It was a mess. What I was doing was wrong, but I was trying to make a point. And if it means a write-up, it means a write-up.

My job now is, I'm looking for things that could cause contamination. Little things that folks don't notice, like tape on equipment: tape is dirty, it holds contaminants that on an open wound, a cut on your hand... We're not only helping out hospital personnel, we're also helping out the patient. We want doors closed, hands washed properly, little things done that can keep from contaminating, and things that lead to infection. It's important, because when these folks go through from the IDPH, the ones that used to go through the Burn Unit with me wore white gloves. [runs finger across table] They would touch *everything*. We had a system where, they're on the sixth floor, they're working their way down, we would get to certain areas and wipe them off just before they got there— to make sure that when they laid that white glove over there, it was clean. We'd call from floor to floor. That's why now, when I make rounds, no one knows what ward for sure. My co-worker and myself just appear: there we are, walking around asking questions.

I've always worked at County. I came across the street from Malcolm X College that morning, started the 28th of June of '71. I've been here ever since, and I just don't feel like going anywhere else. There's the right way, and there's the County way. We're close to the right way, but because we don't have enough equipment and stuff, we have to impro- vise. This is why we can work anywhere in the world: because we've been at County, we know what to do, we know what not to do, and it works.

There's certain things that County has to do that it looks like other hospitals don't have to, and that sort of hurts me. I don't know if it's because this is a public institution—they want it really up-to-snuff—or if it's a political thing. We get looked at a lot harder than the rest of these institutions. You go to these other places and they're lax. They *claim* they do a good job, but I know better. About three months ago, I was in my friend's mother's room at a private hospital. We *have to* put bed tags on all the beds; there was no bed tag on her bed. We *have to* put certain drips and things on the IV infusion pump; they didn't have to. It's little things like that I noticed. I noticed the way they kept their charts up—not that I looked in it—but I could just see from little things there that these folks aren't up-to-snuff like us.

The first thing I'm going to do, if anyone asks, is to talk about County. When I broke my wrist, I got in the car—stickshift—my friend and myself, and drove to County. It never dawned on me that I was in this PPO, HMO—whatever that stuff is—plan, and that I should have gone to another hospital. I should have called them, gotten the number. But I came straight here, I came home. And home took care of me. [holds wrist out] I mean, it looks kind of funny, it's deformed. [laughs] But home took care of me.

Legacy of the Seventies

Dr. Jorge Prieto

FORMER CHAIRMAN OF *Family Practice. He is seventy-four and recently retired. We speak not long after the death of his friend Cesar Chavez. "Before I went to join the 300-mile march with Cesar Chavez, I thought I was doing a great job just seeing my patients and making hospital rounds, delivering babies day and night, making house calls. Then I went on that march, and that changed my whole life. It's not enough to be a good doctor."*

FIRST OF ALL, I'M A MEXICAN, AND I'M MARRIED TO A MEXICAN girl. We have nine children.

Although I came from a Third World nation and I'd done an internship in the poor people's hospital in Mexico City, that hospital was much better than County was in 1950 when I arrived here. I didn't know how terribly equipped, how poorly supported Cook County Hospital was. It was horrible. It was a place where they dumped the poor and the Black. They had police at the entrance—the entrance was very difficult to get through. There were no telephones for families to call their homes, or patients to call their homes—no telephones at all, anywhere. And they were treated like animals. They were treated more as medical experiments, with of course some exceptions—there's always doctors with sensitivity and compassion. But the Cook County Board was driving it, and they really didn't care too much about people that would come to the hospital.

It's changed greatly now. The administration at County Hospital is a very good administration, and they can get most of the apparatus and technology that they need; but they don't get it easily, ever. I would tell young students to go to a place like Cook County today, but not in 1950. Not before civil rights.

I was a resident at Columbus Hospital in '50, and had a private practice in Pilsen [a predominantly Mexican-American neighborhood] from '52 to '74. I had to close down my private practice. It was very hard, but many of my patients followed me out to County. I gave, as a condition of accepting the chair of Family Practice, that I would not take the position if the residents were trained only at the hospital. I said that I'd take it only if I was allowed to pick a location out in the neighborhoods I knew. Nobody was worried about the Hispanics, and I think that's generally still true. The other condition was that I be allowed to pick an administrator outside the group that the patronage group at Cook County Hospital had. I picked a very wonderful, intelligent person, Carmen Mendoza. It was a blessing that she was unemployed and came as administrator of the program because, you know, the administration of a program at County Hospital can drive you crazy. Mostly because—if I'm going to be candid—many of the people working there are pure patronage beneficiaries. They're there not because they're competent, but because they're Black. I know that they're going to resent that, but that's the truth. I have never seen more discourtesy than I saw at County all those years, from Black clerks toward Black patients. They're extraordinarily indifferent, poorly trained. They're not there because they're competent—with some shining exceptions.

Now there's good administration for the whole hospital, but when I came it was under George Dunne [the president of the Cook County Board of Commissioners]. I met with the abandoned residents—they'd had a chairman who'd run away after six months. Nobody wanted that position, because they knew that County is inefficient; it's inefficient because there is no accountability. Even some nurses, they don't seem to feel accountable.

When I first came to County in '74, the Department of Obstetrics was a charnel house. They routinely did cesarean sections without telling the patient why, or anybody in their family—the husband, the father. It never came up! One of my nephews was a resident in Internal Medicine, and his wife was having their first baby there. She had a cesarean section, but they didn't come out and tell him. I forced him to go in. They were shocked when they saw that this young girl actually had a husband waiting—they never considered that. The patients were clinical material.

But things have improved, and yet you only hear the bad things in the press, when there's a mistake or an unexpected death at County. You don't hear about the unusual and good things done at County, the extraordinarily good care patients get in every department. Now we have a clinic out on the near West Side that's going to go from four thousand square feet to twenty thousand. I called it the South Lawndale Health Clinic, but somebody decided to give it my name. I thought it was premature—they usually do that after you die—but anyhow...Not that it displeases me. Everybody has a little bit of ego.

They're going to enlarge the clinic and give more service, the kind of service that is desperately needed—comprehensive. And only family doctors can do it. There are so many things that a family doctor does, and does better and at a better time. The majority of people with diabetes don't go to an endocrinologist. In fact, the majority of people don't even know there *is* an endocrinologist. The majority of people with a chronic cough don't go to see a pneumonolgist, and a well-trained family doc can and does diagnose and treat pulmonary tuberculosis. It's wise, of course, to ask for help. It's a very foolish family practitioner who never asks for help from a specialist.

I retired because my rheumatoid arthritis was too far advanced to continue. I called my staff in one Monday morning and on the blackboard I put: [says it in Spanish and translates] "An old love is never forgotten and never forsaken because it never says good-bye." And that's how I feel about County. And I thanked them for enriching my life. I wish the patients had been there, because in my private practice and the clinic at South Lawndale, the patients have enriched my life.

You'll find that most of those who have been at County express some frustration, of course, at the deficiencies that are inevitable, but mostly a great...The right word is love. It's a wonderful place. But the ones with the best, accurate appraisal are the ones who've had legs amputated, diabetes treated, high blood pressure treated, serious accidents well treated. You know, that Trauma Unit is a marvel—I'm sure that God looks down on that Trauma Unit and smiles. And I'm sure it's not the only place at County that the good Lord smiles on.

Dr. Stan Harper

CHAIRMAN OF FAMILY *Practice. He has a calm manner and a sweet face behind large aviator glasses. His residency was at County. "I felt at that time, and I still feel today, that once you've trained at County, in whatever discipline, you can do a good job wherever you choose to go in the future—whether it's in a big city, a rural area, or an underdeveloped country."*

I GREW UP IN ROBBINS, A SMALL, PREDOMINANTLY BLACK, southern suburb of Chicago. It was during, probably, my second year of college, when I pondered what I wanted to do with my life, that I decided to pursue medicine. I remembered those days when I was growing up, because there were no physicians per se based in Robbins, and we would all, just before school, get together in this huge auditorium. The one physician from a nearby town would actually come and give immunizations and vaccinations for all of us.

I wanted to do something to help people—that old altruistic zeal—because, you know, growing up was not easy for anybody in my family. And, certainly for most people who lived in Robbins—it was a relatively poor community, basically poverty-stricken. Once I decided medicine, I decided it had to be family practice, and I stuck to that.

I had been to County when I was a kid. I sat in the Pediatric Emergency Room with my mom and my sister. I remember sitting there for hours and hours and hours with this awful sore throat. I must have been about five years old. We had to take the bus, so that was like one and a half, two hours just to get to County. This was mid- to late fifties. There was no Medicare or Medicaid, and at that time most hospitals in Chicago did discriminate against African Americans. The only hospital that embraced African Americans was County.

A year earlier, my brother had died. My mother actually did take him to St. Francis: they basically refused to deal with him, refused to treat him. By the time she got him here to County he was pretty much dead. That was reality in the fifties. And when you look at the African Americans that use Cook County's services now, many of them are really tied to this hospital. Most could go somewhere else if they chose to, but they like this place, and a lot of that comes from years and years of discrimination in the thirties, forties, and fifties.

County was always the number-one place where I wanted to train. It forces you to use your clinical judgment. You can't get a CT scan within thirty minutes of the decision being made to get one. You can't get a result of a certain test within fifteen minutes, because every system is overwhelmed, because there's a long waiting list for many of these more esoteric tests. You have to use your clinical intuition, and I think that really helps people down the road, when they get into practice. Because if you're in a rural area and the hospital is two hours away—if a woman presents with pregnancy-induced hypertension to your office—you have to be able to manage that right then and there: assess the fetus, stabilize her, and then transport her.

The system right now is overwhelmed, as are many other public hospitals around the country. We basically have to ration the resources that are available here, just like HMOs *ration* resources. They refuse to admit it, but that's what they do. We're always under the microscope by everyone: small things that go wrong here are usually brought up by some of the members of the Cook County Board of Commissioners. And many things are exaggerated, blown way out of proportion—picked up by the press and the next thing you know, big headline—and that indeed triggers some inspection by a host of agencies that regulate hospitals. I think the direction that we should move in over the next few years is the direction that many large public hospitals took around the country twenty years ago: that is, there was a separate and distinct board dealing specifically with health issues in that metropolitan area.

A place like County, and in family practice especially, it can't just be about pushing pills or pushing medications. You have to learn how to deal with the whole patient and to be an advocate for the patient, and sometimes be a case manager. It wasn't unusual during training, and it's not unusual now, for many of the residents to make sure that the young families that come through can access WIC, or to help them with housing. Because many of the patients would come here looking for that type of assistance from providers, you have to know what resources are out there. I think more primary care training programs—certainly those in the inner city—are moving in that direction: actually teaching people how to access those kinds of resources.

Also, it's our job as teachers of family medicine, specifically, to sensitize our providers—regardless of their background—to patients' sense of their disease. During our residency retreats, we do a lot of soul-searching, we do role-playing, vignettes. One role play had a Mexican American patient here at Fantus and an African American physician: there are certain things that the Mexican American had done for their illness before they reached the physician, including going to see what's called a *curandero*—sort of a spiritual healer. Unless that African American physician was sensitive to the fact that these folk healers exist in that particular community, that's something that ordinarily would be missed. And many patients are a bit reluctant to say, "Well, I went to a faith healer"—because, from a physician's point of view, a faith healer is nonsense. In the role play, you sensitize the provider to some of these other resources that patients use when they develop an illness.

We have three family practice clinics, but each is a different operation, and each is a different population. At Jorge Prieto Clinic, the population is predominantly Mexican American; it's younger, because that community has the highest fertility rate in the city. At Englewood the population is predominantly African American; the population is a little bit older, the health issues in that particular community are different from South Lawndale. In Fantus, the community that we have here is predominantly older and it's a mixture of different ethnic groups.

We have not focused on that base of primary care providers in this country, and that's basically contributed to the mess that we're in today. We focused on hospitals, high-tech. You had all the medical universities that focused on the high-tech, *no*-touch, and they produced a lot of high-tech, no-touch physicians. Which then contributed to policies that supported high-tech, no-touch. Now we're forced to change that, and to turn it around is not going to be easy: we've created a monster.

There are a couple of times in this country that a critical decision was made—and because that decision was made, we ended up where we are today. One of those critical points, as I see it, is the Hill-Burton Act. During World War II there was a significant movement to establish, basically, national health insurance for everybody—to reward the veterans returning from World War II. You had a group of representatives and senators that wanted to push for universal health insurance for everybody; national health insurance, or whatever you want to call it. Then another group that opposed it. The group that opposed it wanted sort of edifices built in their particular district—a building that they could show their constituencies: "Yeah, I'm Representative So-and-so, I put this here." The AMA at the time lobbied very hard against the universal health insurance group but supported the edifice group, because they felt universal access somehow would result in control of physicians' practices by the government.

The compromise was the Hill-Burton Act, which was the Hospital Construction Act of 1947 or something. And what happened was, the government spent billions of dollars over the next thirty-five to forty years building hospitals, not community health centers. There was another little blip during the Carter era with the Health Planning Act. There were regional health planning centers, regionally supported. But when Reagan came on board he deleted it. We made a conscious decision fifty years ago and it was a *bad* decision. Clinton's reforms will probably look good on paper, but given the dysfunctional Congress, whatever he proposes is going to get whittled down. [wearily] The Senate has become akin to the House of Lords of the U.K.: it's ridiculous. Our Congress is not representative of the population of this country. A bunch of rich White men, basically. I don't have too much faith in the ultimate package that is passed by Congress, no matter what it is.

There will still be populations left out that still need to be served. I think that a good proportion of poor people will be left out in the cold. A good number of undocumented people in the country are probably not going to be covered. We see a lot of that here; we don't ask those questions, we just take care of them, whatever the issue is—it's not our job to serve as an INS agent. They come to us, we help them as much as we can. So I'm sure there will be large populations left out of this package, whatever package eventually passes—if it passes at all. [He sounds so despairing that oddly, we both start laughing.]

The catastrophic health insurance package from a couple of years ago should teach us a good lesson. People simply do not want to pay any more taxes. I thought the intent of that law was a good one, but people just didn't want to pay those few extra dollars. I have to say that most Americans are relatively selfish—most of us don't care about what happens to the common man, to our neighbors. And that's a sad commentary on the state of American society.

Somehow, we have to overcome that if we're going to survive as a country. I think the next ten years will tell the tale. If we don't turn things around in this country in ten years, we're going down the tubes.

Dr. Carole Warshaw

IS FROM NEW YORK *and has a New Yorker's air of urgency and hustle. She came to Chicago for medical school in 1972.* "My medical school experiences were very alienating—the attitude towards patients, the attitude towards women, the attitude towards everything. I remember, going on rounds, where there'd be eight guys and they'd talk about the patient like they weren't there, and leave the bedclothes strewn around and the railing down. I'd go back and put things back together, and then they'd have their discussions and act like I was weird for being concerned about the patient."

I WAS INVOLVED IN THE WOMEN'S MOVEMENT AND A LOT OF other things when I came to Chicago. A friend and I would venture out and try to meet others with similar interests. There was a group of us, we were all at different medical schools, but we sort of found each other and ended up starting a study group and a women's group. We all came to County together—because it was a public hospital, it was a much more progressive institution—and many of us have stayed.

County doesn't have the same kind of sterile hospital environment that a lot of hospitals have. There's so much more life here, and the people who are the staff are, in certain ways, much less constrained by the hierarchy of medicine. The house staff who do the bulk of the doctoring work are always changing. The people who are the clerks and the nurses, and faculty—people who are here for the long haul—feel like it's more theirs.

I came initially as a resident in Internal Medicine, and, after finishing, worked in the ER for eight and a half years. I liked the intensity. During that time I went back and did a psychiatry residency at Michael Reese, so now I get to integrate those experiences. I direct the Behavioral Science curriculum for a small, grant-funded, primary care internal medicine residency. It's been going for maybe five, six years.

What we have, which I think is exciting, is a very extensive psychosocial curriculum, which deals with issues of race, class, gender, sexuality, death and dying, chronic illness, violence, substance abuse, doctor-patient communications, psychodynamics, recognizing common psychiatric disorders, et cetera. Part of what's different about this program is the emphasis on learning to see from the patient's point of view. That means learning to listen, learning to recognize the more subtle forms of communication, and allowing ourselves to be taught by our patients' experiences.

Nobody routinely asks people what is going on in their lives. It's not just that primary care physicians tend to miss depression and anxiety; even if they "diagnose" those disorders, they often miss what's really going on in the person's life that may be contributing to what they're feeling, or what the experience they're having means to them. So this program is this pilot, working with a small group of people. And we may be able to expand it to the whole Department of Medicine, or something like that, the psychosocial aspects of medicine. I think that's going to be very important when we push to have better-trained primary care physicians who have a much more comprehensive approach to patients.

The other thing I do is codirect a Domestic Violence Program at County, which is a collaborative project with a grass-roots community agency, the Chicago Abused Women Coalition. There are about five domestic violence programs like this in other hospitals in the country that I know of, but a lot of places are now trying to start them. We train health care providers about domestic violence, and about the importance of asking, how to ask and what to do. We have advocates on site who will do the interventions. One of the things we found was that a very high percentage of women who were HIV-positive or were substance-abusing, pregnant women, are in abusive relationships—their partners don't let them use condoms. Often, substance abuse escalates dramatically after the battering begins. If you try and prevent any of those, but you don't deal with the violence, you're not going to be able to do it.

Around '84 we wrote the sexual assault and domestic violence protocols for the ER. There was a standard policy that was mainly about how to use the evidence collection kit, and that nurses were supposed to stay with a woman who was a rape victim. But we developed it further in terms of how to treat someone, and how to not revictimize someone who's already been victimized. It was the same thing with domestic violence: nobody was really dealing with the issue at all. There were a couple of studies showing that between 22 and 35 percent of women who walked in the door of an emergency room were in fact being battered at that time, and that very few doctors asked about it. We did a study and also found that people weren't asking, so we wrote the protocol and trained the ER staff, and people were better for a while. But then they stopped asking again, except in the most obvious situations; I repeated that study in '87 and found, again, that there was only one case out of a two-week period where somebody actually asked.

I think behavior change is hard, and it's a difficult issue. It really challenges people to deal with things that are upsetting to them. Personally, it's upsetting to hear someone talk about the horrible things that have happened to them and to realize that they're happening to large numbers of the people we see and care for every day. It's hard to listen to each individual story and stay in your efficient, high-control mode. Now that cutting health care costs has become a national priority—and the danger of losing so-called nonessential services is imminent—it's important to realize that the time spent on repeated visits for the undiagnosed causes of violence is far greater than the time it would take for appropriate intervention.

But given the prevalence of abuse and violence, many people—especially those in high-control professions—probably have their own experiences that they don't want to have evoked when they're trying to function in a professional capacity. I think that within the hierarchy of medicine, which is quite abusive itself, people deny what their own experience is like and identify with being more in the powerful position. It's very hard to empathize with someone who is being victimized when you're struggling to identify with being in a position of power.

Some of the structural problems are the time pressure, and that emotions aren't valued. Another aspect of this problem involves the theory of medicine, the way people are trained to think in the medical model. They narrow the focus to pathophysiology, to something that's going on in the patient's body: the context and the framework in which their symptoms have developed is left out. So, the way people are afraid to face their own personal issues, the way they're socialized as professionals, the abusive heirarchy in which medical training takes place, all contribute to the non-recognition of abuse in people's lives. People feel like part of what it means to be a good doctor is to be able to diagnose problems and fix them; so when you're faced with a situation you can't fix right away, you get frustrated. It makes you feel inadequate, and you get angry at the patient for not making you feel like you're doing a good job. Since domestic violence isn't something you can fix—"it's *her* choice"—it creates conflicts.

I think the issue of domestic violence really challenges the way we think about practicing medicine, and that's why it's such an important issue. Because there's so much to do, it becomes easier to do the things you feel you're good at. The current economic structure of medicine puts people into a time-money framework, which makes it very hard to deal with anything that has to do with talking. What internists say is that they don't get reimbursed for talking to patients: because it's devalued in terms of the insurance industry reimbursement structure, physicians feel they can't afford to do it. It's a serious issue for health care reform, because the current plans are so based on immediate cost, and not on what's cost-effective in the long run.

The whole idea of prevention is so difficult. One of the things that I feel very strongly about is mental health—that if you want to invest in having a healthy society, you want to end violence, you want to stop substance abuse, if you don't invest in people's mental health…In learning how to understand and talk about feelings, rather than having to act in destructive ways to get rid of them—it's not going to change.

The other thing that we're talking about doing is starting a women's program, or a primary care track in women's health that would train clinicians to learn the things that they don't usually learn about women. These are ideas that have been eloquently expressed by two doctors— Karen Johnson and Eileen Hoffman—in their work on the need to develop a primary care speciality in women's health. It's usually Ob/Gyns who do birth control and office gyn, but they don't necessarily know about hypertension and diabetes and all the other medical issues that women have to deal with. So if an Ob/Gyn is their primary physician they miss a whole lot of what's comprehensive, and the same thing if their primary physician is an internist. They miss out on a lot of gynecological care. Women tend to get fragmented care. We end up being seen in terms of organ systems, rather than as whole people with complex lives.

One of the things that's also wonderful about County is that it's a very international group. It's a much richer place to be, and people learn from each other's experiences. One of the things that happens in our seminars is that people really talk about how it's different in their country or their culture, and what are the things that they have to deal with when they come here that are different. I always learn a tremendous amount just from listening to the residents. One of the things I feel very strongly about is that you can't expect residents to be able to be sensitive and thoughtful and empathetic towards their patients, if nobody treats them that way. If you don't create an environment that supports their capacity to be human and to feel, then you train out that capacity for them to be that way with their patients. We really try to do that, at least within primary care, and hopefully we'll be able to do this on a larger basis.

But all that could change with health care reform. I'm really concerned about the current health care plans. Managed care is a disaster for health care, and lack of choice is a real serious problem: it has the potential to destroy health referral networks. If you find somebody who's good, who you would trust, and you don't have a choice anymore...For mental health it's a *total* disaster: there's *no way* you can have therapy with someone where it's not a good fit, and when it's interrupted after twelve sessions...Managed care is designed to discourage people from getting the health care they need.

People don't understand how important the relationship with a doctor is. Most of the damage that's done to people psychologically is done through abusive and neglectful relationships. The undoing of that also has to come through relationships that can be consistent, understanding, empowering, and safe over time. So managed care is absolutely antithetical to what is required to turn around the effects that abuse and violence have had on a significant number of people in this country. To reduce the psychological impact of victimization to the symptoms—to this mechanistic, diagnosis-driven approach—is dehumanizing in exactly the way people's experiences have been that have caused them problems in the first place.

Dr. Steve Hessl

CHAIRMAN, OCCUPATIONAL MEDICINE *Department. His office is decorated with attractive, framed posters. "I try to collect things for my office that are related to work. Like that Lewis Hines photograph poster—that's a pipe fitter, and he's adjusting something on a turbine." A print of the Chicago Picasso hangs near his desk. "Oh..." [chuckles] "That one I can't explain. But I can explain the Brueghel. See, that's a work scene."*

My FATHER WAS A SURGEON WHO EMIGRATED HERE DURING the Second World War from Czechoslavakia. He was in solo practice. I used to joke that he was like the corner grocery store, about to become extinct. I never felt any pressure to become a physician—but he was a very important role model.

I ended up going into the army during the Vietnam era, but I was lucky enough to be placed in Germany. I gave them three years as a result too. But it's interesting, everything you do in life has an influence on you. And while I can't say that I was particularly happy being in the military— because I felt I was forced, and it was not a part of my career plan—on the other hand, I gained a fair amount of appreciation for preventive medicine in the military. They have a captive group of people, and they can institute a lot of preventive measures in terms of being sure that everybody gets their inoculations, and that the soldiers are fit.

Of course, exactly *what* they're trying to assure that they're fit for, I have a problem with to some extent—but it's an interesting analogy between the military and occupational medicine, which is what I'm in now. There are a lot of interesting parallels. How do you approach keeping workers healthy and how do you approach keeping soldiers healthy? The other thing that's ironic about the military is that, in a sense, they have socialized medicine: the military provides not only for the soldiers, but they provide for their families. I always found that as kind of an interesting irony in our society.

Occupational medicine is an area of medicine which deals with the health of working people. In this country it's considered part of preventive medicine, it has a preventive focus; but we also deal with people who already have established disease—occupationally related injuries or illnesses. Things like carpal tunnel syndrome, lead poisoning, or asthma related to occupations. The interesting thing about it is that many occupational diseases imitate diseases that are common in our population. There are a lot of people suffering from asthma in our population, and a small but significant proportion of them have their asthma either caused or aggravated by their employment. If that's the case, then it's actually occupational asthma.

If I'm a crusader about anything, it's to get the physicians in our society to recognize occupational diseases when they actually occur. The biggest problem is the fact that they turn out *not* to be recognized, which has a lot of ramifications. I'll just stick to the asthma problem, because it's a common one: If it's not recognized as work-related, number one, the person may not know to avoid exposures that make it worse. In other words, instead of treating the person with medication, there's another approach, which is to remove them or somehow get them to avoid the exposures that are triggering the condition. By not recognizing it as occupational, there's a missed treatment opportunity to prevent the illness from getting worse.

The second aspect is, where does the medical cost get paid? If it's not recognized as occupational, it comes out of this, what is it, $810 billion medical care bill we have, which Clinton is hopefully going to fix. It comes out of that instead of out of workers compensation—which, in our country, is a whole different insurance scheme. Furthermore, some of these patients end up getting their medical care provided by the County. Medicaid may be paying for it, or the County in part is paying for it, and then they may be getting social security disability, because they're too ill to work. And yet who should be bearing the cost of that? In my opinion— if you recognize it as occupational—then the company, or the company's insurance carrier for workers compensation, ought to.

The other ramification of all this is that if workers are getting sick because they're overexposed in the workplace, and yet it's not costing the company anything, there isn't a lot of incentive to correct the problem. They very often use the argument that the worker already had asthma, but we have plenty of patients that never had asthma until they were working at a particular place where, we feel, it was triggered. That's an interesting area of occupational medicine, because there are these gray zones where one physician might believe it's not related to occupational medicine, another physician believes that it is. Because of the workers compensation and the product liability aspects, it is sometimes a very contentious, litigious area of medicine.

We have an Occupational Medicine Clinic here that we started in 1976. Patients can refer themselves there if they think they have an occupational disease. Very often they're referred by other physicians within the West Side Medical Center here; they also get referral by attorneys who want an opinion as to whether or not this is an occupational disease case. I think OSHA has helped: I think workers tend to be a little more knowledgeable, they have better access to information.

When I started in this area, for example, workers did not have what's called a "Right to Know": there was no obligation for employers to notify workers as to what the hazardous substances were that they were exposed to. And so we had to go to great lengths sometimes to find out what their exposures were. For instance, we would ask patients to bring in labels or copy labels; we had one patient take some of the material with him from his workplace and we had it analyzed—though we were worried that we were going to get in trouble for that with the company...We were even concerned that we might be accused of stealing and stuff. We had to go through all these conniptions to get information which was vital to make an appropriate diagnosis and give treatment.

We first got word out about the clinic through several organizations. Quentin Young and others started the Chicago Area Council for Occupational Safety and Health. CACOSH is a group that is supported in part by local labor unions as a resource for workers. They can call CACOSH, for example, if they need information about hazards in the workplace, or if they think they have an occupational illness or injury. The other was the Chicago Area Black Lung Association. They've been a very active group of former coal miners here in the Chicago area—they would complain to us about other medical providers in the city who didn't believe that chronic bronchitis could be related to working in the coal mines, things like that. They would send us patients, and we developed a rotation so that, for example, the Internal Medicine residents could spend some time with us, get some introduction. They began to recognize problems here on the wards in the hospital, and in the other clinics too.

A graphic example of that is, one of the interns in 1976 was working in the Emergency Room one day, and a gentleman came in who was complaining of headaches, difficulty sleeping, and loss of interest in sex. He said that he had been diagnosed as being depressed—and those *are* very common manifestations of depression—and had been treated, in fact, at a university hospital here in Chicago for depression. He wasn't getting better, and he didn't have money, so he ended up at the County screening clinic. This doctor, who had a little introduction to occupational medicine, asked him about his job. He said, "I work in a battery factory." She said, "Are you exposed to lead?" He said, "Yes"—she got a blood lead level on him, and it was sky high. That was the reason that he was having these complaints. She referred him to us, and then it was just like word spread like crazy.

This battery factory had 120 workers, total, and we ended up seeing forty-two of them. Needless to say, the company was *very* upset with us. We had to remove most of the workers from exposure—which meant they couldn't work, and they started applying for workers compensation. [chuckles] It turns out that this company was a subsidiary of a large corporation, and that some high-level person—this is what I heard, I wasn't there in the executive director's office when the telephone call occurred—but I was told that this high-level person for this corporation called the executive director of the Governing Commission, Jim Haughton, and said, "What are you guys doing here?" You know, cease and desist. Fortunately, he didn't bend to that kind of threat, and we continued to see these patients.

We still sometimes see some flagrant occupational diseases, but they tend not to be as severe. We see a lot more of the cumulative trauma–type patients: carpal tunnel syndrome, tendonitis, things like that. We're seeing what the rest of the country is seeing. I personally think that it's mostly improved recognition—before patients just suffered with it—but it could also be changes in the work practices. We're also beginning to see more patients with so-called multiple chemical sensitivities, which can be work-related, and often are environment related. That's a new sort of a syndrome that we didn't see much of before. But again, maybe we weren't good at recognizing it.

I think our program is an example where County will start and be in the forefront of programs that are of value to the public that it serves. It's a court of last resort for people, but it also fills real public health needs that aren't met by other institutions in the city. The satisfaction I get out of working here is providing a service that probably somebody wouldn't get otherwise, and the opportunity to influence a lot of other physicians.

And then there is what I would call a "support group." The other physicians that I work with here have the same goal, to a large extent the same ideology, and we tend to support each other. There's an esprit de corps that exists—and at a lot of places, that doesn't exist. It's people just making a living, a very good living sometimes, and that's the trade-off. But I'm comfortable, and I'd rather not make those sacrifices just to make more money.

Dr. Terry Conway

ACTING CHAIRMAN OF *Internal Medicine. Though he's neatly suited and tied, his longish salt-and-pepper hair lends him a distinctly nonestablishment air. When we meet, he's just moved into his new office, which, filled with furniture of substance, speaks of authority. He merely apologizes for its lack of personality—he's not had time to put up his own things.*

I NEVER THOUGHT REALLY I COULD BE A DOCTOR OR ANY-thing like that. I was in the Jesuits. I didn't get ordained, but I was in the novitiate for a while. At the Jesuits, I also worked a little bit as an orderly, and I liked it. When I was in college, I used to drive an ambulance at nights. [shrugs] It was a job. I applied and got conscientious objector status, and I started working at County—that was in 1970. At that time, I decided that I kept being drawn back to this medical stuff, and I took the pre-med courses that I needed to go to medical school.

I started working in the psychiatric hospital here, first as an orderly, then I worked as a transportation orderly, and then I worked in the Intensive Care Unit as a lab tech. I went from there into medical school. I got a scholarship from the U.S. Public Health Service in medical school, which paid my tuition—it was just like manna.

When I was a resident here, there were a lot of people of different political parties. When I was head of the House Staff Association, sometimes the major issue at meetings was how to keep the members of the RCP [Revolutionary Communist Party] off of the Communist Party members. And there would be some motions made by other people from the Progressive Labor Party about how we really should be denouncing what's going on in Albania. [smiles] Now, not everybody was in a party—but there was really a lot of talk, a lot of process. People were not so worried about their careers, about making a bundle of money—they really wanted to change things. A lot of things that have come to pass we really asked for, pushed for. They're now—especially now that we have this new administration—making more relationships with community groups, trying to aggressively plan for things that are coming, like TB epidemics, AIDS. I mean, it's a tough institution to turn around.

There are three types of employees. Maybe 80 percent of them are in the middle—they're regular people, they're just like anybody, they're pretty decent workers. But then you have two other groups, and they're the 5 to 10 percent each: the saints and the sinners. You get the saints, and you run into them here, especially. You run into a ward clerk or a nurse, and *no matter what* they will take care of these patients—there are just incredible odds they'll go through. And then you get the sinners. What you have to do, primarily, is pay attention and reward the saints and move the whole mean up. You also have to take care of the sinners, but they're usually quite good at resisting. But if you take care of them, it isn't motivating the middle to work better, it just frightens them: it's chilling when people are punished. So instead you've got to motivate. The other thing is to pay attention—by giving people direction, giving them training, and trying to listen to them. Not just listen, but try and get them involved in what is the solution. And then also make them feel like in their area they *own* this work, it's their work. Make it so that what they do and what they think is important to this. That's what I believe in. It's worked in other areas I've worked in here. I'm not cynical at all about the people who work here, and I've been here many years.

Another thing is that County people have a great sense of humor, which I really like. You go to other places, the doctors are stuffy, sour, arrogant. You don't run into too much of that here: the physicians here don't make anywhere near the salary that they do in other places. They may not be doing it for the money, but you don't want to insult them either. I know people who work here who are world-renowned, and who are moonlighting in the Emergency Room because their kids are in college and they need a little bit more money. So you'll see an expert in diabetes for the rash under your arm.

I'm in Internal Medicine. It's the largest single category of doctors, and yet nobody knows what you're talking about. They say, "Is that an intern?" or "Is he taking care of things inside?" It's somebody who takes care of adults, but doesn't do surgery to deliver babies. That's what an internist is. So if you have a heart attack, an internist takes care of you. A doctor who's a cardiologist or a diabetes specialist, they're all internists. And then, to be a specialist, they take a little bit more training. I stayed a general internist and became interested in Primary Care.

In Primary Care, you're supposed to be comprehensive, you're supposed to be able to take care of most of the patients' problems. It should be continuous, you see the same person. We're supposed to coordinate all your care, supposed to be the person that you first go to when you have a problem. You know: "Doc, I'm getting a little pain in my left arm." It might be arthritis, muscle strain, it might be heart disease. Family practitioners can see children and adults, but they focus on the family. One of the reasons that the U.S. is so costly is that specialists have a tendency to do specialized things, to do tests and do work-ups that are expensive, but not comprehensive. They may take care of, and spend $10,000 on, a heart problem that I might be confident not spending as much on. This is what they do—so they do what they do, but they may not do pap smears, or they actually may not even check your cholesterol—even though it's related to heart disease—because they're more into treating heart disease rather than in preventing it.

It's like they say, in many people 85 percent of the health care costs, they'll incur in the last year of their life. Well, that's kind of grim, looking at it, and it doesn't say exactly what you should do—but it gives you an idea that things are a little bit skewed—out of balance. A lot of times people will be in that last year of life with something that is essentially irreversible because they didn't get anything earlier.

I think County has to be part of a health system, not just a hospital as an island. We've got to move out where we can intervene a little bit earlier so that the primary care for the patients can be closer to their home, and can be part of their community—can be related not just to the health of the people who happen to walk into the clinic, but related to the health of the whole community. You have to keep in contact with the health of those communities, because it could change: epidemics come up, immigrations happen. A community and its health are dynamic: it gets older, people age. County needs to move in that direction, and I think it is. Even if there is a national health program, it will be a few years before it really affects anybody, the way I see it. There may be legislation and things, but it's going to be a while, and it probably will come in phases. I'm sure our patients will be the last to be included anyhow, so...And even though we have insurance, we're still going to have populations that have tremendous ill health.

The Women and Children HIV program is an example, and the community ought to know that we have—Mardge Cohen did it, but with a lot of people's help—built something that is very culturally sensitive, very humane, extremely high quality medical care, and connected to the community in a hundred ways. It's sensitive to the community: as issues come up and need to be met, they are. We as a hospital want to *be* that, we want to be recognized as that—and show that it can work. You don't have to completely reinvent the wheel: this *has* worked other places—not so much in the U.S., but it's worked other places. It's got to be a solution that's really our own, but nobody questions what will work. They question how you're going to pay for it and who's going to control all the powerful forces in health care right now.

Being a public institution, we almost aren't supposed to say our goal is to survive. "What do you mean to survive?" You're not supposed to be self-perpetuating. Well, I think if you do as good a job as County does, you deserve it—and you should advocate for it, you should blow your own horn some. If anything goes wrong at County, it's on the front page of the newspaper. We have really good mortality statistics here. HCFA [Health Care Financing Authority] does it: they look at all Medicare, they adjust all the patients so everybody's at a level field. If a certain level of patient went in somewhere, where would they be most likely to do well? And in the city of Chicago, it was Cook County the two times they've done it in the recent past.

The other thing is, just something about County—it grabs people's interest more. They know we treat people who've worked all their lives, who don't have two nickels to rub together, and then we also treat people who are the castoffs of society. I think people in the mainstream kind of have a voyeuristic interest in that. It's all right, but I wish that the media would do that responsibly. That's what's so crazy. I've been at the best institutions in the city of Chicago and seen the same things as at County, and it's not even news. It's no news.

Dr. Arthur Hoffman

DIRECTOR OF THE SECTION *of Early Detection and Prevention.* "*I don't know that I had a long-haul view that I would stay at County for a long time. It was much more the immediacy—it seemed very important to take care of people who were there. It seemed personally enriching to be there, just from the people I met when I would go there in medical school. I remember the first day that I went to the Admitting Ward. I walk onto the ward and this nurse who was six-foot-one, and 250 pounds—who had met me at Rush—runs up to me and [wraps arms around himself] grabs me and welcomes me to the ward. It was that kind of passion that was missing elsewhere.*"

MOST OF MY PATIENTS I'VE BEEN TAKING CARE OF SINCE 1975. Most of my patients are older, but even people in their forties and fifties, it's very intimidating to go to the doctor, and that's not particular to County. I see a lot of passivity, and one of the exciting things about this preventive medicine program that I'm doing is the fact that people get to be active.

People being treated with dignity and respect is missing in a day by day way in our lives at County. I think it's the single most important thing that I'd like to see change. If we're going to succeed and survive as anything except a hospital for the unwanted people of this country, then County is going to have to deal with treating everyone with more dignity.

When I was a resident, I remember so many times talking to people who work at the hospital and saying, "How'd you end up at County?" People would always ask *us* that question because we were these White doctors. People would say, "You know, when I first came to County I came because it seemed like it would be a different kind of place to work; it would be a job that had some meaning." Some of them had worked in this factory or that factory; most of the people I remember talking to were LPNs or housekeepers, dietary. They said that County seemed like a place where they could take care of other people from their community, or a place where their work could have some meaning. I'd be surprised if people come with that expectation anymore. And most of the people who I spoke to felt saddened by the fact that that expectation was hard to fulfill, although there were moments of it.

In those days there was much more of a tendency, if there was a crisis or whatever the situation, to pull together, to really work together—to make the best of a situation that was really oppressive.

Come the eighties and the PATCO strike, followed by everything else that Reagan did to undermine the fabric of our culture…That it was OK to make things better—the message was, *"Don't* try and make anything better. This is it, and what you've got is going to get worse from here on out." When you send that message out to all of America—"tighten your belts"—when you sent that out to people who are thin, and meanwhile there's all these stockbrokers making all this money, you create an environment where people really don't see a future. I saw that reflected in the staff's attitude, the staff that's from the community that we serve. There was a lot less hope.

In terms of physical ugliness, I think things are not worse and maybe in some areas a little better. In terms of personal ugliness, I think they're worse. People are exposed to more negative interactions with people now than they were back when I was a resident. I remember the institution running out of medicine, but I don't remember people being treated like they were animals in the way that I see if I stand by the pharmacy window now. The same with the lab or EKG: sometimes you'd send a patient up to the lab, and they would get sent back for some stupid bureaucratic thing. But it wasn't with the kind of vengeance that it seems like it is now.

I've seen old people who are treated by some young person, some twenty-year-old treating a ninety-year-old like, [hostile] "Well, whadda you want?" That harshness—who knows what it is? I think it's related to the violence in our society. We see another level of violence, of young people being rude to their elders. *Rude.* Mean. Heartless. Mindless. It's not everyone, not even most of the time; it's just that it happens too often, by too many of us, to too many patients. I don't want to paint a picture that that's all that happens, because there's a lot of other stuff; but, you see, where you told me the story about the housekeeper who got in trouble for being nice to somebody! [loudly] But you can yell at somebody, [whispers] and nothing happens. We've got to change that.

In Preventive Medicine there's primary, secondary, and tertiary prevention. Primary is before somebody has the disease, secondary is before the disease is symptomatic, and tertiary is preventing progression of the disease after it is established. Mostly, in my section, we do primary and secondary prevention. Most of that is in cancer and coronary artery disease because those are the biggest epidemics that exist today.

The first prevention program we did was a flu vaccine program. I did it as a political organizing effort—I think almost all of our preventive medicine programs have that aspect to them. We went first to the patients with brochures and handouts, and we went to the doctors and told them why they should give the shots. We went to the nursing staff and had meetings with all the nurses in the clinic and talked about public health and what it was about, and about saving lives. The nurses were interested, but passive. In the beginning, people didn't want to do it because it was extra work. What happened, and this was the most exciting thing, is that as a few years went on and this approach worked—at least in General Medicine—the nurses were more and more invested in this program being *theirs.*

The second program, the colon cancer screening program, I think the most poignant vignette about that was the site visit from the grant, the American Cancer Society. A physician came and was extremely scornful of us and our patients. He said, "These patients at County don't want to do early cancer detection, they're just going to come here for gunshot wounds," and this and that. It really captures the external world's perception. People from the outside don't realize, they don't think about, they don't want to think about, the people who come to Cook County, the human beings who come. It's too painful.

You hear stuff all the time about how poor people aren't going to come for preventive medicine because they've got other problems that are more important to them, and there are endless studies that will show that. [angrily] It's crap! You talk to anybody and you ask, "What's the most important thing to you?" You don't have to be Black or White or rich or poor: you don't want to be unhealthy. But no matter how much we do at County, no matter how much we show our successes, people don't believe us because their bias is so great. So that's been one of our big battles in prevention.

Then there's how medical science works. We had another site visit, and at one point this mean-spirited site inspector said, "You all have to understand, NCI [National Cancer Institute] funds research to stop cancer, it doesn't provide care." And another doctor, Richard Cooper, said, "Maybe that's why the rate of cancer has gone up." It's a little oversimplified, but I think that's one of the issues in prevention. We talk about mass epidemics, but we have to have ways to take things we find and *apply* them—and there's no mechanism for that. That's another reason why County is so unique.

We also started the smoking cessation programs, and we've added the nutrition program, and the stress-reduction/relaxation program, and we need to add an exercise training program. We've got a very broad program of cancer detection and prevention, and cardiac risk reduction and heart disease prevention. I think that that brings us to the nineties, and into what's happening in preventive medicine right now. My feelings about that are that there's a lot of talk about prevention, but we're still in a period where cost is determining everything: there's a lot of talk about prevention, but nobody wants to pay for it. People haven't really concretized what preventive medicine *is*. To me, what it means is battling epidemics, taking epidemics and the causes of those epidemics and trying to change the burden of those exposures, whether they be cigarettes or diet or environmental exposures. What we do at County has been much more in terms of the personal one-on-one, because it's a health *care* institution, it's not a public health institution.

What preventive medicine is, one-on-one, for patients, means really helping people figure out how to make these changes. These programs are really important for helping people to learn the tools of self-care, of health. Working with stress is a way to deal with smoking, eating, exercise, and every other practice—not to mention the benefit of working with stress in and of itself. That's why we're now trying to incorporate stress-reduction into our programs. We live in a world that we're not really made for. Evolution takes a hundred thousand years to change, but capital development has turned us from an agrarian to an urban environment, worldwide, in a matter of two hundred years. Our genes have not caught up: the brain centers that are the stress-response centers are overactivated.

The role of preventive medicine in the future of County or health care, it's a very exciting time, but a very unclear time. It costs money to do these things: you can't take the necessary time to teach people how to change their diet in five minutes. We forget that medicine is not all that complicated. But it's moving into the monopoly system—this is a lot of what is going on in the health care debate—and the people who are going to control that are the insurance companies. The absurdity of that...It's not wrong to have health insurance reform, but the absurdity of calling that health care reform is just mindlessness.

Prevention is a funny breed. It stands in the face of this capital development, because prevention is not about technology, it's about changing your lifestyle and changing the environment. There's tension within the business community over what to do about health: they *talk* about cost-cutting, but all those technology-oriented subspecialists getting all those high salaries are using up equipment left and right—they're using up products that were produced by businesses that want to produce more. Those businesses are going to go out of business if those doctors no longer have a reason to do all those surgeries.

You know those studies that have come out that look at the thing that best predicts what treatment you're going to get? It's insurance. They had this article in the *New England Journal of Medicine* last week about how HMOs do less catheterizations than private insurers, and Medicaid does even less. The authors said that they thought that HMOs are probably the best balance. I'll tell you something: working people with HMOs don't have the best health. The best health still belongs to the upper-middle class, OK? And *maybe* that's because of their health care—but I doubt it: it's probably because of their lifestyle. So the story of prevention is unfolding. I think we're pretty unique. It's like nobody can even imagine that this is going on at County, and yet we've got this whole huge section of Preventive Medicine.

As I was thinking about what to say about County and what animates me, I was thinking that I believe that prevention is unequivocally the best bang for a buck. But the thing that makes me want to work at County is that it seems to offer very special opportunities for bringing dignity to the whole process of health care. I don't know that I can tell you exactly why, but that's where my love for it really comes.

Quentin Young—Part 3

To look at county in retrospect in a national context, there are several issues. First and foremost is, what is the role of public medicine beyond public health? Prevailing and conventional wisdom would have it that this is an unpleasant alternative that's grown up, and we have to have it as a safety net, or to take care of *those* people, et cetera. I have a completely opposite view: I think for what it does County is superior to any other arrangement that's been devised in the U.S., certainly the urban U.S., for care of the poverty sector of all races.

It doesn't merely do an OK job or an alternate job, it does a *better* job. And better means several things: the patients do better, it means that better research is done—when you consider that it typically gets the large-scale responsibility for tough problems like massive burns or like AIDS or a huge, huge responsibility for premature babies. There's a difference between having a neonatalogy unit for three or six kids and having one for sixty. There's a difference between taking care of one burn and taking care of twelve. And they do that. Trauma. These are always brought out, and I'm doing it now, to give the melodramatic, easily understood example. But that really doesn't get down to it. County is the preferred place of care for most of its clients.

County needs to be replaced. It's eighty years old—the oldest public hospital in the country—and we need to find the money to replace it. Not because it did so good for all those years, not certainly because even though the private hospitals could absorb the patients, they won't—they can't absorb them. It should be done because County is the best way to deliver care to this particular sector for the foreseeable future. And this becomes genuinely irresistible when what's happening at County under Ruth Rothstein becomes reality, and it's doing that. The long delayed march into the community, the establishment of primary care clinics—both County-run and a not insignificant number of historic, community-based, non-profit clinics—to weave them into a network and use the County Hospital, and now it's sister hospital Provident, as the hospital backup, is to not merely meet some needs. This is the model for the future if as is true—and it is absolutely true—that we have to break the back of hyper-specialism and change the ratio of 20% primary care, 80% specialist to 50/50.

If we do a forced march we can do that in about ten years. And as it was the magnificent and huge trainer of specialists for the first half of this century, County can become the mass trainer of primary care docs with a proper balance between hospital experience and community-based care. So I'm not one who defends the County out of sentimentality, or because nobody else will do it. I think it does better what it does than anybody else. Beyond that you get into the whole question of public and private, which is very large, but County is one of the many shining examples of how public medicine, public health, government activity works.

One of the legacies of the Reagan era is that government can't do anything. We're told we can't have health reform: would you like the efficiency of the post office and the compassion of the IRS? These cynical, market-driven fallacies...What about the National Institutes of Health, the most magnificent way of organizing research, with billions of dollars to allocate, ever devised. It's the envy of every civilized country in the world. And yes, the public hospitals, of which County is an outstanding example, doing better what they do than anybody. And even the public health system in this country—the boards of health, the departments of health, on the state and local levels. They're always underfunded. The culture within medicine has treated the professionals, doctors and others, as if they're second-class citizens.

Despite all of these unearned inequalities, there's no question at all that 80% of the improvement of life expectancy in this country in the last century—from roughly forty to roughly seventy-five years—is due to public health triumphs, in the face of all this adversity. If you believe, as I do, that you're going to do future planning, whether it's health or housing or any other field, you better deal with it real fast. The American public has got to get its head screwed on right about what the public sector in medicine can do, has done, and will do if it's permitted.

Dr. John Barrett

As we speak, the nation is debating the future of health care, and health care reform is much on the minds of legislators. Many would argue that with reform there will no longer be a need for public hospitals; that with universal coverage patients will have freedom of choice and the public hospitals will collapse.

But public hospitals provide access to care that will not and cannot be duplicated in the private sector. These public institutions see millions of outpatients a year, and the private sector simply doesn't have the capacity to deal with them. In addition, the public hospitals have a history of experience in dealing with the problems of the poor. Public hospitals provide a culture that is friendly to these patients, and have also developed great expertise in dealing with some of their concerns: trauma, burns, neonatology, and diseases of addiction, among others.

Our society will always need this safety net of public hospitals, and we should all struggle to support and nurture them into the 21st century.